TOOLS FOR TEACHING COMPREHENSIVE HUMAN SEXUALITY EDUCATION

TOOLS FOR TEACHING COMPREHENSIVE HUMAN SEXUALITY EDUCATION

Lessons, Activities, and Teaching Strategies Utilizing the National Sexuality Education Standards (Grades 6–12)

Dominick Splendorio
and Lori Reichel

JOSSEY-BASS™
A Wiley Brand

Cover design by Wiley
Cover images (from left to right): © Compassionate Eye Foundation/Justin Pumfrey/Getty, © Vstock/Getty, © sturti/Getty, © zhang bo/Getty

Published by Jossey-Bass
A Wiley Brand
One Montgomery Street, Suite 1200, San Francisco, CA 94104-4594—www.josseybass.com

Jossey-Bass books and products are available through most bookstores. To contact Jossey-Bass directly call our Customer Care Department within the U.S. at 800-956-7739, outside the U.S. at 317-572-3986, or fax 317-572-4002.

Wiley publishes in a variety of print and electronic formats and by print-on-demand. Some material included with standard print versions of this book may not be included in e-books or in print-on-demand. If this book refers to media such as a CD or DVD that is not included in the version you purchased, you may download this material at http://booksupport.wiley.com. For more information about Wiley products, visit www.wiley.com.

Library of Congress Cataloging-in-Publication Data
Splendorio, Dominick, 1949-
Tools for teaching comprehensive human sexuality education : lessons, activities, and teaching strategies utilizing the national sexuality education standards / Dominick Splendorio, Lori Reichel. —First edition.
pages cm
Includes bibliographical references.
ISBN 978-1-118-45303-2 (pbk.) — ISBN 978-1-118-45615-6 (pdf) — ISBN 978-1-118-45616-3 (epub)
1. Sex instruction—Study and teaching—Handbooks, manuals, etc. 2. Family life education—Study and teaching—Handbooks, manuals, etc. I. Reichel, Lori, 1966- author. II. Title.
HQ56.S757 2013
613.9071—dc23

2013030390

Printed in the United States of America

FIRST EDITION

PB Printing 10 9 8 7 6 5 4 3 2 1

CONTENTS

THE AUTHORS

Dominick Splendorio received his bachelor's degree in health education from the State University College of New York at Brockport and his master's degree in humanistic studies from the State University of New York College at New Paltz. He taught middle and high school health education for over thirty years in the Clarkstown Central School District in Rockland County, New York, and also served as Clarkstown's district health education coordinator.

Dominick is past president of the health section of the New York State Association for Health, Physical Education, Recreation, and Dance (NYS AHPERD) and has twice been selected as New York State Health Teacher of the Year by the New York State Federation of Professional Health Educators in 1994 and by NYS AHPERD in 2001. Dominick presently runs his own education consulting company, Prime Time Health. He has presented at the national American Alliance for Health, Physical Education, Recreation and Dance conference, and at the American School Health Association conference.

Dominick is available for teacher in-service training, curriculum writing, student and teacher workshops, and assembly programs and keynote presentations. Dominick's first book, *Tools for Teaching Health* (Jossey-Bass), was published in 2007 and is presently being used in many school districts and by many health educators across the United States.

He can be contacted at domsplendid@yahoo.com.

Lori Reichel is a New York certified K–12 health educator with twenty-plus years' experience. She received her bachelor's and master's degrees from Stony Brook University of New York, and her doctorate of philosophy in health education from Texas A&M University. Her experience includes teaching health education courses to K–12 students as well as health education undergraduate and graduate courses. In addition, Lori obtained her administrative degree and became a health coordinator for two school districts. Within these positions, Lori participated in the first NYS Healthy Schools Leadership Institute. She is currently an assistant professor in the Department of Health Education and Health Promotion at the University of Wisconsin–La Crosse.

Lori has presented over forty workshops at local, state, regional, and national conferences, demonstrating her passion for effective health education programs. She has attended numerous workshops and curriculum trainings, strengthening her skills as an educator and presenter. She was also recognized as the recipient of the following: the Health Education Professional of the Year Award in 2011 from NYS AHPERD; Health Education Professional of the Year from the American Alliance for Health, Physical Education, Recreation, and Dance (2010); Health Educator of the Year from the Eastern Division Association of AHPERD (2009); Health Educator of the Year from NYS AHPERD (2007); and Health Educator of the Year from Nassau County, NYS AHPERD (2004).

She can be contacted at lreichel@uwlax.edu.

NOTES TO THE TEACHER: HOW TO USE THIS BOOK

Tools for Teaching Comprehensive Human Sexuality Education is a compilation of classroom-tested lessons designed for use with middle and high school students. It is not presented in a traditional textbook format, and the lessons are, with few exceptions, nonsequential. You can select those activities that are most appropriate for your students.

The book is divided into seven chapters. Each chapter includes learning experiences that are aligned with one of the seven topic areas chosen as the minimum, essential content and skills for sexuality education, as described in the 2012 National Sexuality Education Standards.[1] Although the chapters are divided into different topic areas, a number of content areas may be addressed in one lesson, and the appropriate performance indicators for each of those topic areas are listed in each instance. Performance indicators note what children should be able to know or do by the end of the specified grade.

The purpose of this book is to offer teachers a chance to "pick and choose" activities and learning experiences to supplement an existing human sexuality curriculum. You can use the lessons in the format provided, or adapt the activities to align with guidelines established by your state department of education and local school district.

It is critical for any individual teacher or supervising body using any of the lessons in this book to have a board-level-approved statement supporting age- and developmentally appropriate sexuality education lessons. You should check with your building administrators, district-level administrators, your school's health advisory committee, your school board, or a combination of these before incorporating any of these lessons into your existing sexuality curriculum.

WHAT IS COMPREHENSIVE HUMAN SEXUALITY EDUCATION?

According to the Sexuality Information and Education Council of the United States (SIECUS), comprehensive human sexuality education programs "include age-appropriate, medically-accurate information on a broad set of topics related to sexuality, including human development, relationships, decision-making, abstinence, contraception, and disease prevention."[2]

Many schools and health professionals look to SIECUS, long recognized as a leader in promoting comprehensive human sexuality education, for guidance in developing comprehensive and developmentally appropriate materials and resources as well as for expertise in creating local curricula focusing on human sexuality. The organization's booklet *Guidelines for Comprehensive Sexuality Education* (3rd edition) was a valuable resource in gathering developmentally appropriate learning experiences and activities for this book.

We recognize that instruction about human sexuality varies greatly from one school district to another, and that no curriculum meets the needs of every community. There may be some schools teaching minimally about human sexuality. Other schools may focus on "abstinence-only" or "abstinence-based" sexuality education. Research suggests a comprehensive approach to human sexuality education to be effective in assisting youth in postponing sexual activity and lowering the number of sexual partners, as well as in helping youth who are sexually active in using contraceptives. Research has also noted that students in comprehensive human sexuality education programs are not at an increased risk of becoming sexually active, not at an increased risk of increasing sexual activity, and not at an increased risk of experiencing negative sexual health outcomes.[3]

In selecting a local curriculum, it is suggested that schools include evidence-based interventions (EBIs). EBIs have demonstrated their effectiveness in achieving desired behavior changes, such as delaying the onset of intercourse and/or increasing condom use, through research and evaluation.[4] More information about these programs may be obtained from the Future of Sex Education (FoSE) website at www.futureofsexed.org/evidence-basedsexed.html.

Recognizing that all people are sexual beings, one goal of comprehensive human sexuality education is to assist youth in developing a positive view of sexuality. Advocating for comprehensive human sexuality education promotes the belief that all humans should have the opportunity to enjoy a safe, consensual, and fulfilling sex life, *when they are ready for it.* It is our hope that the lessons in this book will assist you in developing a comprehensive approach to teaching human sexuality that provides students with the information and skills to make respectful, healthy decisions about their sexuality, now and in the future.

NATIONAL SEXUALITY EDUCATION STANDARDS (NSES)

The NSES are the result of a cooperative effort by the American Association of Health Education, the American School Health Association, the National Education Association Health Information Network, and the Society of State Leaders of Health and Physical Education, in coordination with the FoSE Initiative.[5] The FoSE Initiative is a partnership between Advocates for Youth, Answer, and SIECUS, three organizations that seek to promote the institutionalization of comprehensive human sexuality education in public schools.

In January 2012 the "National Sexuality Education Standards: Core Content and Skills, K–12" was published in the *Journal of School Health.* This document's purpose is to "provide clear, consistent, and straightforward guidance on the essential minimum, core content and skills for sexuality education that is developmentally and age-appropriate for students in grades Kindergarten through 12."[6] Performance indicators for what students should know and be able to do are presented in these National Sexuality Education Standards, and separated into seven topic areas. The chapters in this book correspond to each of the seven topic areas:

1. Anatomy and Physiology
2. Puberty and Adolescent Development
3. Identity
4. Pregnancy and Reproduction
5. Sexually Transmitted Infections and HIV
6. Healthy Relationships
7. Personal Safety

The full text of the NSES may be downloaded from the FoSE website, www.futureofsexed.org. For a detailed explanation of how to read the performance indicators, you may refer to page 11 of the NSES document.

The NSES are based on a theoretical framework that includes the social learning theory and the social cognitive theory, as well as the social ecological model for prevention.[7] This framework recognizes that before a behavior is "taken on," a person has both individual and environmental factors to manage. Individual factors include what teenagers perceive as relevant information, their perceptions of possible consequences for partaking in certain behaviors, their ability to act in a particular manner (self-efficacy), personal skill development, and affective and emotional aspects of learning.

Environmental factors pertain to the social and physical world around the individual.[8] This includes "social norms," or the behaviors perceived as typical among members of a group or within society at large. For teenagers, the environment can include their family as well as friends, peers, school, and the media. By watching the behaviors of the surrounding world, people "experience" potential consequences of or responses to those behaviors. These consequences or responses can be positive or negative.

These individual and environmental factors interact with one another, leading individuals to readjust their behaviors according to the consequences or responses received. Furthermore, the ecological model recognizes that an individual begins with himself as a center core and has layers of influence surrounding him.[9]

NATIONAL HEALTH EDUCATION STANDARDS (NHES)

First published in 1995, the NHES were developed to establish and promote health-enhancing behaviors for students at all grade levels. The NHES are written expectations for what students should know and be able to do to promote personal, family, and community health. They provide a context for curriculum development and selection, instruction, and student assessment in health education. With support from the American Cancer Society, the Joint Committee on National Health Education Standards was formed to develop the standards. *National Health Education Standards: Achieving Excellence* (2nd edition) was published in 2007 by the American Cancer Society.[10] The NHES have become an accepted reference on health education, providing a framework for the adoption of standards by most states.

Within this book, every lesson references one or more of the NHES, focusing not only on health knowledge but also on important health skills. These standards, included in the 2007 NHES book,[11] read as follows:

Standard 1: Students will comprehend concepts related to health promotion and disease prevention to enhance health.

Standard 2: Students will analyze the influence of family, peers, culture, media, technology and other factors on health behaviors.

Standard 3: Students will demonstrate the ability to access valid information and products and services to enhance health.

Standard 4: Students will demonstrate the ability to use interpersonal communication skills to enhance health and avoid or reduce health risks.

Standard 5: Students will demonstrate the ability to use decision-making skills to enhance health.

Standard 6: Students will demonstrate the ability to use goal-setting skills to enhance health.

Standard 7: Students will demonstrate the ability to practice health-enhancing behaviors and avoid or reduce health risks.

Standard 8: Students will demonstrate the ability to advocate for personal, family and community health.

BOOK FORMAT

We developed the lessons in this book by drawing on our over fifty combined years of classroom experience in teaching human sexuality at all levels. The learning experiences are designed to engage students in stimulating discussions to reflect not just their knowledge of human sexuality but also their personal beliefs, opinions, and values.

Each individual lesson is broken down into the following components:

- Title of the lesson
- Appropriate developmental level (middle school, high school, or both)
- Approximate time or duration of the lesson or activity
- Reference to the appropriate National Health Education Standards
- Reference to the appropriate National Sexuality Education Standards and performance indicators
- Rationale for the lesson
- Required teacher preparation and materials
- Procedural steps for facilitating the lesson
- Suggested questions for processing the lesson
- Suggestions for diagnostic, formative, or summative assessments

The majority of lessons involve an opening activity to immediately engage students, followed by discussions and student-centered learning experiences. The lessons include assessments that range from constructed response questions to authentic assessments, as well as journal writing, simulations, demonstrations, role-plays, and other tangible products and performances. Health skills to be practiced are also recommended within specific lessons. Some sample rubrics are included to assist you in assessing students' acquisition of health knowledge and skills.

A teacher's supplement is available at www.josseybass.com/go/splendorio. Additional materials, such as videos, podcasts, and readings, can be found at www.josseybasspublichealth.com. Comments about this book are invited and can be sent to publichealth@wiley.com.

Also, if definitions of terms are needed, you can access the glossary of terms from the National Sexuality Education Standards by going to the FoSE website www.futureofsexed.org.

HOME-SCHOOL CONNECTION

Effective communication between parents or guardians and their child about sexual health has many positive effects for teens, including delaying the initiation of sexual intercourse and reducing risky sexual behaviors. Positive communication helps young people establish individual values and make healthy decisions. Some families are already talking about sexual issues, but for other families open communication may be more difficult.

Each chapter in the book contains a Home-School Connection activity that relates to the unit under study. Such activities are designed to open the lines of communication between parents or guardians and their child by raising potentially challenging topics for discussion. In addition, the activities provide parents or guardians with the opportunity to share their knowledge, opinions, and personal values with their child.

In some cases, students are not comfortable discussing sexuality issues with parents or guardians. In these instances, you should encourage students to complete the activity with one or more trusted adults, such as a relative, coach, counselor, or clergy member.

On the day the Home-School Connection worksheet is due, you can ensure that the activity has been completed and signed by the student and at least one adult by noting the signatures. *This worksheet will not be collected or graded.* Students and parents or guardians have the option of passing on any parts of the activity in which they do not feel comfortable sharing.

Follow-up class discussions should focus on clarifying information, and on sharing and respecting the diversity of opinions and values parents or guardians may have in regard to human sexuality. All information in the Home-School Connection activity will remain private, and students do not have to share any of their personal opinions or values (or those of their parents or guardians) that they wish to keep confidential.

Note: Some sexuality curricula have similar optional "parent or guardian homework." You should use your own judgment in deciding how best to incorporate such assignments.

REFERENCES

1. Future of Sex Education Initiative, *National Sexuality Education Standards: Core Content and Skills, K–12; A Special Publication of the* Journal of School Health (Bethesda, MD: American School Health Association, 2012).
2. National Guidelines Task Force, *National Guidelines for Comprehensive Sexuality Education: Kindergarten–12th Grade,* 3rd ed. (New York: Sexuality Information and Education Council of the United States, 2004), 39, www2.gsu.edu/~wwwche/Sex%20ed%20class/guidelines.pdf.
3. Douglas Kirby, *Emerging Answers 2007: Research Findings on Programs to Reduce Teen Pregnancy and Sexually Transmitted Diseases* (Washington, DC: National Campaign to Prevent Teen & Unplanned Pregnancy, 2007), www.thenationalcampaign.org/EA2007/EA2007_full.pdf.
4. "Evidence-Based Sex Education: Compendiums and Programs," Future of Sex Education, accessed July 12, 2013, www.futureofsexed.org/evidence-basedsexed.html.
5. Future of Sex Education Initiative.
6. Ibid., 6.
7. Ibid.
8. Mark Edberg, *Essentials of Health Behavior: Social and Behavioral Theory in Public Health* (Sudbury, MA: Jones and Bartlett, 2007).
9. Ibid.
10. Joint Committee on National Health Education Standards, *National Health Education Standards: Achieving Excellence,* 2nd ed. (Atlanta, GA: American Cancer Society, 2007), www.cancer.org/healthy/morewaysacshelpsyoustaywell/schoolhealth/national-health-education-standards-2007. Permission was granted from the National American Cancer Society to reproduce the NHES standards.
11. Ibid., 8.

GENERAL GUIDELINES FOR ADAPTING HUMAN SEXUALITY EDUCATION LESSONS FOR STUDENTS WITH SPECIAL NEEDS

Darrel Lang, EdD
Kansas State Department of Education

For a variety of reasons, parents or guardians and educators find teaching about human sexuality a difficult task. It is even more challenging when teaching students with special needs. All students, including students with special needs, should be provided with comprehensive human sexuality education, but students with intellectual and developmental disabilities are often exempted from class when the topic of human sexuality is discussed. Usually this exemption is granted because most educators have had little or no formal education in the teaching of human sexuality to students with special needs. On a personal level, the discussion of sex and sexuality with any group of students can make most educators uncomfortable, and this is particularly the case when students have special needs. Cultural, ethical, religious, and moral issues influence human sexuality education, and human sexuality education is a "red flag" that causes considerable controversy in communities across the United States. Some parents or guardians believe that education about human sexuality should be done in the home and only by them. Research has shown, however, that 90 percent of parents with children in grades seven through twelve think that schools should do more on the topic of human sexuality.[1]

Parents or guardians are the primary sexuality educators of their children. However, it is very difficult for them to be the *sole* sexuality educators of their children, unless they do not allow them to watch TV, listen to music, read a book, or talk to anyone!

One of the main reasons students with special needs should be taught about human sexuality is that these students are two to three times more at risk of sexual abuse compared to the general population. Students with special needs may not have adequate education about human sexuality because of several areas of deficiency that may lead to vulnerability. The areas of deficiency are

- **Knowledge.** Students with special needs often have less knowledge than other students about their body and their sexuality. These students are also often more prone to having received misinformation.
- **Social skills.** Students with special needs may have limited opportunities for social development. This may result in their exhibiting improper behaviors, such as inappropriate hugging or inappropriate demonstration of affection. In addition, students with special needs may not have the ability to resist negative peer pressure. Appropriate social skills can be developed through activities that address communication, refusal skills, and decision making.
- **Judgment.** Many times, students with special needs demonstrate poor judgment and an inability to control their impulses when making decisions.
- **Self-esteem.** The keystone of human sexuality education is self-esteem. Students who have low self-esteem are often more likely to participate in risky behaviors in an effort to be accepted by their peers. Many students with special needs have low self-esteem and are easily coaxed by their peers to perform risky behaviors.

When planning a human sexuality education program for students with special needs, one should consider four questions:

1. How do students' particular disabilities affect their social-sexual development?
2. How does the disability affect their needs?
3. How does the disability affect their ability to learn the information?
4. What other or extra information or materials may be needed or used to address their disability so that they can learn the information?

The student with special needs can usually be successful if given appropriate time to assimilate the information, complete the assignments, build a foundation of knowledge and skills from each proceeding lesson, and practice the appropriate skills. Accommodation and modification should always be kept in mind when planning lessons for children with special needs. These terms are defined as follows:

Accommodation—a change made to the teaching or testing procedures to provide a student with access to information and to create an equal opportunity for the student to demonstrate knowledge and skills.

Modification—a change in what a student is expected to learn, demonstrate, or both. Although a student may be working on modified course content, the subject area remains the same as for the rest of the class.

Modifications and accommodations for general education should be made in regard to (1) instruction, (2) assignments, (3) content and materials, and (4) assessments.

Modifications and accommodations for *instruction* include

- Peer teaching
- One-on-one instruction
- An adjusted pace of the lesson or lessons
- An adjusted amount of material taught
- Hands-on instruction
- Review and practice
- Reteaching of basic concepts
- Cooperative learning
- Pre-assessment of needs
- Use of student-focused learning strategies:
    - Graphic organizers
    - Highlighting
    - Study guides
- Direct instruction

Modifications and accommodations for *assignments* include

- Shortened assignments
- Alternative choices
- Extra time for completion
- Breaking down assignments into smaller steps
- Directions given both in written format and orally
- Framed assignments
- Text alternatives
- Alternative grading
- Use of technology

Modifications and accommodations for *content and materials* include

- Use of audiotapes or CDs
- Use of Braille or larger print
- Use of books that are off grade level
- Use of visual aids

- Fewer problems given, and fewer words on a page
- Highlighting text to teach the most important concepts

Society places many obstacles to healthy sexual development and expression for students with special needs. When working with these students, we need to guard against negative attitudes as well as myths and misconceptions. Sexuality education for students with special needs requires a certain degree of individualization. The student's Individualized Education Plan (IEP) can be used as an instrument for adapting the sexuality curriculum for the student. If human sexuality education is written into the IEP, it is more likely to be designed and delivered according to the specific needs of the individual student. As health and sexuality educators, it is our responsibility to make sure that we provide for the sexual health of students with special needs.

REFERENCE

1. "Sex Education in America: General Public/Parents Survey," National Public Radio, Henry J. Kaiser Family Foundation, and Kennedy School of Government, January 2004, www.npr.org/programs/morning/features/2004/jan/kaiserpoll/publicfinal.pdf.

ACKNOWLEDGMENTS

We would like to thank our friend and colleague Robert Winchester for his advice and support in designing the Up Close and Personal lessons in each of the chapters in this book.

Sentence stems to be completed have been used by health educators for many years to stimulate critical thinking and affectively based discussions. However, the concept of using these sentence stems in a structured, organized manner was adapted from Robert's book, *Up Close and Personal: Effective Learning for Students and Teachers.* Robert is an award-winning, highly respected health educator with over thirty years of experience as a classroom teacher. He has also presented workshops in New York State as well as at national and international conferences. Further, he has been an active member in several health education organizations and a true advocate for high-quality health and sexuality education. Robert can be contacted at trustinbob@aol.com.

We would also like to thank Darrel Lang for writing the supplementary material on teaching human sexuality to students with special needs. Darrel was the program consultant for HIV/AIDS and Human Sexuality Education for the state department of education in Topeka, Kansas. Darrel presently serves on the board of the Sexuality Information and Education Council of the United States.

We would like to thank proposal reviewers Elissa Barr, Sarah Beshers, Gary English, Joanna Kain Gentsch, Graham Higgs, Gary Kelly, Dorothy Van Dam, and Laurie Wagner, who provided valuable feedback on the original book proposal. Elissa Barr, Kurt Conklin, Gary English, Barbara Huberman, Laura Pietropaolo, and Laurie Wagner provided thoughtful and constructive comments on the completed draft of the manuscript.

A special thanks to all of our friends and colleagues in the field of health education who shared their ideas and expertise in workshops and conferences, inspiring us to continue to grow as health education professionals. Finally, we also thank our former students, who through their participation and feedback have motivated us to create the skills-based, interactive activities and lessons in this book.

1 Anatomy and Physiology

An effective sexuality program provides a comprehensive view of sexuality, beginning with medically accurate information. The lessons and learning experiences in this chapter establish a baseline of appropriate terminology as well as a foundation for understanding more complex issues found in subsequent chapters. By participating in student-centered, interactive activities within a supportive classroom environment, students will learn accurate information and develop their skills. These lessons serve as a starting point for sexuality discussions, leading to lessons on pubertal changes found in Chapter Two.

TIPS ON HOW TO TEACH STUDENTS EFFECTIVELY

Creating a safe, nonthreatening environment is essential for the success of any sexuality education program. The most effective sexuality educators are those who are comfortable with talking about sexuality, knowledgeable about the subject, and honest and nonjudgmental in their responses to students. Facilitation of student-friendly discussions is also needed.

To help educators acquire or strengthen their skills, professional development conferences and workshops are available. There are also online courses and webinars to keep teachers up to date on the latest research, effective teaching strategies, national and state standards, and advances in technology. It is recommended that you refer to local and state organizations for information on available trainings and resources.

Other tips to consider when teaching sexuality education lessons include

- Addressing both the positive and negative aspects of sexuality, rather than simply using "scare tactics."
- Talking on the students' level. If students only know "slang" terms (not vulgarity) when asking legitimate questions, you can initially accept their questions while encouraging the use of medically accurate and classroom-appropriate terminology for future discussions.
- Being cautious of using terminology that implies heterosexuality. Many of the lessons in this book use the word "partner" rather than "boyfriend" or "girlfriend," particularly in scenarios or role-plays. By using "gender-neutral" names ("Chris" and "Pat"), you are less likely to disenfranchise students who are gay, lesbian, or bisexual.
- If possible, arranging chairs in a semicircle or "concentric horseshoe" setup so that students can see one another during class discussions.
- Allowing for both sexes to participate in activities equally. Although it may sometimes be appropriate to separate males and females for certain topics or activities, allowing lessons to be coed encourages open lines of communication, the sharing of feelings, and different points of view.
- Not moralizing or judging. A teacher's role is to encourage health-enhancing behaviors, not to impose personal values on students. Set personal boundaries for the sharing of personal information and encourage students to do the same.
- Being sensitive to students' personal histories. It is possible that some issues raised during class discussions (for example, sexual abuse, unplanned pregnancy, or STIs) may create discomfort for some students. Inform students of available trusted adults within in the school and community for counseling and referrals.
- Taking a positive approach to sexuality education, focusing on what is sexually healthy rather than sexually unhealthy, and acknowledging that sexual feelings are normal and natural.

Most of the lessons in Chapter One are designed for middle school students, providing basic information on the female and male reproductive anatomy. Some lessons, however, may be used as a review with high school students or as a diagnostic assessment of what students know and are able to do.

Also, as with all lessons presented in the classroom setting, you need to evaluate these lessons before integrating them into an existing curriculum. You should follow state mandates and local guidelines, and should obtain approval of a district advisory committee or curriculum review panel to determine which lessons are most appropriate for the intended population.

LESSON 1: PEOPLE SEARCH

Level: Middle school

Time: 30–40 minutes

National Health Education Standard

1. Core Concepts

National Sexuality Education Standards: Performance Indicator

- Describe male and female sexual and reproductive systems including body parts and their functions.

Rationale

Sometimes people do not feel comfortable talking about their sexual body parts. This interactive activity introduces students to the skill of communicating respectfully and without embarrassment about reproductive anatomy. It will also serve as a diagnostic assessment of what students already know and do not know about the male and female reproductive systems.

Materials and Preparation

Copies of "Reproductive Anatomy People Search" worksheet

Copies of "Reproductive Anatomy and Physiology Vocabulary" worksheet

Procedure

1. Explain to students that they are going to be playing a game similar to bingo. It will be a people search in which they will try to find classmates who can answer questions or who fit particular descriptions. The topic will be male and female reproductive anatomy. Ask students to be respectful of their classmates, whether they can answer a question or not.
2. Distribute the "Reproductive Anatomy People Search" worksheet, and ask if students understand the task. Reinforce that they should not print their name on someone's paper unless they can justify what is written. Also, tell them that the activity is being timed, and that they will have five minutes to get all the boxes filled in. If someone does, that student should yell out "BINGO!"
3. If someone gets all sixteen boxes filled with names and yells "bingo," that student should come to the front of the room. If no one gets all the boxes filled in after five minutes, call "TIME!" and have all students sit down. Ask how many people *almost* got all the boxes filled. Find the student who got the *most* boxes filled in and have her come to the front of the room. If there is a tie, have both students come to the front of the room.
4. Begin going over the sheet by asking the "bingo winner" who signed the first box (top left). When that person's name is given, call on him to give the answer. In this case, the answer should be "fallopian tubes." Ask the person who signed that box to explain what he knows about the fallopian tubes and fertilization. Check for understanding and accuracy. Expand on the answer by asking the class to add anything not mentioned by the person who signed his name.

5. Continue with the same procedure given in the previous step, going over all boxes and statements. Facilitate discussions and clarify any misinformation.
6. At the end of the game, when the last box has been discussed, thank the bingo winner and the class for participating in the activity.
7. Hand out the "Reproductive Anatomy and Physiology Vocabulary" worksheet.
8. Pair off students or form small groups. Based on the information discussed in the people search, students should complete the worksheet by reading each definition and choosing the correct vocabulary word from the word bank to match the definition with the correct term. For your reference, the worksheet's answer key is as follows:
    1. Fallopian tubes
    2. Clitoris
    3. Uterus
    4. Testes
    5. Penis
    6. Menstruation
    7. Breasts
    8. Cervix
    9. Scrotum
    10. Labia
    11. Semen
    12. Vagina
    13. Urethra
    14. Erection
    15. Ejaculation
9. Conclude the lesson by asking the processing questions.
10. For an optional assignment, any student who wishes to do so may bring his people search sheet home and discuss the activity and content with a parent or guardian. If the adult signs the sheet, confirming she discussed the answers with her child, the student obtains five extra credit points on the next test or quiz.

Processing

1. What is one thing you learned today that you did not know or understand before?
2. Where did you learn about your body? Where did you learn about the bodies of members of the opposite sex?
3. Who has spoken with a parent or guardian about sex? What was it like? Comfortable or uncomfortable? Who brought up the topic?
4. How many of you talked about this topic in elementary school? Who taught it? Was the conversation comfortable or uncomfortable? Why?

Assessment

- Students correctly provide information on the male and female reproductive systems during the people search.
- Students accurately complete the "Reproductive Anatomy and Physiology Vocabulary" worksheet.
- Students complete the optional assignment and have it signed by a parent or guardian, to receive extra credit points.

Name: ______________________________

Reproductive Anatomy People Search

Directions: Find out what other people in this room know about reproductive anatomy and physiology by completing this people search. Walk around the room with this paper and a pen or pencil and find others who "fit" with the statements in the boxes that follow. When you find someone, have that person **print** his or her name in that box. No person may sign your sheet more than once. *You are allowed to sign one box yourself.* The objective is to get all boxes filled in with the names of different peers. If you get all sixteen boxes filled before the five-minute time limit is up, yell "BINGO!"

Note: Do not sign your name if you cannot honestly answer the question!!!

Find Someone Who . . .

1. Knows where an egg gets fertilized in the female reproductive system	2. Knows the name of the gland in males that secretes a chemical forming part of the fluid that carries sperm	3. Can name the male organ of intercourse by which urine and semen are discharged from the body	4. Knows the name of the male reproductive glands where sperm are produced
5. Knows what the cervix is, including its location	6. Knows the difference between an erection and ejaculation	7. Knows the name of the organ where the baby grows during pregnancy	8. Knows the name of the white fluid sperm live in
9. Knows the name of the folds of skin that surround and protect the external sex organs in the female	10. Knows the name of the opening in the female that serves as the organ of intercourse, the passage for menstrual discharge, and the birth canal	11. Knows the name of the small, sensitive, erectile organ located at the upper end of the vulva (external genitals)	12. Has a urethra
13. Knows where the mammary glands are located in the female	14. Knows the name of the sac holding the testes	15. Is a male and can explain what menstruation is	16. Has had a discussion about sex with a parent or guardian

Name: ________________________________

Reproductive Anatomy and Physiology Vocabulary

Directions: Working with a partner or in small groups, complete this worksheet by writing the correct vocabulary word for each of the definitions provided. A word bank has been provided to assist you in completing this worksheet.

Word Bank		
Scrotum	Vagina	Urethra
Ejaculation	Penis	Menstruation
Breasts	Cervix	Fallopian tubes
Labia	Semen	Clitoris
Uterus	Erection	Testes

1. ______________________: where an egg is fertilized in the female reproductive system
2. ______________________: the name of the small, sensitive erectile organ located at the upper end of the vulva (external genitals) in females
3. ______________________: the name of the hollow, muscular organ where the baby grows during pregnancy
4. ______________________: the name of the male reproductive glands where sperm are produced
5. ______________________: the name of the male organ of intercourse by which urine and semen are discharged from the body
6. ______________________: the monthly discharge of blood and other fluids from the uterus
7. ______________________: the external sex organs of the female where the mammary glands are located
8. ______________________: the lower end or "neck" of the uterus or womb
9. ______________________: the name of the sac of skin holding the testes
10. ______________________: the name of the folds of skin that surround and protect the external sex organs in the female
11. ______________________: the name of the white fluid sperm live in
12. ______________________: an opening in the female that serves as the organ of intercourse, the passage for menstrual discharge, and the birth canal
13. ______________________: found in both sexes; in females, the tube through which urine is discharged from the body; in males, the tube through which both urine and semen are discharged from the body
14. ______________________: the name of the change that occurs in the male during sexual excitement, whereby the penis fills with blood and becomes firm or hard
15. ______________________: a discharge of semen from the male penis

LESSON 2: WORD ASSOCIATION ACTIVITY: "SEX"

Level: Middle school

Time: 30–40 minutes

National Health Education Standard

1. Core Concepts

National Sexuality Education Standards: Performance Indicator

- Describe male and female sexual and reproductive systems including body parts and their functions.

Rationale

Students will be involved in an anonymous word association activity to identify what words come to mind when they hear or see the word "sex." Once a master list is complete, discussion will follow, centering on the positive and negative connotations of words associated with sex. The brainstorm list will include more than anatomical terms, and this serves as a good introductory activity to illustrate how sex involves more than simply the act of intercourse. At the conclusion of the lesson, the term "sexuality" will be defined. Students will be able to distinguish between the terms "sex" and "sexuality."

Materials and Preparation

Front board or newsprint and markers

Small squares of paper, all the same size and color

Small box or other container to anonymously collect slips of paper

Procedure

1. Ask students if they have ever played a word association game. Give a simple example: if someone says the word "up," one student may think of the word "down," whereas another student may think of the word "sky." Give some other simple examples.
2. Explain that for the lesson, a word association game is going to be played in which everyone will have the same word to think about. That word is "SEX"!
3. Hand out the pieces of paper. Tell students to anonymously write down at least three to five words that come to mind when they hear or see the word "sex." Explain that this word can mean many things to different people, and that there are no right or wrong answers.

4. It should be emphasized that there may be some "slang" or "street" words associated with the word "sex." Explain that the goal in class is to use acceptable language. If a "scientific" word is not known, students are allowed to write down the word they know or may have heard. They should not share what they write with anyone else. Allow a few minutes for students to write their responses. Then tell them to fold their paper in half two times. Go around and collect the slips of paper in a box, a hat, or some other container.
5. Ask for a student to volunteer to serve as the recorder on the front board (or newsprint). In large letters near the top of the board, he should write "sex". You will then begin to open the slips of paper and read the terms out loud. As they are read, the recorder will list the words on the board. Basing your decision on the developmental level and particular makeup of the class, you should determine which words can be written as is and which words need to be modified.

   For example, if the word "boobs" is written, you may say the word out loud, but then ask the class for the more acceptable scientific word ("breasts"). "Breasts" would then be the word written on the board. In some instances, students may write words that are not appropriate to say out loud, but that can still be added to the list if they can be modified. One way to handle this would be to say something like, "The word written on this paper is a slang word dealing with the mouth of one person coming into contact with the sex organs of another person. Rather than write that word on the board, we will simply write the words 'oral sex.'"
6. As you open and read more slips of paper, and words are mentioned more than once (which will definitely happen), instead of writing the entire word again, ask the recorder to simply put a check mark next to that word.
7. Continue until all words on all slips of paper have been read.
8. Have students look at the list and discuss the following questions:
   a. Are there any items whose meaning you do not know?
   b. Are there any items you do not think belong on the list (because of inaccurate information, because they are not related to the topic, and so on)?
9. Continue the discussion by asking students the processing questions. Allow them to discuss how common slang terms are used on a daily basis and whether or not they are appropriate.
10. Write the word "sexuality" on the board. Ask students: "What does the word 'sexuality' mean? How is it different from the word 'sex'?" After a brief discussion, write the definitions of sex and sexuality on the board. Have students copy them in their notebook.

    Sexuality—everything about you as a male or female. It is how you see and express yourself as a sexual person. It is an important part of your total personality, and includes your knowledge, attitudes, values, and behaviors. Everyone is a sexual being, starting at birth and ending at death.

    Sex—refers to whether a person is male or female. It also is commonly used as an abbreviation to refer to sexual intercourse.

11. To conclude the activity, inform the students that the day's discussion on human sexuality included most of the terms and concepts to be further explored within a family life and human sexuality unit. In this unit, students will
    - Learn the difference between "sex" and "sexuality"
    - Receive correct, up-to-date information about male and female reproductive anatomy
    - Have the opportunity to ask any legitimate questions and to share knowledge, opinions, and values with each other
    - Participate in open, honest discussion about the important topic while also being encouraged to communicate with parents or guardians
    - Contribute to an atmosphere of trust while respecting themselves and others
    - Understand their responsibility for their actions as sexual beings and that sexuality is a normal and healthy part of our lives
12. As a closure activity, read the following scenario aloud to the class: "In third-period study hall, your friend Alex says, 'So, I heard you talked about sex in health class today. How can you spend a whole period talking about having intercourse?'" Give students a few minutes to reflect on the scenario. Then have them answer Alex's question in their notebook using at least five words from the brainstorm list that do not involve sexual intercourse. After students share their answers and have a brief class discussion, summarize the activity by explaining to the class why there is a lot more to being a "sexual being" than just the act of intercourse.

Processing

1. Which words were mentioned the most (had the most check marks next to them)? Why do you think many students in class associated these words with the word "sex"?
2. How many words needed to be changed to the "scientific" or appropriate terminology?
3. Where do young people hear inappropriate or slang terms? (peers, the media, music, and so on)
4. Which words have a "positive" connotation? Which have a "negative" connotation? Can some have both?

Assessment

- Students correctly distinguish between the words "sex" and "sexuality" in their notebook by writing two words that specifically relate to sex (intercourse, gender) and two words that relate to the much broader term "sexuality" (interpersonal relationships, gender roles, sexual orientation, affection, intimacy, body image).
- Students copy the master list of words from the board into their notebook.
- Students respond to the closing scenario in their notebook.

LESSON 3: MYTHS OR FACTS?

Level: Middle school

Time: 30–40 minutes

National Health Education Standards

1. Core Concepts
3. Accessing Information

National Sexuality Education Standards: Performance Indicators

- Describe male and female sexual and reproductive systems including body parts and their functions.
- Identify accurate and credible sources about sexual health.

Rationale

Students believe they know correct information about female and male reproductive systems. This activity allows students to explore what facts they do know and some of the myths they may also have heard.

Note: Prior to teaching this lesson, you should be prepared to accurately answer *all* of the myth or fact statements included at the end of this lesson. The answer key is provided.

Materials and Preparation

Teacher copy of "Myth or Fact Statements," with individual statements cut apart

Large envelope for individual statements to be placed into

Three small signs reading "Myth," "Fact," and "Not Sure" to be placed in three different sections of the room

Copies of "Accessing Reliable Information on the Internet" handout

Procedure

1. Explain to the students that they will be reviewing information they may already know about the female and male reproductive systems. Stress that the activity is not about competition, but rather about exploring what truths and myths people have about the human body and human reproductive systems.
2. Ask each student to take one of the slips of paper out of the envelope *without telling any other students what the statement reads.* If a student feels uncomfortable with his statement, allow him to choose another one from the envelope.
3. Explain that students will have five minutes to mingle with their peers and read each other's statements. Their goal is to have a correct statement at the end of the activity. To do this, each student will need to respectfully approach another student, at which point the following interaction should occur:
   a. Student A asks his peer (Student B) to read her statement aloud.
   b. Student B reads her own statement aloud.

c. The students jointly decide which one is more likely to be a true statement.

d. If either student wants to exchange statements, he or she can ask to do so. If a student believes her statement is a fact rather than a myth, she *does not* have to exchange with her peer. (Again, the goal is to end up with a factual statement.)

e. Next, the students each go to another peer and repeat the reading of statements. They should repeat this process with several other students.

4. After five minutes have passed, ask students to stand in one of the three areas of the room—marked by a sign reading "Myth," "Fact," or "Not Sure"—depending on the statement they are left holding.
5. After all students are standing under the appropriate sign, ask them to read their statement aloud, one at a time. As the students are doing this, you can decide to correct misinformation by having other students in the class state if they agree or disagree with their reasoning. After brief discussion, you should verify whether all answers are myths or facts.
6. After all statements have been read and discussed, ask the students to return to their seat.
7. Distribute the "Accessing Reliable Information on the Internet" handout. Discuss the main points with students, stating that anyone can post information on the Internet, and that often the information may be inaccurate or deceiving. Explain to students that in future lessons they will be using the information in this handout to access reliable information on a variety of topics related to human sexuality.

Processing

1. How comfortable were you completing this activity?
2. What statements did you feel comfortable about? Uncomfortable about?
3. What is one thing you learned today that you did not already know or understand?
4. Which statements were many people unsure of?
5. What information do you think the class is lacking about the male and female reproductive systems?

Assessment

- Students state whether their statement is a myth or a fact, with peers or the instructor validating or correcting their answers.
- Students identify accurate and credible sources pertaining to sexual health based on the information provided in the "Accessing Reliable Information on the Internet" handout.

Answer Key

1. M	4. F	7. F	10. M	13. M	16. F	19. F	22. M	25. M	28. M
2. F	5. M	8. M	11. F	14. F	17. M	20. F	23. F	26. M	29. M
3. F	6. F	9. M	12. M	15. F	18. M	21. F	24. M	27. M	30. F

Myth or Fact Statements

1. Females need two ovaries to have a baby.
2. If a male has only one testicle, he can still get a female pregnant.
3. An egg is about the size of a poppy seed.
4. Some females can start getting their menstrual periods as early as the fourth grade.
5. Males can control nocturnal emissions (wet dreams).
6. If she has unprotected sex, it is possible for a female to get pregnant at any time during her menstrual cycle (including when she is having her period).
7. Pre-seminal fluid from a male has enough sperm in it to get a female pregnant.
8. In a male's body, the testicles are always the same size.
9. A male can urinate and ejaculate at the same time.
10. Only males can experience a hernia.
11. Sperm can live for up to five days in a female's reproductive system.
12. Both females and males have a prostate gland.
13. Identical twins occur when two different sperm fertilize one egg.
14. Each fallopian tube is about four inches long and has a diameter as wide as a piece of spaghetti.
15. A healthy male makes one hundred million to three hundred million sperm per day.
16. The uterus is about the size and shape of an upside-down pear.
17. Only males have a urethra.
18. A baby grows in a female's vagina.
19. Only females have fallopian tubes.
20. Most male babies born in the United States are circumcised.
21. The male epididymis stores mature sperm.
22. Sperm and semen are the same thing.
23. Sperm cells have tails to help them move.
24. Egg cells have tails to help them move.
25. If a female has not gotten her first period, she cannot get pregnant.
26. A female urinates and releases the menstrual lining through the same opening in her body.
27. Males are not able to reproduce after they turn seventy years old.
28. Females usually release two eggs per menstrual cycle (each month).
29. The coccyx is the narrow bottom part of the uterus extending into the vagina.
30. There are three openings to the outside from the female pelvis.

Accessing Reliable Information on the Internet

Accessing information is a basic health skill. Intelligently navigating the Internet can bring you credible health information and access to services. Unfortunately, not all Internet sites are reliable. The following questions can assist you in determining whether a site is a legitimate source of information:

1. Is the site from a nonprofit organization (.org), government agency (.gov), or educational institution (.edu)? These sites tend to be more reliable than sites from commercial organizations (.com).

2. Is the information based on research and scientific evidence? How do you know?

3. Are the author or authors clearly identifiable, with provided credentials and contact information?

4. Some .com sites do have valuable and credible information. How can you ensure that the site is providing correct information?

5. Is the site selling something, rather than simply supplying information?

6. Be suspicious of sites that consist of personal opinions and testimonials. If the site relies mostly on testimonials rather than scientific research, you should not trust these sites to be accurate and legitimate.

7. How up to date is the information on the site? How do you know?

LESSON 4: THE HUMAN SEXUAL RESPONSE CYCLE, PART 1

Level: High school

Time: 40 minutes

National Health Education Standards

1. Core Concepts
4. Interpersonal Communication

National Sexuality Education Standards: Performance Indicators

- Describe the human sexual response cycle, including the role hormones play.
- Demonstrate respect for the boundaries of others as they relate to intimacy and sexual behavior.

Rationale

Often, the reason young people get themselves into risky situations is that they are not taught how to recognize signs and symptoms of sexual response and the accompanying physical and emotional changes in their body. By being aware of the signs and phases of sexual response, teens can decide how comfortable or uncomfortable they may feel in regard to physical intimacy. This can help empower them to make the conscious decision to discontinue what they are doing at any point by assertively communicating their wishes to their partner.

Many sexuality education curricula focus on the role that sexual intercourse plays in the reproductive process. Unfortunately, those same curricula often neglect to discuss the pleasurable feelings that can be associated with sex, and that those feelings are normal and natural. For those students who make a conscious choice to be sexually active, information on sexual communication, arousal, and response can contribute to a more positive, healthy view of sexuality. This lesson attempts to provide such information and includes a handout summarizing clinically accurate information about the phases of the human sexual response cycle. Because the brain is involved in these responses, no two people will experience the human sexual response cycle exactly the same way.

Note: As with any controversial topic, you should modify the learning experiences so they are within district and state guidelines and are developmentally and age appropriate.

Materials and Preparation

Four sheets of newsprint, taped around the room, and a marker

Copies of "The Human Sexual Response Cycle" handout

Set of 21 index cards, each listing one of the changes that occur in males or females during any of the four phases of the human sexual response cycle (sample statements included at the end of this lesson)

Masking tape, preferably cut into one-inch pieces

Copies of "Teens and Sexual Behavior: What Do You Think?" homework

Procedure

1. Introduce the lesson by asking students, "Why do people have sex?" Although responses may vary, the two most common reasons students will give are "to reproduce" and "for pleasure."
2. Write the word "pleasure" on the newsprint. Have students brainstorm ten things, including activities, that may bring them pleasure. (Some examples may be food, being with friends or family, pets, sports or games, listening to music, chatting on the computer, kissing or other sexual behaviors). After a brief discussion on why these things are pleasurable, have students record them in their notebook.
3. Explain that abstinence from intercourse has benefits for teenagers and adults, especially because of possible negative consequences. Note to the students that most people decide to engage in sexual behaviors to bring them pleasure at some point in their lives.
4. Give a brief overview of research into the human sexual response cycle by saying, "William Masters and Virginia Johnson, two pioneers in the field of sexuality research, provided the most thorough information about how human bodies respond to sexual stimulation. Although there is some controversy among researchers about the validity and relevance of their research, the Masters and Johnson model is one of the most widely held theories to explain this aspect of human sexuality."
5. Distribute the "The Human Sexual Response Cycle" handout to each student. Because this information is clinical, there may be some words that students are not familiar with or have questions about. Allow time to go over the provided information and answer questions.
6. Begin the index card activity:
   a. On four separate sheets of newsprint taped around the room, write the four phases in the human sexual response cycle in large letters—"EXCITEMENT" (also referred to as the arousal phase), "PLATEAU," "ORGASMIC," and "RESOLUTION."
   b. Hand out the index cards with the male and female sexual response changes written down. In a large class, each student may only get one card. In a smaller class, some students may get more than one card.
   c. Explain that students are to read the statement on their index card and decide (1) if the change occurs to males, females, or both; and (2) what phase of the human sexual response cycle the information represents. If they are not sure, they can ask other students in the class for advice.
   d. On making a decision, students should tape each index card under one of the four phases written on the newsprint. Masking tape, cut into small pieces, should be available for students to use.
   e. When they have completed this task, they may return to their seat.

f. Have the class look over the four categories to determine whether all of the cards are placed in the correct category. Students may refer back to their handout to assist them with this review. If cards are placed incorrectly, have students explain why each is incorrect and what changes they would make. Note that cards occasionally may actually fall under more than one heading.

Note: Explain that not all phases are the same for everyone, and that sexual response is experienced differently by all individuals, depending on a variety of factors.

g. When all cards have been placed correctly, end the index card activity.

7. Ask the class the processing questions.
8. Hand out copies of the "Teens and Sexual Behavior: What Do You Think?" homework for students to complete according to the directions provided. During the next class session, students should be prepared to share their opinions with their peers and hand in the completed assignment.

Processing

1. What new information did you learn from the handout on the human sexual response cycle?
2. Many of the terms discussed today have been medical or in scientific language. Which terms were you familiar with? Which terms were you unfamiliar with?
3. Refer to the first piece of newsprint, dedicated to the Excitement phase. Why might some couples never reach the first phase? (There is no attraction or "chemistry," they see each other more as friends than as romantic partners, they are turned off, and so on.)
4. If one or more partners decide to stop after the Excitement phase, is this okay? What might be some reasons for this? (He likes the other person, but wants to "take it slow"; she is not ready to move or comfortable moving on to the next phase; he recently got out of a failed relationship and needs time to sort out his feelings; she wants to remain abstinent; and so on.) Does the other partner have an obligation to respect that decision?
5. Which phase or phases involve the most physical or sexual contact?
6. If one partner forces or coerces another partner to do something against his or her will, what might some of the consequences be? (There can be emotional or physical harm, lack of trust in your partner, lack of trust in future relationships, legal consequences for sexual assault and rape, and so on.)

Assessment

- Students provide correct responses in the index card activity involving the description of the human sexual response cycle.
- Students complete their homework assignment.

The Human Sexual Response Cycle

In the 1950s and 1960s researchers William Masters and Virginia Johnson developed something that they called the human sexual response cycle. Since that time, there have been other models and descriptions of what actually happens during a sexual act, but the Masters and Johnson model is still widely accepted by most researchers.

Within their response cycle, Masters and Johnson divided the sex act into four phases:

1. Excitement
2. Plateau
3. Orgasmic
4. Resolution

The following descriptions are based on their model, outlining what happens during the physical act of sex. Although the response is similar for both males and females, there is much variation among individuals.

1. The **Excitement** phase marks the beginning of sexual arousal. Sexual arousal usually begins in the brain and occurs in response to words, images, senses, or physical contact, like kissing or hugging. Several things happen during this phase in anticipation of sexual interaction. Pulse rate, blood pressure, and breathing rate all increase. Blood is sent to the penis in males, causing an erection. In females, blood causes the clitoris to swell, the labia expand and open more, and the vagina becomes lubricated. The female's breasts may also enlarge, making the nipples erect and more sensitive. In both sexes, the body becomes more sensitive and receptive to touch.
2. In the **Plateau** phase, physical arousal builds as pulse and breathing rates continue to increase. The penis becomes fully erect and sometimes secretes a few drops of pre-seminal fluid (which often contains active sperm). The clitoris remains sensitive to stimulation. Vaginal lubrication continues. The degree of arousal may fluctuate during this phase. This phase is often referred to as "foreplay," or the kissing, hugging, touching, or other forms of sexual stimulation that precede coitus, or intercourse.
3. The **Orgasmic** phase is the third and shortest phase of the cycle. It is usually described as the high point of sexual arousal. During orgasm, blood pressure and heart rate reach their peak. The muscles in the vaginal walls and the uterus contract rhythmically, as do the muscles in and around the penis as the male ejaculates. Occasionally, one or more partners may not reach the phase of orgasm. Although this is frustrating for some, most people can still experience sexual pleasure and intimacy without having an orgasm.
4. During the **Resolution** phase, both men and women tend to experience enhanced intimacy and a sense of well-being. Arousal slowly subsides and returns to normal. The males experience a refractory period, during which they are unable to achieve another erection or orgasm. The length of the refractory period varies; for one man it may last a matter of minutes, and for another it may last several hours.

It is important to keep in mind that the brain and related structures are responsible for the secretion of hormones influencing sexual feelings and response. The major hormones involved include androgens, estrogens, progestin, oxytocin, dopamine, vasopressin, and serotonin. Most researchers and scientists agree that the brain is considered the most important organ involved in sexual response.

Index Card Activity

Sample Body Changes and Teacher Answer Key

Excitement Phase

- Increased muscle tension
- Slight increase in heart rate and blood pressure
- Swelling of the clitoris and labia
- Erection of the penis
- Increased vaginal lubrication
- Slight swelling of the breasts, making the nipples more erect
- Sexual thoughts and feelings
- Stimulation caused by thoughts, words, images, senses, or physical contact

Plateau Phase

- Fully erect penis
- Testes engorged with blood
- Fluid appearing at the tip of the penis
- Sometimes referred to as "foreplay"

Orgasmic Phase

- Sudden release of muscle tension in series of contractions followed by relaxation
- Spike in pulse rate, breathing rate, and blood pressure
- Ejaculation or discharge of semen
- Usually the shortest phase of the cycle
- The high point, or "peak" of sexual stimulation
- Possibly a phase not experienced by one or both partners

Resolution Phase

- Swelled and erect body parts return to normal
- General sense of relaxation and enhanced intimacy
- Loss of erection of the penis, followed by a refractory period

Name: ______________________________

Teens and Sexual Behavior: What Do You Think?

Directions: Choose two of the following six statements dealing with teens and sexual behavior. For each of the two statements you choose, (1) indicate whether you agree or disagree with the statement, and (2) give two specific reasons, two specific examples, or a combination of both to back up your opinion.

1. Abstinence from intercourse has benefits for teenagers and adults.
2. Young teenagers are not mature enough for sexual relationships that include intercourse.
3. Teenagers in romantic relationships can express their feelings without engaging in sexual intercourse.
4. Teenagers who date need to discuss sexual limits with their dating partners.
5. Teenagers considering sexual activity should talk to a parent or guardian or other trusted adult about their decisions, including those related to contraception and disease prevention.
6. Individuals need to respect the sexual limits set by their partners.

Response to statement ________:

Response to statement ________:

LESSON 5: THE HUMAN SEXUAL RESPONSE CYCLE, PART 2

Level: High school

Time: 40 minutes

National Health Education Standards

1. Core Concepts
4. Interpersonal Communication

National Sexuality Education Standards: Performance Indicators

- Describe the human sexual response cycle, including the role hormones play.
- Demonstrate respect for the boundaries of others as they relate to intimacy and sexual behavior.

Rationale

In this lesson, students will be given the opportunity to ask questions related to human sexuality using an anonymous Question Box format. Lesson 4, "The Human Sexual Response Cycle, Part 1," used clinical and scientific terminology related to intercourse and intimate sexual behavior. The Question Box activity allows students to ask questions related to any aspect of human sexuality "in their own words."

The anonymous nature of the Question Box enables students to feel more comfortable asking questions related to any aspects of human sexuality. You can provide support to students by letting them know that most kids their age have similar questions and worries. Let students know that if they want to ask questions privately, they are able to do so during certain periods of the day. In some cases, particularly those pertaining to sexual abuse, harassment, "textual harassment," or "cyberbullying," teachers are legally obligated to refer students to counselors, psychologists, or administrators, and possibly to report the information to authorities.

Materials and Preparation

Small box with an opening large enough to insert small, folded pieces of paper, which will serve as the Question Box

Small, identical pieces of paper for each student

Procedure

1. Review the homework assignment from Lesson 4 for twenty minutes. You should ensure that all students have completed their homework and adequately responded to at least two of the six statements from their take-home assignment.

2. Engage students in a discussion of their varied responses to the take-home assignment. Because these are values-based statements, students are entitled to their personal opinions. However, you should attempt to guide the discussion toward the most health-enhancing behaviors. For example, if a student does not agree with statement 6, "Individuals need to respect the sexual limits set by their partners," you are obligated to explain the potential ethical and legal issues involved with that decision.
3. After all statements have been discussed, collect student papers. You can use these as a formative assessment by checking students' comprehension of Lesson 4's basic objectives.
4. Begin the Question Box activity:
   a. State to students:

      In the previous lesson, you were given a fact sheet on the human sexual response cycle. Some of the terms and words used in this clinical explanation may not have been familiar to you. In the follow-up to that lesson, you are going to have an opportunity to ask questions about the phases of the human sexual response cycle. You will also be able to ask any questions related to male and female reproductive anatomy, hormones, thoughts and feelings about becoming sexually mature, dating, what is "normal," and any other concerns you may have. This will be done by using an anonymous Question Box.

   b. Explain that questions may have a specific answer, or they might be open-ended questions that different people might answer differently, depending on their religious beliefs and their family or personal values. Then outline the rules in regard to appropriate and inappropriate questions by stating:

      Here are some rules to determine which questions are acceptable: first, a question is not okay if it has a person's name on it or in it. Second, it is not okay if the question makes fun of or puts down anyone or any group. Third, a question is not okay if I believe it is not appropriate for students of your age to discuss. This does not mean that it is not a good question—it may instead be a question to be discussed with a parent or guardian or school counselor. Finally, if a question uses slang or street language, yet is otherwise legitimate, I will change the wording so it is more acceptable to say in class.

   c. Hand an identical small slip of paper to each student. Ask students to write anonymously any questions pertaining to the subject on the paper, and then to fold it in half so that no one can see it. If a student has more than one question, he should write additional questions below the first one. Remind students that questions are to be anonymous and that no one should know who wrote which questions. You are the only person who will see the questions. Allow students about three to four minutes to come up with questions. If a student does not have any questions, she is to write, "I do not have any questions at this time" on the slip of paper.
   d. When all students have completed their questions, collect them in the Question Box.

e. After all questions are collected, take out one of the slips of paper. If the question is acceptable to read as written, read it aloud. Then ask if anyone has an answer or opinion related to the question. If no one does, answer the question yourself. If you do not know the answer to a question, inform the class of this, and then find out more information pertaining to the question and inform the class at a later date.

f. Continue going through the Question Box until all questions have been answered, if time permits. Some questions may be answered during the next class.

5. State the following, and then ask the processing questions:

   The previous day's lesson on the human sexual response cycle included a very clinical description of what actually happens physiologically and emotionally during sexual arousal. The reality is that sexual and physical relationships are different for everyone. All people, whether they are having sex or not, are sexual human beings. Your sexuality is an important part of who you are as a total person. Having a close physical relationship with someone you care about and who cares about you can be one of life's most enjoyable and satisfying experiences. It is important, however, to be aware of the potential negative consequences of engaging in sexual behaviors.

Processing

1. What are some possible negative health consequences of becoming sexually active? (Possible answers may include an unplanned pregnancy or a sexually transmitted infection, guilt, and loss of self-esteem.)
2. "Being involved in a consensual, respectful sexual relationship can be a healthy expression of affection and caring when it is with the right person, at the right time, and for the right reasons." What does this statement mean to you? Do you feel that most teens are mature and responsible enough to have a sexual relationship? Why or why not?
3. "Sexuality education classes should provide teens with the knowledge and skills to make healthy decisions about their sexual health." Do you agree or disagree with this statement? Explain.

Assessment

- Students actively participate in the in-class discussion of the previous lesson's homework assignment, demonstrating the ability to verbalize appropriate rationales for their opinions on the two statements they chose to write about.
- Students participate in the Question Box activity and follow-up discussion.

LESSON 6: WHAT TO EXPECT AT THE DOCTOR'S OFFICE

Level: Middle school, High school

Time: 40–50 minutes

National Health Education Standards

1. Core Concepts
3. Accessing Information
4. Interpersonal Communication
8. Advocacy

National Sexuality Education Standards: Performance Indicators

- Identify medically-accurate resources about pregnancy prevention and reproductive health care.
- Identify accurate and credible sources about sexual health.
- Identify the laws related to reproductive and sexual health care services (i.e., contraception, pregnancy options, safe surrender policies, prenatal care).
- Advocate for sexually active youth to get STI/HIV testing and treatment.
- Demonstrate communication skills that foster healthy relationships.

Rationale

This lesson covers basic medical care, including exams for males and females, dealing with the reproductive system. With this knowledge, teens develop a better understanding of their individual rights related to accessing information and resources for sexual health. In addition, having students of both sexes learn about each other's exams and procedures supports understanding and healthier relationships between them.

Materials and Preparation

Copies of "What Should You Expect at the Doctor's Office?" worksheet

Diagrams of female and male reproductive systems on large wall charts or Smart Boards. (Alternately, 3-D male and female reproductive system models may also be used—some district science departments have these.)

Nonlatex medical glove

For examinations on females: breast self-exam (BSE) model, Pap smear (HPV) test swab, empty specimen tube, and speculum

For examinations on males: testicular self-exam (TSE) model, empty specimen or blood tube, and swab

Additional resources from local clinics, doctor's offices, or health departments (optional)

Copies of "Fact Sheet: Reproductive Health Services for Teens" handout

Procedure

1. Begin class by placing students into mixed-sex groups of four to five. Students can also be placed in same-sex groups if requested. Distribute copies of the "What Should You Expect at the Doctor's Office?" worksheet, one copy per student.
2. Give groups five to ten minutes to answer the questions on the worksheet. Any questions they do not know can be left blank to be completed after the class demonstration and discussion of the "Fact Sheet: Reproductive Health Services for Teens" handout.
3. As students are completing the worksheet, circulate from group to group to note when students have finished writing down what they know, and to get a sense of which questions certain groups have answered correctly.
4. After group time is done, ask the students to face toward the diagrams or models of the female and male reproductive systems. With guidance from you, groups will complete their worksheets, filling in any missing information through the class discussion.
5. Begin the discussion by starting with the "Females" portion of the worksheet, explaining why it is important for teen girls and adult women to seek medical care for the reproductive system. Then, follow the same process for the "Males" part of the worksheet. If you noted earlier that a group had correct information for any question, ask that group to share their answers. Although this lesson can be easily led by you, allowing students to share information with one another supports effective communication skills and the acceptance of going to medical professionals to maintain one's health.
6. When discussing specific examinations, you or a student can refer to a diagram or model for a better representation of what a patient can expect. Also, when discussing the examinations for males and females, show the props used, if available. (Also, please ensure your school or department supports the use of these props.) For example, when explaining the Pap smear or HPV testing procedure, the speculum can be shown and explained.
7. When explaining the breast and testicular self-exams, you can pass the BSE and TSE models around the room so that students can note possible nodules. You can also distribute additional handouts or brochures covering proper BSEs and TSEs.
8. When students have completed the worksheet, ask them the processing questions. After all questions are answered, distribute the "Fact Sheet: Reproductive Health Services for Teens" handout, asking students to read the information to themselves. Ask if they have additional questions from the fact sheet.
9. For homework, assign extended response questions. Ask students to answer the following questions based on the day's lesson and the information in the "Fact Sheet: Reproductive Health Services for Teens" handout. Tell them that responses should be clear and concise, and that any questions involving personal views, values, or opinions should be backed up with rationale statements.

a. Based on the state you live in, what are three laws (county, state, or federal) pertaining to reproductive and sexual health care services (contraception, including emergency contraception; pregnancy options; safe surrender policies; prenatal care; and so on)? Note the source from which you received your information. If it was from the Internet, did the URL end in .org, .edu, or .gov? (These sources are not going to sell you a product, and are usually reliable, up to date, and unbiased.)

b. How do you feel about these laws? Do you think they are necessary? Fair? If you were a parent and your teen needed to use these confidential services without your knowledge or consent, do you think you would feel differently? Why or why not?

Processing

1. What is one thing you learned today that you did not already know or understand before?
2. When do people need to go to a medical professional when it comes to their sexual health?
3. What would you tell a friend who was hesitant about going to a medical professional about his or her sexual health?
4. How can learning about the examinations for members of the opposite sex affect personal relationships?

Assessment

- Students correctly complete their worksheet from the small group and class discussions.
- Students provide valid answers to the extended response questions.

Name: ______________________________

What Should You Expect at the Doctor's Office?

Directions: Answer the following questions to the best of your group's ability.

Females

1. List and explain some reasons why a female might go to a doctor's office or clinic (specifically dealing with her reproductive system).

____

____

____

2. What type of doctor could a female go to?

____

3. Following are some common exams. What would each entail?

   a. Breast exam:

   ____

   ____

   ____

   b. Pap smear (most young women usually get their first Pap smear around the age of twenty-one, or earlier if they are sexually active):

   ____

   ____

   ____

   c. Pelvic exam:

   ____

   ____

   ____

   d. Sexually transmitted infection (STI) tests:

   ____

   ____

   ____

(continued)

Name: ________________________

What Should You Expect at the Doctor's Office? (*continued*)

Males

1. List and explain some reasons why a male might go to a doctor's office or clinic (specifically dealing with his reproductive system).

2. What type of doctor could a male go to?

3. Following are some common exams. What would each entail?

   a. Hernia exam:

   b. Testicular exam:

   c. Prostate exam (the American Cancer Society usually recommends that men get their first prostate exam around the age of forty-five):

   d. Sexually transmitted infection (STI) tests:

Fact Sheet: Reproductive Health Services for Teens

What Are Reproductive Health Services?

Reproductive health services help maintain your sexual health. Reproductive health services include

- Sources of information on reproductive health
- Counseling related to pregnancy options, abuse, rape, and sexually transmitted infections (STIs)
- Prenatal care
- Birth control
- Screening and testing for STIs
- Screening for cancers of the reproductive organs (breasts, ovaries, uterus, cervix, and testicles)

Where Can Teens Go for Reproductive Health Services?

Across the United States, a small percentage of schools offer health resource centers where teens can go for confidential health services. If one is not available in your school, there are many clinics, doctor's offices, hospitals, and voluntary health agencies offering reproductive health services to teens. Most county health departments also provide free, confidential services and screenings. Reproductive health counseling can help teens decide about sexual activity, become better informed about contraceptive options, and reduce the risk of unplanned pregnancies and STIs.

Although state and local laws vary, at many clinics, reproductive checkups and exams, contraceptive options, and testing and treatment for STIs are free or offered for a sliding-scale fee to teens under eighteen years of age. (Planned Parenthood [www.plannedparenthood.org/health-center/] makes it easy to find a health center near you by simply typing in your zip code on its website.)

Do Teenagers Need Permission from Parents or Guardians?

In general, teenagers can receive pregnancy counseling, birth control, pregnancy tests, and screening for STIs without the knowledge or consent of their parents or guardians. In the case of abortion, some states require the permission of at least one parent or guardian if you are under the age of eighteen. In other states, notification of a parent or guardian is required. If a teen feels she cannot tell a parent or guardian, a judge can grant her permission for an abortion through a process called *judicial bypass.* The judge will meet confidentially with the teen to discuss her circumstances to decide whether to allow the abortion.

Why Do Teens Need Reproductive Health Services?

The national teen pregnancy rate has declined almost continuously over the last two decades. Between 1990 and 2008 the teen pregnancy rate declined by almost 42 percent. According to recent national data, this decline is due to a combination of the increased percentage of teens waiting to have sexual intercourse and the increased use of contraceptives by teens.* Giving teens better access to sexual health information and making reproductive services available to teens can help lower the risk of unplanned pregnancies and sexually transmitted infections.

*Kathryn Kost and Stanley Henshaw, *U.S Teenage Pregnancies, Births, and Abortions, 2008: National Trends by Age, Race, and Ethnicity* (Washington, DC: Guttmacher Institute, February 2012). www.guttmacher.org/pubs/USTPtrends08.pdf

LESSON 7: ANATOMY MATCHING GAME

Level: Middle school, High school

Time: 40 minutes

National Health Education Standards

1. Core Concepts
4. Interpersonal Communication

National Sexuality Education Standards: Performance Indicators

- Describe male and female sexual and reproductive systems including body parts and their functions.
- Demonstrate communication skills that foster healthy relationships.

Rationale

This lesson serves as an introduction to reproductive anatomy for middle school students. It may also be useful for high school classes for reviewing information previously learned in middle school health or biology.

Within the lesson, students will be able to identify anatomical parts of the male and female reproductive systems; state whether a given body part can be found in the male, the female, or both; and describe the function of each part. Students will participate in a matching game in which they are given a card with a body part and must attempt to find another student who "matches" their card in a variety of ways.

Materials and Preparation

Set of twenty-nine cards (or enough cards for everyone in the class to have at least one) with a reproductive organ or other term on each card. (A list of possible terms used in this activity is included at the end of this lesson.) Cards should be large enough for the entire class to see clearly from the back of the room. (*Note:* In a small class, each student can be given *two* cards. Students then have to "trade" with someone to end up with two cards that match in some way.)

Anatomical charts, 3-D models, or other projected pictures of the male and female reproductive systems for students to use as a reference

Procedure

1. Hand out one card to each student. Explain that the lesson's objective is for students each to match up with someone else who has a card that relates to their own. Tell them that some cards of the same sex can match up, and some cards of the opposite sex may match up. Further, there are no exact right or wrong answers. Every time the activity is done, slightly different matches may occur.

Explain that matches may be based on any of the following criteria:

- The cards represent comparable anatomical structures in males and females.
- The cards represent body parts that are near to one another within either the male or the female reproductive system.
- The cards represent items performing the same physiological function.

2. Tell students to walk around the room to find someone whose card matches theirs; once they have paired off, they should sit down together. Students who have not found a partner should meet in the center (or at the front) of the room, where you can assist them in making a match. Occasionally, it may be necessary to have a triad or to rematch students who may not know the true meaning of their cards. When students have paired off and are sitting down, give them two minutes to discuss the following questions:
   a. Describe the body part on your card as if you are that body part. (For example: "I am the testes. I am a gland.")
   b. What sex are you found in?
   c. Where are you located in the body?
   d. What is your job or function?
   e. How or why are you matched up with your partner?
3. Ask volunteers to share the answers for their pair. For this, the partners will stand, show their cards to the class, and answer the discussion questions just given. When they have offered their rationale for why they paired off, ask the class if they have any questions.
4. To conclude the lesson, ask the processing questions.

Processing

1. What terms were the easiest to pair with?
2. What terms were the most difficult to pair with?
3. How well does the class seem to understand the female reproductive system? Explain.
4. How well does the class seem to understand the male reproductive system? Explain.
5. When do people need to use the terms reviewed today?

Assessment

- Each student pair shares correct information, including what different parts are and how they function.
- Students demonstrate assertive communication.

Suggested Terms for Reproductive Anatomy Cards

Penis	Testes	Epididymis	Prostate gland	Estrogen
Vas deferens	Urethra	Seminal vesicle	Semen	Breasts
Sperm	Testosterone	Foreskin	Y chromosome	Vaginal fluids
X chromosome	Vagina	Labia	Vulva	Menstruation
Hymen	Clitoris	Cervix	Uterus	Ovulation
Fallopian tubes	Ovaries	Endometrium	Ovum	

LESSON 8: UP CLOSE AND PERSONAL

Level: Middle school

Time: 40 minutes

National Health Education Standards

1. Core Concepts
4. Interpersonal Communication

National Sexuality Education Standards: Performance Indicators

- Demonstrate communication skills that foster healthy relationships.
- Demonstrate effective ways to communicate personal boundaries and show respect for the boundaries of others.
- Describe male and female reproductive systems including body parts and their functions.

Rationale

Health is affected by a variety of positive and negative influences within society. This Up Close and Personal (UCP) lesson will stimulate discussion about some of the internal and external influences in society affecting attitudes and behaviors among youth. In addition, students will practice positive communication skills, including using appropriate anatomy and physiology terminology.

Note: It is unlikely that you will get through all sentence stems in one class session. You can decide which statements would be most appropriate for your students. Choices may be based on background information discussed in previous lessons, students' developmental level, restrictions you may have concerning what topics *can* and *cannot* be discussed, and your own comfort level in facilitating discussion.

Because UCP lessons deal mainly with the affective or emotional domain, they have a greater potential for personal disclosure on the part of students. You should be aware of and prepared to handle this. Sometimes it simply involves reminding the class that what is said in class stays in class. At other times, it may involve discussing issues with students privately to offer advice, resources, and support.

Materials and Preparation

Small lamp (optional)

Up Close and Personal sheet with several UCP sentence stems. (*Note:* Prior to teaching this activity, you should familiarize yourself with "Facilitating a UCP Session," which can be found at the end of the lesson.)

Procedure*

1. Ask students to form a circle with their chairs. Turning off the overhead lights and using a lamp may make the environment more conducive to an informal discussion.

*Unfinished sentences have been a useful learning tool for many years. The specific format used in this lesson has been adapted from the book *Up Close and Personal: Effective Learning for Students and Teachers* (Raleigh, NC: Lulu Press, 2007), by teacher, colleague, and friend Robert Winchester. Robert can be contacted at trustinbob@aol.com.

2. Introduce the activity in the following manner:

   Today we are going to do an activity called Up Close and Personal. It is simple to do, but for it to go smoothly, there are some rules to follow.

   First, understand this is not group therapy. Instead it is an opportunity for you to talk about how you feel about yourself, relationships, likes, dislikes, things that have come up in class, memories, and life in general. Although I will be facilitating the activity, I will also be sitting in the circle and participating along with everyone else.

   The activity is in the following format: I will read an unfinished sentence. Each of you will think about how you would finish this same unfinished sentence. Someone in the circle will then raise his or her hand and state his or her completed sentence. He or she will point to his or her right or left to determine which way around the circle we will proceed.

   When going around the circle, there should be no talking by anyone else. If something is said that you want to respond to or comment on, you must wait until we have gone all the way around the circle. If you cannot think of anything to say, or choose not to respond when it is your turn, you may simply say, "Pass" or "Come back to me." Everyone, including the teacher, is allowed to pass.

   When we have gone around the entire circle, I will ask anyone who passed if he or she would like to respond at this time. I will also ask for any questions or comments about anything that was said when going around the circle. At this point, there can be open discussion.

   Please note that during this activity, no names should be mentioned at any time. Instead, say something like, "I know someone who . . ."

   In addition, as with other lessons, what is said in class stays in class. However, please do not share anything that is too personal, that makes you feel uncomfortable, or that you wish to keep to yourself.

3. Once the rules have been explained and agreed on, read the first sentence stem aloud. After allowing a few moments for reflection, ask a student volunteer to start by stating his completed sentence. That student will then point to his left or right to note in which direction the remaining students will be given a chance to complete the sentence. Students then give their responses until everyone around the circle has spoken or passed.

4. At times, a student may simply not be ready to respond to a particular question. When this happens, remind her to pass, noting that she can answer after everyone else has spoken. It is also not unusual for many students to have the same response to a question or statement. "Repeats" reinforce the important concept that although all people are unique, they often share many of the same thoughts, feelings, and values.

5. After all students have responded, open up the discussion by asking if anyone has any questions or comments about anything that was said. Encourage students to talk in more detail about why they completed the sentence the way they did. Students may also ask others in the circle, including the teacher, to expand on their answer. Students may do so, or they may choose to pass.

6. Continue the circle discussion for as long as it is viable, constantly monitoring and enforcing the rules. When the discussion on a given sentence has run its course, move on to the next unfinished sentence.
7. Share the processing statements.
8. All UCP sessions should end with some brief closure in the form of another unfinished sentence. Examples include the following: "Today I learned . . ." "I learned that I . . ." "Right now I feel . . ." and "Something I want to say to one of my classmates is . . ."
9. Conclude the day's activity by summarizing what occurred in the session, making appropriate connections to the subject matter and curriculum. Then thank the class and say, "This ends our Up Close and Personal class for today."
10. Specific to this particular UCP session, assign homework in which students must write a reflection paper (of at least two to three paragraphs). A possible prompt is, "Based on what I learned about anatomy and physiology during today's UCP discussion, one thing I will consider changing about my attitudes, my future behavior, or both is . . ."

    This assignment allows students to reflect on and develop changes in attitudes and behaviors over time. When shared with the class in a subsequent lesson, it further allows the student, the class, and the teacher to observe changes in knowledge, attitudes, and values.

Processing

1. If anyone has any concerns or questions about what was discussed during our UCP session today, he or she can speak to me privately after class or can bring it up for discussion during our next class session.
2. There are many people, including teachers, coaches, counselors, or school psychologists, who can assist you with any personal issues that you may want to share with them. Keep in mind that these individuals, as mandated reporters, *must* report any verbalization or indication that you may want to hurt yourself or hurt others, or revelations of abuse of any kind, to the appropriate authorities for follow-up and counseling services.

Assessment

- Students actively participate in the UCP activity. Even though some students may decide to pass on one or more questions, as long as they are actively listening and following the ground rules, they are "actively participating."
- Students complete the homework assignment and share their response in a future class session.

Facilitating a UCP Session

- Facilitation is a skill that you can improve with practice.
- Silence is not a negative phenomenon. Silence often indicates that higher-level thinking is taking place.
- Going over ground rules at the beginning of each session is a needed and helpful technique to prevent inappropriate behavior.
- Unacceptable behavior should be stopped the moment it is recognized. To do this, pause the activity and point out the offense to the individual. For example, say, "What was just said is a put-down (or personal name), and it is not allowed in the circle discussion. Please do not do it again," or "Please do not talk to your neighbor when you should be listening to the one person who is supposed to be talking."
- If a student persists in breaking the activity's rules, talk to him one-on-one after class. Let the student know that if his behavior continues, he may not be able to participate in the future. This almost always stops the offensive behavior.
- Remind students of the information teachers *must* report if shared:

  1. If they are going to hurt themselves
  2. If they are going to hurt others
  3. If they are being abused

Possible UCP Sentence Stems: Anatomy and Physiology

1. Right now, I feel . . .
2. Sex is . . .
3. One thing I learned from my parents or guardians about sex and where babies come from is . . .
4. It may be embarrassing for some people to talk about sex because . . .
5. One thing I do not understand about my body is . . .
6. One thing I am curious about or do not understand about the bodies of members of the opposite sex is . . .
7. During our discussion this week about reproductive anatomy, one thing I was surprised about or found interesting was . . .
8. When we were learning the names of different body parts and what they do, I . . .
9. Abstinence is . . .
10. Someone is ready to have sex when . . .
11. Something I learned from friends or peers about sex and growing up is . . .
12. One thing I learned today is . . .

LESSON 9: SEXUALITY PRETEST

Level: Middle school, High school

Time: 35–40 minutes

National Health Education Standards

1. Core Concepts
2. Analyzing Influences
3. Accessing Information

National Sexuality Education Standards: Performance Indicators

- Describe male and female sexual and reproductive systems including body parts and their functions.
- Identify accurate and credible sources about sexual health.
- Define sexual abstinence as it relates to pregnancy prevention.
- Examine how alcohol and other substances, peers, media, family, society, and culture influence decisions about engaging in sexual behaviors.
- Identify prenatal practices that can contribute to a healthy pregnancy.
- Define STIs, including HIV, and how they are and are not transmitted.

Rationale

This group activity is designed to serve as a diagnostic assessment of what students *already know* in regard to human sexuality. This will be done by administering a questionnaire with thirty-three multiple choice questions at the start of a sexuality unit. By working in mixed-sex groups, students can pool their knowledge, learn from each other, and begin to feel more comfortable communicating about sexual issues with their classmates.

Materials and Preparation

Copies of "Sexuality Pretest" worksheet

Procedure

1. Divide the class into mixed-sex groups of four to six students each. Have each group choose one person to serve as the group leader. Arrange desks so groups cannot hear each other.
2. Hand out a copy of the sexuality pretest to each student. Read the directions aloud to the class to review rules, and then set the fifteen-minute time limit. Remind students to speak quietly so as not to share answers with the other groups. Tell them that because this is to serve as a diagnostic assessment, students are not allowed to use textbooks or other resources to look up answers.

   Note: You may give some sort of incentive ahead of time, such as extra credit points or a free homework pass, to encourage all students to do their best. Students can also be rewarded if an average class score of at least twenty-five correct answers is recorded.

3. Next, the group leader should read each question quietly to the rest of the group members. As groups are working, circulate around the room to ensure that all students are participating in the group decision-making process. Every few minutes, remind the class of the remaining time.
4. At the end of the fifteen minutes, collect the papers from each of the group leaders.
5. Process the activity by having a volunteer from each group read a question and her group's answer. You will then give the correct answer. For each question, students will write down the correct answers on their sheet while you make corrections on the group leaders' sheets. Here is the answer key for your reference:

1. c	5. d	9. a	13. d	17. c	21. d	25. d	29. b	33. d
2. c	6. c	10. a	14. c	18. d	22. b	26. c	30. d	
3. c	7. d	11. a	15. b	19. a	23. a	27. c	31. c	
4. a	8. d	12. d	16. c	20. a	24. b	28. c	32. b	

6. Ask the processing questions.
7. At the conclusion of the activity, record the number of correct responses for each group and return the sheets to the group leaders.
8. For homework, students can write in their notebook or journal three facts, statistics, or concepts about sexuality they learned from their peers while working in their group. They can also write down any answers that surprised them. Their responses can be discussed in the next class session.

   Note: If students have any questions or concerns about any of the questions or topics that they do not wish to share in class, they can discuss them privately with you. They also have the option of placing them in an anonymous Question Box, which should always be available somewhere in the classroom.

Processing

1. Which questions did most groups answer correctly? Where do you think you learned about this—parents or guardians, school, the media, other sources?
2. Which questions did several groups answer incorrectly? Why do you think these questions were more difficult to answer?
3. How did you feel working on this pretest with a coed group? Do you feel your group would have done just as well or better if it had been composed of all males or all females? Was it helpful to have opinions from both males and females when coming up with a group answer?
4. What are some things you learned in your group discussions that you found interesting or never knew much about before?

Assessment

- Students provide correct answers on the test.
- Students participate in the class discussion of the processing questions.
- Students complete the homework assignment and participate in a discussion in the next class session.

Names: ______________________________

____

Sexuality Pretest

Directions: Your group has fifteen minutes to complete this pretest while working cooperatively. You are not expected to know all of the answers.

For each question, discuss the choices and decide on the best answer. Mark your group's answer in the blank space next to the question number. If there is disagreement in the group, the **group leader** makes the final decision. Please discuss your possible answers quietly while in your groups, so other groups cannot hear you. When the time is up, the group leader's sheet will be turned in to the teacher as the "official" answer sheet for your group. At that time, all the correct answers will be given, and all students should make any corrections to their own worksheet. The corrected group leader's sheet will then be returned, and the group with the most correct answers will be the "winner."

____ 1. Which of the following medical doctors specializes in the diagnosis and treatment of disorders of the female reproductive system?

a. Optician
b. Pediatrician
c. Gynecologist
d. Dermatologist

____ 2. Approximately how many teenage girls get pregnant in the United States each year?

a. One hundred thousand
b. Five hundred thousand
c. Just under one million
d. Just over ten million

____ 3. "Monogamous" refers to

a. the presence of only one testicle in the scrotum.
b. a mound of fatty tissue located over the female's pubic bone.
c. having a sexual relationship with only one person.
d. removal of a single lump rather than the entire breast to treat breast cancer.

____ 4. The most effective method of preventing pregnancy and sexually transmitted infections (STIs) is

a. abstinence.
b. the birth control pill.
c. contraceptive foam.
d. condoms.

Sexuality Pretest (*continued*)

____ 5. Advantages of sexual abstinence include which of the following?

a. It is free.
b. You do not need a doctor's prescription.
c. You do not have to worry about an unplanned pregnancy or STIs.
d. All of the above

____ 6. How many sperm are released during an average ejaculation?

a. One hundred thousand to five hundred thousand
b. Five hundred thousand to one million
c. One hundred million to five hundred million
d. Over one billion

____ 7. Women who drink alcohol and smoke cigarettes regularly during their pregnancy increase the chances of giving birth to which of the following?

a. A premature baby with a low birth weight
b. A baby with fetal alcohol syndrome
c. A baby with certain types of birth defects
d. All of the above

____ 8. Which of the following is believed to be the most common STI in the United States?

a. HIV
b. Syphilis
c. Gonorrhea
d. HPV (genital warts)

____ 9. Which STI can generally be cured with antibiotics?

a. Chlamydia
b. HPV (genital warts)
c. Genital herpes
d. HIV

____ 10. An STI that can cause precancerous cells on the cervix is

a. HPV (genital warts).
b. syphilis.
c. gonorrhea.
d. pubic lice.

____ 11. In most girls, menstrual periods usually last about

a. three to six days.
b. three to six hours.
c. twenty-four hours.
d. twenty-eight days.

Sexuality Pretest (*continued*)

_____ 12. Which of the following statements is true?

a. Sexual intimacy is generally more satisfying and fulfilling in a loving relationship.
b. A person has the right to refuse any sexual behavior.
c. People with disabilities have sexual feelings and the same need as all people for love, affection, and physical intimacy.
d. All of the above

_____ 13. The advantage of using condoms as a birth control method is that they

a. can be bought in drugstores easily.
b. do not have dangerous side effects and can reduce the risk of STIs.
c. do not need a prescription to be purchased.
d. All of the above

_____ 14. Estrogen, which causes changes in girls' bodies during puberty, is produced by the

a. thyroid gland.
b. pituitary gland.
c. ovaries.
d. uterus.

_____ 15. Testosterone, which is responsible for changes in boys' bodies during puberty, is produced by the

a. scrotum.
b. testes.
c. pituitary gland.
d. liver.

_____ 16. Which of the following would be the best source of accurate information about puberty, growing up, and sexual development?

a. Friends
b. TV shows
c. A health teacher or school nurse
d. Teen magazines

_____ 17. Which of the following changes at puberty does NOT occur in boys?

a. A growth spurt
b. A deepening voice
c. The beginning of ovulation
d. Hair growth on the face, under the arms, and in the pubic area

_____18. Which of the following is true about abortion in the United States?

a. People's beliefs about abortion are based on their religious, cultural, and family values.
b. People who are "pro-choice" support the right of a woman to choose whether or not to carry a pregnancy to term.
c. People who are "pro-life" oppose abortion on the grounds that it is taking a human life.
d. All of the above

_____19. Which of the following statements about birth control is false?

a. You can purchase the birth control pill without a doctor's prescription.
b. It is advisable for young people who are considering sexual intercourse to talk with a parent or another adult about their decision to use contraception.
c. Each contraceptive method has advantages and disadvantages.
d. Emergency contraception, which is a pill taken after engaging in unprotected sex, works by preventing a woman's ovaries from releasing eggs.

_____20. In regard to STIs and HIV,

a. the organisms causing STIs and HIV are usually found in the semen or vaginal fluids and blood of an infected person.
b. you can tell if someone has an STI just by looking at that person.
c. HIV can be spread by casual contact, like shaking hands with an infected person.
d. use of latex condoms can eliminate the chance of getting an STI or HIV.

_____21. "Oral sex"

a. refers to when partners talk to each other during sex.
b. is a form of sexual behavior practiced by some people, whereby the mouth of one person is used to stimulate the sex organs (genitals) of his or her partner.
c. can spread certain types of sexually transmitted infections.
d. Both b and c.

_____22. Approximately what percentage of American high school students have had sexual intercourse?

a. 30 percent
b. 50 percent
c. 75 percent
d. Over 90 percent

Sexuality Pretest (*continued*)

_____23. Being under the influence of alcohol or other drugs

a. increases the risk of teens' having sex because it may affect their judgment.
b. decreases the risk of teens' having sex.
c. has no effect on the possibility of teens' having sex.
d. increases the percentage of teens who use condoms during sex.

_____24. John is pressuring Nancy to have sex. Nancy responds by saying "no," giving a reason, and walking away. These are all examples of

a. decision-making skills.
b. refusal skills.
c. goal-setting skills.
d. passive behavior.

_____25. Which of the following statements is true?

a. Believing all boys or all girls are or should be alike is a stereotype.
b. Boys and girls receive messages about how they should behave from their family, their friends, the media, society, and their culture.
c. There are laws that protect a woman's or a man's right to participate equally in athletic activities.
d. All of the above

_____26. "Homophobia" refers to

a. the fear of being gay.
b. a disease whereby the blood has difficulty clotting.
c. the strong negative attitude and irrational fear of someone who is gay.
d. someone born with sex organs of both sexes.

_____27. Couples in healthy, intimate relationships

a. have sex just about every day.
b. spend all their free time together.
c. maintain separate interests as well as shared ones.
d. never have disagreements or arguments.

_____28. Soap operas, commercials, talk shows, music, and other forms of media

a. always give accurate information and advice about sex and relationships.
b. often show realistic and healthy role models and relationships.
c. often present an unrealistic image of what it means to be male or female, what it means to be in love, and what parenthood and marriage are like.
d. never stereotype the roles of men and women.

Sexuality Pretest (*continued*)

____29. Gabriela gets a text message from her ex-boyfriend, Carlos. He is upset that she broke up with him. He threatens to spread a rumor on his social networking site that she has engaged in oral sex with a lot of different guys. This is an example of

a. date rape.
b. sexual harassment.
c. sexual abuse.
d. a healthy relationship.

____30. Dating helps people experience and learn about companionship and intimacy. Which of the following is true about dating?

a. Families may have different standards and rules about dating for boys and girls.
b. When couples spend a lot of time together alone, they are more likely to become sexually involved.
c. Gay and lesbian youth, like heterosexual youth, may or may not date.
d. All of the above

____31. When it comes to making good decisions, which of the following is true?

a. Alcohol or drugs help you make healthier decisions.
b. The best way to make a decision is to just go with your first instinct.
c. People should carefully evaluate the consequences, advantages, and disadvantages of each choice when they make a major decision.
d. Your individual and family values do not play a major role in your decisions about sex.

____32. With respect to effective communication, which of the following is false?

a. Males and females may sometimes communicate differently, which may cause miscommunication.
b. Couples should not talk openly and honestly about their relationship and sex because it is embarrassing.
c. Communication may be improved by listening well, stating feelings, and trying to understand the other person's point of view.
d. Being assertive and using messages beginning with "I" are helpful in communicating your thoughts and feelings to another person.

____33. Some agencies, like local health departments, help teens with problems related to sex, relationships, or both because

a. sometimes teens need to talk with an adult other than their parents.
b. they can provide birth control and other services not requiring parental permission.
c. their services are confidential and often cost little or no money.
d. All of the above

LESSON 10: HOME-SCHOOL CONNECTION

TALKING ABOUT ABSTINENCE

Level: Middle school

Time: Varies

National Health Education Standards

1. Core Concepts
2. Analyzing Influences
4. Interpersonal Communication

National Sexuality Education Standards: Performance Indicators

- Define sexual abstinence as it relates to pregnancy prevention.
- Analyze influences that may have an impact on deciding whether or when to engage in sexual behaviors.
- Demonstrate the use of effective communication skills to support one's decision to abstain from sexual behaviors.

Rationale

Parents or guardians are the primary sexuality educators of their children. The role of the school is to supplement family teaching by providing students with accurate information as well as engaging them in practicing interpersonal skills. It is the parents or guardians' responsibility to communicate family values and beliefs. The main purpose of the Home-School Connection activities is to provide teens and their parents or guardians with the opportunity to privately discuss issues related to human sexuality.

After completing the assignment, parents or guardians are requested to sign on the bottom. All responses from teens and parents or guardians on the Home-School Connection activity will be kept confidential. It will not be turned in to the teacher or graded. On the due date, students will be asked to *voluntarily* share any interesting comments or insights they learned or observed by participating in the assignment. Students *and* parents or guardians can choose to pass on any discussion they wish to keep private.

With family input and support, the overall goal is to encourage teens to become well-informed, caring, respectful, and responsible adults.

Materials and Preparation

Copies of "Talking About Abstinence" worksheet

Procedure

1. Explain to the class that they are going to have an assignment to complete with one or more parents or guardians.
2. Distribute the worksheet to all students and assign a due date.
3. On the day the assignment is due, check if students have completed the assignment by noting whether or not the sheet has been signed on the bottom. The assignment should not be collected or graded.
4. Ask for student volunteers to share results of the discussion they had with the adult or adults they interviewed. Do so using the processing questions, bearing in mind that all student comments and contributions should be voluntary.

   Note: Although students are encouraged to share what they learned by interviewing parents or guardians, they are not required to do so. Sharing and follow-up discussion are strictly on a voluntary basis.

Processing

1. Which family members did you choose to speak with?
2. How did you feel talking to family members about this topic? Were you comfortable with this discussion? Were your family members comfortable with this discussion?
3. Is it easy or difficult to talk to family members about issues related to human sexuality? Explain.
4. What stops or hinders people from communicating about sexuality? What can help people communicate effectively about sexuality?
5. What were some of the messages you received about abstinence and growing up to be a sexually responsible adult?
6. How did you feel about the messages or advice that your parents or guardians shared with you?
7. Did anything surprising come up during the conversation?
8. What did you learn from doing this assignment?

Assessment

- Students complete the assignment and bring a signed copy of the worksheet to class.
- Students participate in the follow-up discussion related to the assignment.

Talking About Abstinence

An important aspect of health education is human sexuality and healthy relationships. Parents or guardians, through their thoughts, personal values, and actions, are the primary sexuality educators of their children. The role of the school is to supplement parental teaching by providing students with accurate information and life skills. With your help, our goal is to encourage teens to become well-informed, caring, respectful, and responsible adults.

Directions: Parents or guardians are requested to sign the bottom of this handout. This is simply to ensure the student has completed the assignment. It will not be turned in to the teacher or graded. All comments from teens and parents or guardians on the Home-School Connection activity will be kept confidential.

With these guidelines in mind, please take a few minutes to discuss the following assignment with your son or daughter. Thank you in advance for your participation.

What Is Abstinence?

A person who decides to practice abstinence has chosen not to be sexually active. Although "sexual activity" can range from holding hands to sexual intercourse, most definitions of abstinence refer to "refraining from any form of sexual activity that may result in a pregnancy or a sexually transmitted infection."

In today's society, peer pressure and media messages can make the decision to practice abstinence more difficult. It is important for those teens who *do* decide to become sexually active to know potential consequences.

As a parent or guardian, what MESSAGES and VALUES do you feel are important for your teen to hear from you about abstinence and growing up to become a sexually responsible adult?

____

____

____

____

____

____

____

____

____

____

Parent or guardian signature(s): ______________________

Student signature: ______________________

Puberty and Adolescent Development

2

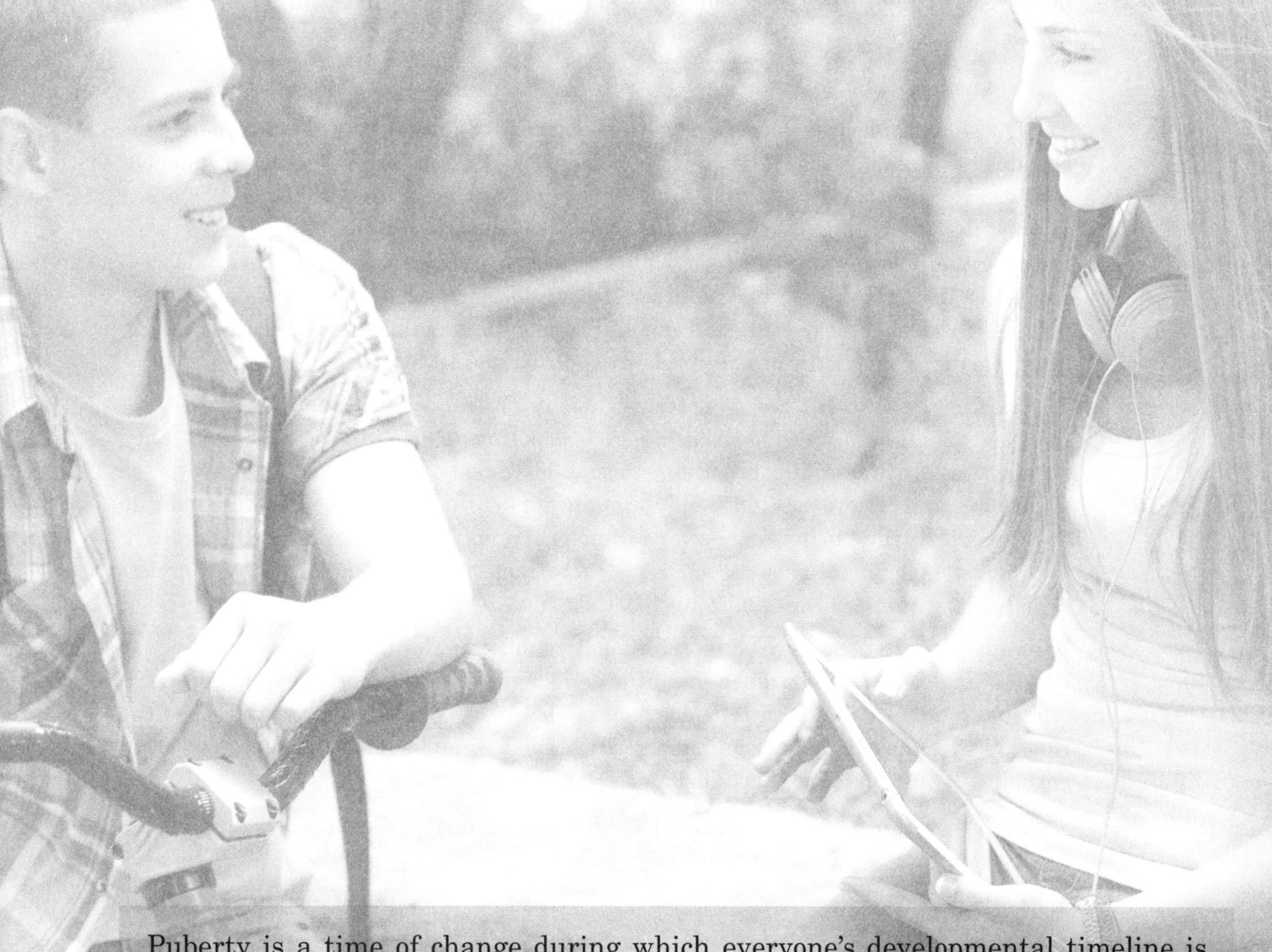

Puberty is a time of change during which everyone's developmental timeline is different. The lessons in Chapter Two attempt to reassure students that changes during puberty are a part of every person's life and are essential in preparing them for adulthood. Further, this chapter stresses the importance of teaching students the physical, social, and emotional changes accompanying this stage of life.

"AM I NORMAL?"

This is the overriding question young people have when it comes to the changes at puberty. Variations in the timing of body changes can cause concern, especially for those students who are developing secondary sex characteristics sooner or later than most of their peers. Several of the lessons in this chapter deal directly with these concerns to reassure students that we all develop at the rate that is healthy for us. Growth spurts and other changes depend largely on each individual's genetic inheritance and the action of hormones.

When discussing pubertal changes in school, males and females may sometimes be separated—with a female teacher, school professional, or outside expert facilitating the discussion with girls and a male teacher, school professional, or outside expert facilitating the discussion with boys. Although this may sometimes be appropriate, all the lessons in Chapter Two can be used with coed groups. In coed groups, students can learn a lot from each other when discussing their questions and concerns about puberty.

QUESTION BOX

The Question Box has been used in health and sexuality education classes for years. This box, in which students can submit questions they may not feel comfortable asking publicly, is placed in a private area in the classroom. Too often, teachers dispense information based on what *they* feel is important for students to learn. A Question Box provides students with the opportunity to ask about what is really on their mind. Occasionally, a student may ask a question that is too vulgar to read as written, or that includes a personal name. In these instances, you should use your professional judgment to determine whether the question is legitimate, or whether it has been asked simply for shock value.

There are generally two types of questions students ask related to sexuality: factual questions and values-based questions. Factual questions may be easier to answer because they require you to give medically accurate information. If a question is asked to which you do not know the answer, you should simply admit to not knowing the answer, but also indicate that you will attempt to find an answer within an appropriate time period and report back to the class. In addition, when responding to factual questions, you should use your professional judgment to determine how much detail to give in your answer.

Values-based questions may be more difficult to answer. You need to be careful not to express your own personal values on controversial topics because these may conflict with a student's familial, cultural, or religious beliefs. There are, however, some universal values that are shared by an overwhelming majority of families and should be supported within sexuality discussions. These include the following:

- Dignity and respect should be promoted for all people, regardless of their race, ethnicity, religion, or sexual orientation.
- Bullying, sexual harassment, dating violence, and sexual abuse are wrong.
- The safest and healthiest choice for teens, especially young teens, is not to engage in sexual behaviors.
- Sexual contact between an adult and a child is wrong.
- A person who knowingly spreads a disease is in the wrong.
- Among young people, sexting—or sending or receiving sexually explicit text messages or photos through a computer, cell phone, or other electronic device—is illegal in most states and can result in serious legal and social consequences.

LESSON 1: THE STORY OF ALEX AND SAM

Level: Middle school

Time: 30–40 minutes

National Health Education Standards

1. Core Concepts
4. Interpersonal Communication

National Sexuality Education Standards: Performance Indicators

- Describe the physical, social, cognitive and emotional changes of adolescence.
- Demonstrate communication skills that foster healthy relationships.

Rationale

Communication is a critical skill that teens can improve through modeling and practice. In the first activity, students will observe and discuss how communication can break down, and consider why this might happen. Follow-up discussion defines the gender roles and sexual stereotypes illustrated in the story featured in the activity.

In the second activity, students pair off to practice the skill of active listening. To assist them, a handout ("Communication Skills: Active Listening") is provided to define effective and poor listening skills, while giving examples of each.

Materials and Preparation

Teacher copy of "The Story of Alex and Sam"

Copies of "Active Listening Activity" handout

Copies of "Communication Skills: Active Listening" handout

Procedure

ACTIVITY 1: COMMUNICATION BREAKDOWN

1. Explain to students that the objective of the lesson is to understand how people can communicate more effectively. Then ask for five volunteers.
2. Give each volunteer a number from one to five. Have Student 1 stay in the classroom. Instruct Students 2 through 5 to wait in the hallway, far enough away from the door that they cannot hear what is occurring in the classroom.
3. Explain to the class that a story will be read. Their job is to listen carefully, observing what happens when the story is retold from one person to another. Make the class aware that this activity is a version of the telephone game, in which one person whispers something to someone else, who whispers it to someone else, and so on. As the story gets passed from person to person, it invariably changes.
4. Read "The Story of Alex and Sam" to Student 1. She cannot interrupt or ask any questions. Read the story fairly quickly and in a monotone.

5. When finished, call Student 2 into the room. Inform him that Student 1 will be telling a story from memory. Instruct Student 2 not to speak or ask questions; instead he should simply listen to the story as remembered by Student 1. When Student 1 has finished telling the story, she may sit down.

   Follow the same procedure with Students 3, 4, and 5.

6. Ask Student 5 to stay in front of the room to repeat the story as best she can remember it. The story will certainly have gotten shorter, and its facts will have changed from the first telling.
7. Allow the rest of the class to note changes within the story. In addition, ask processing questions 1 through 8.

ACTIVITY 2: PRACTICING COMMUNICATION SKILLS

1. Ask students to form groups of two.
2. Distribute copies of the "Active Listening Activity" handout, and go over the instructions as a class. Inform students that they will participate in a brief activity in which they will practice effective listening skills.
3. Distribute the "Communication Skills: Active Listening" handout. Define the term "active listening" and discuss the importance of good listening skills. Read the directions aloud, with the students quietly reading the same directions on their handout. Then give students approximately eight to ten minutes to complete the active listening activity.
4. As students are working in pairs, monitor the time and wander around the room, observing how effectively the students are practicing the communication skill of active listening.
5. After about eight to ten minutes, bring the whole class back together and ask processing questions 9 through 13 to allow students to discuss their experiences. Reinforce the importance of good communication skills. The following can be stated to summarize the activity: "Being able to receive a message is just as important as sending a message. With today's technology, we are constantly communicating on the Internet, on social networking sites, and on cell phones. Unfortunately, because these forms of communication are not face-to-face, the messages can sometimes be misunderstood. Effective communication involves not only hearing or seeing the words but also trying to correctly interpret the meaning and feeling behind the words."
6. End the lesson by asking students to reflect on the day's activities in their journal.

Processing

1. What happened when the story was told by the different students? (It gets shorter, changes.) Why do you think this happened?
2. Why did the story change? Who did a good job of listening? Who didn't do so well?
3. What could have been done to make the communication more effective?
4. How did you feel about the characters in the story? What do you think happened next?
5. In your mind, did you picture Alex as a boy or a girl? What about Sam? Pat? Why?

6. What does the term "gender role" mean? What does the term "stereotype" mean? (A *stereotype* is a prejudiced attitude that assigns a specific quality or characteristic to all people who belong to a particular group; a *gender role* refers to the way society expects someone to behave based on his or her biological sex.)
7. Would you feel differently about the people in the story if the sexes of the characters were different in each case? If so, how? For example:
   - If Alex, Sam, and Pat were all male?
   - If Alex, Sam, and Pat were all female?
   - If Alex were male, and Sam and Pat were female?
   - If Alex and Sam were male, and Pat were female?
   - If Alex were female, and Sam and Pat were male?
   - If Alex and Sam were female, and Pat were male?
8. How do gender roles and stereotypes change how you perceive the story?
9. In the active listening activity, was it easier for you to listen or to speak?
10. Which skills came easily to you? Which were more difficult?
11. How did you feel about the experience?
12. What is one thing that you can practice to improve your listening skills?
13. What is one thing you learned from today's lesson on communication?

Assessment

- Students identify at least three reasons why there was a breakdown in communication in the reading of the "Alex and Sam" story.
- Students demonstrate effective listening skills in pairs.
- Students write a reflection statement in their journal.

The Story of Alex and Sam

Alex and Sam are both fourteen and have been friends since first grade. Although they are still friends, Alex has developed into a skilled tennis player, spending a lot of time with other kids on the tennis team. Sam is not very athletic and is more into listening to music and spending time on the computer.

Now that they are teenagers, their bodies have been changing. Alex grew five inches between seventh and eighth grade. Sam hasn't really experienced a growth spurt yet and is shorter than a lot of kids in middle school. But Sam *has* gone through many of the other changes of puberty, including changes in body proportions, growth of pubic and underarm hair, and an increased sex drive. Sam has also noticed more facial pimples and blackheads.

One day in physical education class, Pat, an unpopular student, called Sam a "zitface." Although Sam was embarrassed, ignoring the remark seemed to be the best thing to do. Unfortunately, Pat, who is a lot bigger than Sam, continued to make comments about Sam's complexion every time they saw each other—in physical education class, in the cafeteria, in the hallways—it was really starting to bother Sam.

On Friday night, Alex called Sam and asked to know if Sam wanted to go to the mall the next day. Sam said, "Thanks for asking, Alex, but I don't think so."

"Why not?" asked Alex. "We always have fun when we hang out there."

"Well, to tell you the truth," said Sam, obviously upset, "I've heard that Pat hangs out there most Saturdays. I just don't want to have to deal with Pat's comments."

"What do you mean? What has Pat been saying?" asked Alex.

"I don't want to talk about it," replied Sam.

"Hey, I'm your friend. What's up?"

"Pat's a jerk. Pat thinks it's real funny making fun of my face and calling me 'zitface' all the time."

"What did you do about it?" asked Alex.

"I've been trying to ignore it, hoping Pat will get tired of bothering me. But it's just gotten worse. Look, I really don't want to talk about this anymore. I gotta go now. Bye."

As soon as Alex got off the phone with Sam, Alex sent a text message to Pat. The text read: "Pat? Alex from school. Wondering if you were going to the mall tomorrow."

A few minutes later, Alex received a text back from Pat. The text read: "Usually go to food court around noon. Why?"

Alex texted back: "Have something important I want to talk to you about."

Pat texted back: "What's the big deal? Just text me."

Alex's final text read, "No, this is something I need to tell you in person. Food court at noon . . . be there!"

Active Listening Activity

Directions: The point of this practice session is to give each student the opportunity to learn how to use verbal and nonverbal communication to become a better listener.

For this activity, you need to pair off with another student. Then assign who is Student A and who is Student B.

Student A will then speak first.

To the speaker: Your task is to talk about something that is important to you—your family, a decision you have to make, or what you like to do in your free time. You will only have ONE MINUTE to speak. You may find yourself in the middle of discussing something important when time runs out. If this happens, you could make an agreement with the person who is listening to continue the conversation during a break or after class.

To the listener: Your task is to practice the skills of an active listener. These include making eye contact; watching for body language; remaining silent; and showing verbal and nonverbal cues (for example, saying "uh-huh," nodding your head, or asking a brief question to clarify something). Concentrate on following the speaker's train of thought.

The listener (Student B) will then paraphrase or summarize the experience of listening to Student A. For this, answer the following questions:

1. What was said?
2. How well did you understand Student A?
3. Did Student A's facial expressions or body language match what was being said?

Next, the speaker (Student A) will share his or her feelings about the listener's listening by answering the following questions:

1. Did you feel listened to?
2. Was Student B able to summarize what you said correctly?
3. Did Student B have any habits you found distracting?

You will then repeat the activity by switching roles. Student B will talk for ONE MINUTE on a topic of his or her choice, and Student A will practice active listening. Then repeat the other step to share the speaking-listening and feedback experience.

Communication Skills: Active Listening

Some disagreements in relationships occur because of poor communication. Good communication skills can help people learn more about themselves and others. **Active listening** calls for the listener to devote full attention to the speaker, genuinely caring what the other person is saying, while encouraging the speaker to keep talking. A common problem for people learning the skill of active listening is that they may be organizing their own thoughts rather than listening to whoever is speaking.

Notes to remember:

Evidence of Good Listening Skills

- Facing the speaker and making eye contact
- Being aware of what the speaker is saying as well as the speaker's facial expressions, body language, and tone and volume of voice
- Waiting for the speaker to pause before asking brief clarifying questions
- Reflecting on the feelings that the speaker is trying to convey (for example, "Seems like that bothered you a lot . . .")
- Giving verbal or nonverbal signs that you are listening (nodding, saying "uh-huh," smiling)
- When the speaker has finished speaking, summarizing the speaker's key ideas

Evidence of Poor Listening Skills

- Interrupting the speaker before he or she is finished
- Looking around the room, being distracted by people or noise
- Continuing to do what you are doing (watching TV, chatting on the computer or cell phone, reading) rather than listening attentively
- Giving advice when all the person wants is to be listened to
- Making unrelated remarks or asking questions about an unrelated topic
- Allowing your mind to wander and only pretending to hear what the speaker is saying

LESSON 2: STIRRING UP HORMONES

Level: Middle school

Time: 40 minutes

National Health Education Standards

1. Core Concepts
3. Accessing Information
4. Interpersonal Communication

National Sexuality Education Standards: Performance Indicators

- Describe the physical, social, cognitive and emotional changes of adolescence.
- Describe how puberty prepares human bodies for the potential to reproduce.
- Demonstrate communication skills that foster healthy relationships.
- Identify medically-accurate sources of information about puberty, adolescent development and sexuality.

Rationale

During puberty, physical and emotional changes occur as a result of increased hormone production. Teens sometimes feel uncomfortable, clumsy, and self-conscious because of the rapid changes in their body. The overriding question that all teens have is, "Am I normal?"

In the first part of this lesson, students will complete a worksheet that classifies whether the changes at puberty happen in males only, in females only, or in both males and females.

In the second part of the lesson, students will develop skits that illustrate one or more changes at puberty and the resulting positive or negative feelings or reactions that may accompany those changes.

Materials and Preparation

Front board

Large pot, bowl, or paper bag with "Puberty" written on the outside

Wooden spoon with "Hormones" written on it

Small, teacher-prepared cards (such as index cards cut into two or four pieces). On each card, write one change at puberty (a list of suggested changes is included at the end of this lesson). Place the cards in the "Puberty" container.

Copies of "Secondary Sex Characteristics: Changes at Puberty" worksheet

Computers, health texts, or brochures for accessing information

Procedure

ACTIVITY 1: "THE PUBERTY FAIRY" AND SECONDARY SEX CHARACTERISTICS

1. Begin class by telling the students about an imaginary figure, the "Puberty Fairy," who comes into their room one night while they are sleeping and sprinkles them with "puberty dust." The next day, they have magically changed from a boy into a man, or from a girl into a woman!
2. After students tell you that there is no such event, ask them, "If you don't believe in the Puberty Fairy, what actually causes boys and girls to go through puberty?" (The answer is *hormones.*) Tell them, "In addition to the changes that you can see on the outside of the body, there are also important changes happening inside the body. The sexual and reproductive systems mature during puberty and prepare human bodies for the potential to reproduce."
3. Write a definition of "hormones" on the front board and have students copy this definition into their notebook: "Hormones are chemical substances produced by glands or organs in the body that travel through the bloodstream to control or regulate other tissues or organs in the body. During puberty, hormones cause the internal and external changes related to growth and sexual maturity. These changes are referred to as secondary sex characteristics."
4. Take out the bag (or other container) labeled "Puberty" and the spoon labeled "Hormones." Explain that you are going to stir up the hormones and see what comes out.
5. Hand out the "Secondary Sex Characteristics: Changes at Puberty" worksheet
6. Ask each student to come up to the front of the room, stir the puberty bag, and pull out a card. Volunteers should each read their card to the class, and then decide whether the change on their card happens to *males only, females only,* or *both males and females.* Discuss each change as a class. Continue the activity until all cards have been discussed. If students are not familiar with a word, provide the correct information, including where the word belongs on the worksheet.
7. As the students are stirring up the puberty cards, you should be keeping on the board a master list of the changes that occur during puberty. Students should keep a list of the changes on their worksheet, categorizing each card under one of the headings provided.

ACTIVITY 2: GROUP SKITS ON CHANGES AT PUBERTY

1. Break students into groups of three to five students, depending on the size of the class.
2. Explain that each group will develop a brief (one- to two-minute) skit illustrating two or more changes at puberty and how kids their age feel about those changes. Skits should deal with a physical or emotional change taking place in males, females, or both. In the skit, students may react positively or negatively to the changes. Appropriate behavior is expected.
3. Characters in the skits may be all female, all male, or a combination, depending on the nature of the skit. Characters in the skit may be peers, parents or guardians, siblings, counselors, or doctors.

4. Tell students that each skit must include at least three accurate facts about puberty, and that they must cite a credible resource (for example, a health textbook, a brochure, or an Internet site ending in .gov, .org, or .edu). Students should be provided with texts, brochures, and computers, if available, to reference accurate information.
5. The skits should conclude on a positive note. For example, a character might give good advice, the changes might be depicted as happening to everyone, the changes might be portrayed as a sign that a character is growing up, or the skit might remind the audience that there are people they can talk to.
6. Students may develop their own skits, but some of the suggestions here could be used or modified:
   - A boy's voice cracking when he gives an answer in class
   - Boys discussing wet dreams, "unexpected" erections, and sexual attraction
   - Girls discussing feelings about getting their period for the first time
   - Being shorter or taller than most of your peers
   - The need for increased hygiene (starting using deodorant, washing hair and showering daily, shaving, and so on)
   - Feelings about the increase in facial and other body hair
   - Complexion problems or being self-conscious about other body changes

   Note: You should stress that all skits should involve fictional, typical teenagers—and that no real names should be used. It is best to rotate through the groups as they are planning their respective skits to ensure that all skits are somewhat different and appropriate. You might also want to make suggestions to make sure skits meet the requirements.
7. Conclude the lesson by discussing the processing questions.

Processing

1. Which skits were realistic? Explain.
2. What did you learn from the skits?
3. What is the main hormone that causes most of the changes at puberty in males? In females?
4. Knowing what the opposite sex experiences during puberty, how do you feel about those changes? Do you think going through puberty is easier for males or for females? Explain your answer.

Assessment

- Students participate in the "stirring up hormones" activity.
- Students actively participate in planning or acting in a group skit—or both.

Suggestions for Index Cards (Changes in Males, Females, or Both)

MALES	FEMALES	BOTH
Broader shoulders	Growth of breasts	Emotional changes
Deeper voice	Wider hips	Increased perspiration
Increased muscle mass	Beginning of ovulation	Acne
Facial hair	Beginning of menstruation	Body odor
Sperm produced	Increased estrogen	Maturation of sex organs
Erections	Increased progesterone	Growth spurt
Ejaculations	Release of eggs (ova)	Hair growth under arms
Nocturnal emissions	Vaginal discharge	Pubic hair
Larger penis	Breast tenderness	Increased moodiness
Increased testosterone		Voice changes
Semen produced		Sexual and romantic feelings

Name: ______________________________

Secondary Sex Characteristics: Changes at Puberty

Males	Females	Both

LESSON 3: ALPHABET SOUP VOCABULARY GAME

Level: Middle school

Time: 30–40 minutes

National Health Education Standard

1. Core Concepts

National Sexuality Education Standards: Performance Indicators

- Describe the physical, social, cognitive and emotional changes of puberty and adolescence.
- Describe male and female sexual and reproductive systems including body parts and their functions.

Rationale

The Alphabet Soup vocabulary game is a fun way to review basic terminology about puberty while separating myths from facts. In addition, by using correct terminology to describe male and female reproductive anatomy, students become more comfortable for future lessons pertaining to human sexuality.

This lesson may be used as a diagnostic assessment to find out what students already know about puberty and sexual development. It may also be used as a summative assessment at the end of a unit on puberty to assess what knowledge students have gained during the unit.

Materials and Preparation

Sack or hat for letters

Four sets of letters of the alphabet (*A* through *Z*). These may be found in dollar stores (foam rubber, magnets, cardboard, and so on), but they can also be made by cutting up index cards into squares and placing a letter on each. Put these in the sack or hat.

Front board or poster paper and markers to keep score

Teacher copy of "Suggested Words and Definitions"

Procedure

1. Explain to the class that the day's activity is called Alphabet Soup because it is a vocabulary game. However, unlike other vocabulary games students may have played, this one pertains to the changes occurring during puberty as well as the male and female reproductive systems.
2. Split the class into two teams and have each quickly come up with a team name. Write each team's name on the board (or poster paper), and then flip a coin to determine which team will begin the game.

3. Explain the following instructions for playing the game:
   a. One person from Team A will reach into the sack (or other container) to pull out a letter. As the game host, you will read a definition of a word related to puberty and sexual development beginning with that letter. The contestant must then come up with the correct vocabulary word that starts with that letter. For example, if the student picks the letter *W*, and the definition "Another name for the uterus" is read aloud, the student needs to answer, "Womb."
   b. The contestant will have fifteen seconds to answer. She may ask people on her team to help, but only the contestant can give the final answer.
   c. If the correct answer is provided, the student's team receives one point (which is marked on the board under that team's name).
   d. If an incorrect answer is provided, members of the other team may confer with each other, and if they believe they know the correct answer, one team member should respond. If that team guesses correctly, the team receives a point.
   e. A student from the other team will then choose another letter from the bag, and the same procedure is followed.
4. Continue playing the game by alternating teams and keeping score. Because the point of the game is to increase awareness of puberty and sexual development, you should ensure that all answers are correct.
5. Conduct a "class whip" in which students each state a quick fact that they learned by playing the Alphabet Soup vocabulary game.
6. Conclude the class by asking the processing questions.

Processing

1. What words surprised you from the game?
2. What terms were known by the class? Were the terms related to one gender?
3. How comfortable were you discussing these terms in a coed class?
4. How important is it for teenagers to be able to describe pubertal changes?
5. Why is it important for teenagers to know the proper terminology to describe the male and female reproductive systems?

Assessment

- Students provide correct terms to match definitions and descriptions pertaining to puberty and reproduction.
- In the class whip, students correctly state one physical, emotional, or social change at puberty and adolescence.

Suggested Words and Definitions

Acne—a common skin condition during puberty in which pores become inflamed, resulting in pimples, blackheads, and whiteheads.

Adolescence—the stage of growth between puberty and adulthood.

Body odor—smell created in the armpit area. This can be problematic for teenagers if they do not practice proper personal hygiene habits.

Breasts—body parts that develop earlier in some girls, and later in others. On giving birth to a baby, the female can feed the baby with milk from these.

Cervix—the lower end of the uterus.

Changes—what kids experience during puberty, both on the inside and on the outside.

Decisions—choices people make that affect their health; as a person gets older, the number of these increases.

Ejaculation—the process by which semen comes out of the tip of the penis.

Erection—the term used when a penis becomes longer and firmer. This occurs when arteries in the penis expand and fill with blood.

Estrogen—in females, a hormone released by the ovaries, controlling several changes during puberty.

Fertilization—the term used when an egg and sperm combine.

Gland—an organ that releases hormones. An example of this type of organ is the pituitary.

Gonads—the scientific name for the ovaries and testes.

Hips—these widen in a female during puberty to prepare her body for the possibility of giving birth in the future.

Hormone—a chemical substance secreted by an endocrine gland to stimulate growth or regulate the body's activities.

Hymen—the thin membrane partially covering the vaginal opening. This opening allows the menstrual fluid to leave the female's body.

Immune—what the letter *I* stands for in the disease AIDS. This is the body system that fights germs.

Kissing—a behavior that is used in most parts of the world to express affection between two people.

Labia—the folds of skin surrounding the vaginal and urethral openings.

Masturbation—the action of a person touching his or her own sex organs for sexual pleasure.

Menstruation—the term used to explain a female's monthly period.

Suggested Words and Definitions (*continued*)

Nocturnal emission—an involuntary discharge of semen as a male sleeps; also called a wet dream.

Oral sex—a type of sex in which a person's mouth makes contact with another person's genitals. It can spread HIV and other STIs.

Ovulation—the monthly release of an egg cell in females.

Penis—the organ in males that releases urine or semen.

Period—a slang term for menstruation. Although most girls get this between the ages of eleven and fourteen, some girls start as early as age eight or as late as age eighteen.

Pituitary—the gland in the brain that controls the growth spurt and other changes during puberty.

Pubic hair—hair that grows around the external sex organs in both sexes. This hair growth is one of the earliest signs of going through puberty.

Reproduction—the scientific term for producing a baby.

Secondary sex characteristics—signs indicating that puberty, or sexual maturity, is occurring.

Scrotum—the soft sac of skin containing and protecting the testes.

Semen—the mixture of sperm cells and other whitish fluids released during an ejaculation.

Shoulders—body parts that become broader and more muscular for males during adolescence.

Tampon—an item that is inserted inside the vagina to absorb menstrual fluid. It can be used instead of a menstrual pad.

Testes—two glands found in males that start to produce sperm cells during puberty.

Testosterone—the hormone responsible for the voice's deepening, muscle development, the growth of pubic hair, and the growth of facial hair.

Urethra—the tube removing urine from the body.

Vagina—the passageway leading from the uterus to the outside of the body.

Voice—something that can become deeper because of an enlargement of the larynx.

Womb—another name for the uterus.

X chromosome—the chromosome responsible for creating a baby that is a female.

Years—the length of time puberty lasts.

Zygote—another term for a fertilized egg cell.

LESSON 4: DR. I. B. HEALTHY

COMMON CONCERNS FOR PRETEENS AND TEENS

Level: Middle school

Time: Two 40-minute sessions

National Health Education Standards

1. Core Concepts
3. Accessing Information

National Sexuality Education Standards: Performance Indicators

- Describe the physical, social, cognitive and emotional changes of adolescence.
- Identify medically-accurate sources of information about puberty, adolescent development and sexuality.

Rationale

Myths abound concerning changes at puberty and sexual development. By taking on the role of an imaginary expert, students will access and share accurate information related to questions and concerns adolescents have about changes at puberty and sexual development. This will be a two-day learning experience. On the first day, students will be broken up into groups and will be given time to research and respond to a query related to changes at puberty.

On the second day, students will share with the entire class the answer to the question that their group researched.

Materials and Preparation

Teacher copy of "Dr. I. B. Healthy Questions," cut into sections

Brochures with information about puberty, health texts, and computers with Internet access (if available)

Lined notebook paper for group answers, one sheet per group

Procedure

ACTIVITY 1: DAY 1—PUBERTY LETTERS

1. Either assign groups or allow students to form groups of four to five students on their own.

2. Explain the task to each of the groups by stating: "During today's class, you will respond to an imaginary letter written by a middle school student. The letter will be addressed to an imaginary expert on puberty and adolescent development, Dr. I. B. Healthy. Your group will have the remainder of the period to answer the letter. To do this, your group will use the brochures, health texts, or computers if available."

   Tell groups that their letter needs to adhere to the following guidelines:

   a. The response needs to be in letter format.
   b. The response must be detailed—not a one-sentence answer. The answer must include a full explanation.
   c. Suggestions of how to handle the situation can also be included.
   d. A reliable resource or resources should be used.
   e. The names of all group members should be listed on the group's response sheet.

   For your reference, here is a possible rubric for grading this assignment:

Letter Rubric (20 Points Total)

CATEGORY	8–10 POINTS	5–7 POINTS	2–6 POINTS
Actual response	A letter was written that answered all parts of the question. The response was well researched and correct. Appropriate terminology was used. Reliable resources were listed.	A letter was written. Some information was supplied, yet was incorrect or too brief. The response was appropriate. A resource was listed, but not referenced for credibility.	The response was too brief, it was inappropriate, it did not directly address the question, or a combination of these characteristics.
Sharing of the letter and its response with the class (use of effective communication and presentation skills)	The group presentation was excellent. All students participated in reading parts of the response. Students could be heard. Any questions posed by the class were addressed accurately.	The reading of the letter was appropriate, but not all group members participated. Students could be heard most of the time. Attempts were made to answer questions posed by the class or teacher, but answers were not completely accurate.	Inappropriate behavior or statements occurred, no additional points or questions were addressed, or both.

3. Let students know that they should designate a role to each person in their group. One person must be responsible for writing the final response from Dr. I. B. Healthy. Another student will be responsible for reading the group's question and response to the class during the next session. *All* group members are expected to contribute ideas and to access accurate information to formulate the final response.
4. Tell students that they need to reference at least one available resource that they used in writing the response. This resource can be an appropriate Internet site, pamphlets or brochures, or a textbook. Internet sites ending in .org, .edu, or .gov are generally reliable sources of information.
5. By the end of the first session, groups should have written a complete response to their assigned question on their piece of lined paper. Groups should be prepared to read their response to the class during the next class session.

ACTIVITY 2: DAY 2—RESPONSES TO PUBERTY LETTERS

1. To begin the class, students should form the same groups that they were in the previous day. Assign a number to each group. Group 1 will start, with each of the other groups presenting their response in numerical sequence.
2. Have the student who was designated by his group read the group's original letter aloud, and then have him read the group's response. After each letter, allow further discussion, answering additional questions students may have pertaining to the situations.
3. To conclude the activity, ask the processing questions as part of a further class discussion.

Processing

1. How realistic were the original letters? Why do you feel this way?
2. Whom can young people talk with if they have questions about puberty?
3. Who taught you about puberty?
4. What resource or resources did you use for your group's letter? Would you recommend the resource or resources to others? Why or why not?

Assessment

- Students work cooperatively in their group, contributing to the final construction of the response.
- Students complete a response written in letter format, including a reference to at least one reliable source of information.

Dr. I. B. Healthy Questions

Dear Dr. I. B. Healthy,

Ever since I got my period in fifth grade, I have used pads. One of my best friends uses tampons, and I am interested in trying them but am afraid. What if I try one and it gets stuck? What if it hurts? What should I do?

Thanks,

Nervous Netty

Dear Dr. I. B. Healthy,

I am an eleven-year-old boy. Some guys in my class have started talking about girls and their bodies. I notice girls, and have some friends who are girls, but I don't feel sexually attracted to them. I prefer hanging out with my guy friends. Does this mean I'm gay or that I will become gay?

Thanks,

Confused in California

Dear Dr. I. B. Healthy,

I've been playing sports for some years, and this spring I have been feeling itchy and uncomfortable in my private area. It's even starting to burn. What is this? And what should I do?

Thanks,

Jock James

Dear Dr. I. B. Healthy,

I've been getting my period for a few years, and all of a sudden, I have been getting this really itchy feeling in my vaginal area and have an unusual discharge. I haven't had any sex so I know it's not a sexually transmitted infection. One of my friends mentioned that I might have a yeast infection. What is this? And, if it is a yeast infection, what do I do?

Thanks,

Itchy Iris

Dear Dr. I. B. Healthy,

I'm in seventh grade. My twenty-eight-year-old uncle has always been healthy and athletic. He was recently diagnosed with cancer of the testes. He is getting treatment, and they said he is going to be okay. I noticed that one of my testicles is a little bigger and hangs a littler lower than the other one. Could this be cancer? What should I do?

Signed,

Concerned Chris

(continued)

Dr. I. B. Healthy Questions (*continued*)

Dear Dr. I. B. Healthy,

I have a friend who wears low-cut jeans and thong string underwear. Every time she sits down, it shows. I have heard a lot of people make fun of her. What should I do? Also, is wearing a thong unhealthy?

Thanks,

Bloomer Betty

Dear Dr. I. B. Healthy,

My older sister is in high school and is very athletic. Outside of school, she likes to hang with some of her close girl friends on the softball team. Sometimes they have sleepovers. The other day she came home very upset. A group of guys and girls in the lunchroom called her "dyke" and "lesbo" when she walked past their table. I don't think she is a lesbian, but even if she is, I still love her, and it wouldn't change how I feel about her. What can she do about this teasing?

Thanks,

Sister Sue

Dear Dr. I. B. Healthy,

I saw this commercial about not feeling "fresh" down there, and it recommended that women douche. What is this? And is this healthy?

Thanks,

Hygienic Helen

Dear Dr. I. B. Healthy,

My uncle recently "came out" and openly admitted that he is gay. He and his boyfriend live together in our neighborhood. I'm kind of confused because neither of them *acts* gay—you know, like, feminine. I thought that gay guys all kind of talked, walked, and acted a certain way. Can you clear this up for me?

Thanks,

Confused Casey

Dear Dr. I. B. Healthy,

Some of my friends were joking in the lunchroom about . . . you know . . . private parts. Like about size and stuff. Should the testicles be the same size? One of mine is lower than the other. Is this normal? Also, why are some guys circumcised and others not?

Thanks,

Bashful Bob

Dr. I. B. Healthy Questions (*continued*)

Dear Dr. I. B. Healthy,

I recently had to go to my doctor for a physical. While there, he asked me to turn my head and cough while he held my testicles. What is this for?

Thanks,

Anonymous in Alabama

Dear Dr. I. B. Healthy,

HELP!!! I am breaking out so much this year! It looks like you can play connect the dots on my face! What is happening to me? What should I do?

Thanks,

Got Zits?

Dear Dr. I. B. Healthy,

Can masturbation hurt me? Will it do any damage to me? Will I grow hair on my palms? Will I need to wear glasses? Will it stunt my growth?

Thanks,

Student "X"

Dear Dr. I. B. Healthy,

Is it normal for guys to have breasts? My uncle was diagnosed with breast cancer, and I didn't think that could happen to a guy.

Thanks,

Worried Walter

Dear Dr. I. B. Healthy,

I'm fifteen. My mom asked me if I wanted to go to a gynecologist for my first exam. What is this? Will it hurt? Will I have to tell the doctor anything?

Thanks,

Private Patricia

Dear Dr. I. B. Healthy,

I sometimes wake up with a wet, sticky spot on my underwear. It's not urine, so what is it?

Thanks,

Stymied Steve

LESSON 5: QUESTION BOX

Level: Middle school, High school

Time: Varies

National Health Education Standards

1. Core Concepts
3. Accessing Information
4. Interpersonal Communication

National Sexuality Education Standards: Performance Indicators

- Describe the physical, social, cognitive and emotional changes of adolescence.
- Identify medically-accurate sources of information about puberty, adolescent development and sexuality.
- Identify parents or other trusted adults of whom they can ask questions about puberty and adolescent health issues.
- Demonstrate communication skills that foster healthy relationships.

Rationale

Middle and high school teens are bombarded with confusing messages about sex from movies, TV, magazines, music, and peers. Parents and guardians are the primary sexuality educators of their children, but they are also confused and often intimidated about what to say and when and how to say it. This activity uses an anonymous Question Box to help answer legitimate questions students have about sexuality. The main goal of this activity is to clarify information about students' changing bodies and other sexual issues in a safe, nonthreatening atmosphere. This activity is most effectively used in classrooms where teachers encourage trust and comfort, and in which ground rules have been established and are enforced.

Materials and Preparation

Small box with a slit large enough to allow small folded pieces of paper through, to be referred to as the "Question Box"

Teacher copy of "Question Box Guidelines"

Small scraps of paper, one per student

Procedure

1. Ask students if they have ever had a discussion with a parent or guardian about the "facts of life." Ask for volunteers to briefly explain how the discussion occurred and what they learned.
2. Raise the point that students may find it difficult to talk about sensitive issues with their parents or guardians. For some adults, it is just as difficult—and sometimes even more so. Allow students to discuss this phenomenon.

3. Ask students where they have seen images and information about sex. Students might respond by stating that images and information are found everywhere, including on TV; in books, magazines, and advertisements; on the Internet; and through peers. Let them know that, unfortunately, the information teens receive from these sources is often inaccurate, and the messages are not health enhancing.
4. Explain to students: "What we are going to do today (as well as other days during the semester) is give you an opportunity to ask questions about puberty, human sexuality, or both. Occasionally, you may have a question that you are not comfortable asking in class. The Question Box activity gives you the opportunity to ask these questions anonymously."
5. Hand out a small sheet of paper to each student. Give these instructions to the class:

   > Think of a question you have about puberty or any other area of human sexuality. Then write it on your paper. If you come up with another question, write it below the first one. Fold the paper in half, and then fold it in half again so no one can see what you wrote. Remember that these questions are to be anonymous, so do not write your name. No one will know who wrote which questions (as long as you do not write your name). I am the only person who will see the questions. You will have about three to four minutes to come up with your questions. Please try to use scientific words, but if you do not know the "acceptable" word, you may use slang. If you do not have any questions, write "I do not have any questions at this time" on your slip of paper.
   >
   > We are going to go over questions asked by your peers. To do this, I am going to open the box and take out one question. I will first read it to myself and determine if it is okay to read. Here are some rules for writing questions:
   >
   > - A question is not okay if it contains a person's name.
   > - A question should not make fun of or put down anyone or any group.
   > - Questions need to be age appropriate. If a question is not read aloud, this does not mean it is not a good question. Instead, the question would probably be better answered at another time or with a smaller group (for example, with a parent or guardian).
   > - If a question has slang or street language in it but is a good question, the wording will be changed to make it more acceptable to say in class.

   When all students have completed their questions, go around the room and collect them in the Question Box.
6. After all questions are collected, choose a question from the box. If it is worded acceptably, read it aloud. On occasion, at your discretion, a question using language that is not acceptable for class use may be read as written, but with the understanding that proper terminology will be used for all class discussions in the future. For example, if a student wrote the term "balls" to describe the testes, then you can first say the term "balls" when reading the question, but should then state the more appropriate term for use in future discussions—"testes" or "testicles." Here are some guidelines for reviewing the questions (see also "Question Box Guidelines" at the end of this lesson):

a. Group common questions together. Tell the class, "There are many questions about [a given topic], so I am addressing them all in this answer." This saves processing time and avoids possible duplication.

b. Acknowledge questions that you could not understand or that seem to be off topic. State, "There are questions that I cannot read," or, "There are questions that do not relate to our current course content." Conclude by saying, "Please see me individually if you do not hear your questions answered today."

c. Be cautious about expressing personal beliefs, opinions, or personal values on sensitive topics.

d. Defer lengthy discussions on questions that relate to future course content. Answer such questions briefly, indicating that the topic will be discussed during an upcoming lesson. For example, you can say, "There are some questions about contraception that we will be discussing next class. If you still have a question or don't understand the correct answer after that lesson, you can resubmit your question at that time."

7. After a question has been read, ask if anyone in class has an answer or opinion on the question. If no one does, you should answer the question. If you do not know the answer to the question, state that you will research the answer and answer the question at a later date. A student may also volunteer to do this research. If it is a "values-based" question, students are encouraged to state their opinions, understanding that not everyone may feel the same way. Students should always be encouraged to discuss these values-based questions with parents or guardians or other trusted adults.
8. Continue going through the Question Box until all the questions have been answered, or as time permits. Also, a few questions may be answered during other lessons.
9. Conclude the lesson with a discussion in which students answer the processing questions.
10. For homework, have students write in their notebook three "I learned . . ." statements based on the class discussion. These statements can be checked and shared in the next or a future class session.

Processing

1. What is one fact you learned today that you did not know before?
2. How comfortable are you discussing these things with a parent or guardian? How comfortable is a parent or guardian talking about these things with you?
3. How does talking about this subject with a parent or guardian differ from talking with a friend?

Assessment

- Students participate in the Question Box activity, following the established rules.
- Students provide medically-accurate information in response to questions taken from the Question Box.
- Students complete the homework assignment, writing three "I learned . . ." statements based on discussions related to the Question Box activity.

Question Box Guidelines

Accessing Accurate Information Using the Question Box

The question box is an excellent way for students to learn the skill of *accessing information.* Generally, Internet sites that end in .org, .gov, or .edu are good sources of information. Although there are numerous legitimate .com sites, many sell products and are not as reliable. As an alternative activity, assign students specific questions from the box. Instruct students to find two legitimate sites to compare the information appearing on both. This is a positive practice to ensure the reliability of both websites and helps students develop consumer skills.

Using the Question Box also serves as an opportunity for you to "plant" certain common questions in the box that students may not think of or may be too embarrassed to ask. Planting these questions in the box allows for these common questions to be answered in a safe manner.

Common Questions Related to Puberty and Adolescent Development

The following are common questions students may have about changes during puberty and other related concerns. You can "stuff" the Question Box with these questions, mixing them in with other student questions.

- Why does my voice sometimes crack when I speak?
- When do teens usually start and stop growing?
- What is happening inside a girl's (or boy's) body during puberty?
- Do breasts or testicles sometimes grow at different rates? Is it normal for one to be bigger than the other?
- Why do erections sometimes happen for no reason? It can be embarrassing!
- How does a girl know when she is going to get her period, especially the first one?
- What is the average size for the male penis?
- If a girl were menstruating and ovulating at age twelve, could she get pregnant if she had sex?
- I woke up and my underwear had a wet spot on it. It was not urine. Is this normal?
- What are some of the first signs of puberty in boys?
- Does eating chocolate cause acne? If not, what does?
- How often should teens shower or take a bath? Shampoo their hair? Use deodorant?
- I heard that masturbation will make you go blind. Is this true? Is masturbation normal?
- I heard that girls are supposed to get their period every twenty-eight days. Is this true?
- What does the term "sex drive" mean? At what age are you supposed to be attracted to others? When should kids start to date?
- I am the shortest kid in my class. Even the girls are taller than me. I have been getting text messages on my phone calling me "shorty" and other names. What can I do about this?
- I feel really embarrassed talking to my mom about the whole "period" thing. Whom else can I talk to about this stuff?
- Should I use tampons or pads?

LESSON 6: DECISIONS, DECISIONS, DECISIONS

Level: Middle school, High school

Time: 40 minutes

National Health Education Standards

1. Core Concepts
2. Analyzing Influences
5. Decision-Making

National Sexuality Education Standards: Performance Indicators

- Describe the physical, social, cognitive and emotional changes of adolescence.
- Demonstrate the use of a decision-making model to evaluate possible outcomes of decisions adolescents might make.
- Analyze the impact of alcohol and other drugs on safer sexual decision-making and sexual behaviors.
- Analyze how brain development has an impact on cognitive, social and emotional changes of adolescence and early adulthood.
- Examine how alcohol and other substances, peers, media, family, society and culture influence decisions about engaging in sexual behaviors.

Rationale

We all make decisions pertaining to our health. Making responsible decisions about sexuality is important. This lesson introduces students to a decision-making model to help them understand the need for effective decision making. Within the lesson, groups will apply the steps in the decision-making model.

Materials and Preparation

Copies of "Decision-Making Guide" worksheet

Four extra chairs to be used as props at the front of the room

Four pieces of blank paper and masking tape

Teacher-developed scenarios pertaining to issues related to growth and development. The scenarios should be separated so that each group has one for which it is responsible (possible scenarios included at the end of this lesson).

Procedure

1. Introduce the concept of decision making by asking students to list five decisions they made the previous day. Decisions could include anything from choosing what clothes to wear to school to deciding whom to hang out with after school, when to call or text someone, or what to have for lunch.

2. Have a "class whip," in which students each quickly read one of the decisions on their list. You may also share a decision you have made.
3. Discuss different ways that internal and external factors may influence people's decisions. These include
   - Simply going with "gut" feelings rather than giving it much thought.
   - Feeling that there is no choice. ("I have to do my homework before dinner, or will get in trouble with my parents.")
   - Asking for advice from a friend, parent or guardian, or other adult.
   - Feeling pressure from peers, parents, or "media messages" when making a decision.
   - Choosing an option because it is convenient or the easy way out.
   - Thinking about possible choices or alternatives. Often there are more than two options when making a decision. Remind students that *doing nothing* is sometimes an option.
   - Gathering facts about the situation to make an informed decision.
   - Thinking about the positive and negative consequences of a decision.
4. Include the following point in the day's discussion: "Although teenagers are becoming more mature, their brains are *not* fully developed until they reach about twenty-five years of age. This delayed development includes the slower growth of the prefrontal cortex, an important part of the brain when it comes to decision making."
5. After this brief discussion about delayed brain development, distribute the "Decision-Making Guide" worksheet. Inform the class that this guide can assist them in making good decisions. Allow students to read the worksheet to themselves.
6. State, "We are now going to demonstrate the steps in the decision-making process by modeling a common decision faced by many high school students." Place four chairs in front of the room, facing the class.
7. Read the following scenario out loud: "You are graduating from eighth grade in a few months. You are looking forward to going to high school because there are many after-school activities you think you might be interested in. You are thinking of joining the school play or playing sports, but you have also considered getting a part-time job to make some money. You will soon have to make a decision about what you will do."
8. Have students look at the decision-making model on their worksheet. (*Note:* Students are not writing on their worksheet at this time. They are simply using it to observe how the decision-making guide pertains to the scenario just given.) Process the given example by going over each step. Ask for a volunteer to stand at the front of the room in close proximity to the four chairs.
9. Have the class assist you in coming up with suggestions for working through the decision-making steps for this scenario.

   Step A: "Clearly state the decision to be made."

      In this scenario, this step is a fairly easy one: "When I get to high school, what do I want to do after school?"

Step B: "List the possible choices or alternatives involved in your decision."

In this scenario three alternatives present themselves: (1) play sports, (2) join the school play, or (3) get a part-time job.

Write each of these options on three of the four sheets of paper and tape them to the front of three of the four chairs. Although these may seem like the only options, ask the class if there may be others that have not been considered. Generally, someone in the class will say, "You could just go home after school and play video games." (*Note:* If students do not come up with this option, you should propose it.) Tape the fourth piece of paper to the remaining chair: "Go home and play video games."

Step C: "Consider the short- and long-term consequences (advantages and disadvantages) of each choice."

At this point the volunteer may ask for assistance from classmates in determining positive and negative consequences of each choice. For example, being in the play might be fun, but several friends are trying out for soccer, and being with them is enjoyable. Getting a job would help save money for a car or college, but a person might miss out on some fun things going on after school. And going home and hanging out might seem relaxing, but it could also start to get boring after a while.

10. When considering the possible consequences, students should also consider things like these:
    - Is it legal?
    - Is it safe?
    - Will it affect my health in a positive or negative way?
    - Does it show respect for myself and others?
    - Does it reflect my personal interests and values?
11. Move on to the next step:

    Step D: "Make a decision, and list your reasons for your choice."

    At this point, ask the volunteer to make a decision by sitting in one of the chairs, based on the choice that was taped to the front. The class may be allowed to call out advice, similar to an audience of a TV game show (peer pressure).
12. Continue to the final step:

    Step E: "Evaluate your decision."

    Once the decision has been made, ask if the volunteer feels the right choice was made, and to explain why or why not.
13. Thank the student volunteer and ask him to return to his classroom seat.
14. Next divide the class into groups of four to five and choose a group leader, who will be responsible for both keeping the group on task and writing down the group's responses. Explain that each group leader will be given one additional worksheet along with a scenario dealing with puberty and the accompanying changes. As a group, they are to come up with the responses that the group leader will input on this separate

worksheet, following the decision-making guide, based on their particular scenario. If all members in the group do not come to agreement on what the "best" solution is, they should poll the group and choose the decision that the majority of the members feel is best. Allow approximately seven to ten minutes for the groups to complete their worksheet and come to a decision.

15. When the time is up, have each group leader read the group's scenario to the class and then discuss how they arrived at the best solution using the decision-making model. Each group should explain what the major influences were when making their final choice.
16. Conclude the class by asking the processing questions and having a follow-up discussion.

Processing

1. What feelings arise when you think about becoming older?
2. Why is the skill of effective decision making important for teenagers?
3. What examples do you have of teenagers making good decisions?
4. What examples do you have of teenagers making poor decisions?
5. How can teenagers ensure that they make the best decisions for themselves?

Assessment

- Students participate in the class whip.
- Students correctly implement the decision-making model, as noted within the worksheet they filled out in their group.
- Students actively participate in answering the processing questions and the related discussion.

Name: ______________________________

Decision-Making Guide

How do you make decisions? This decision-making model may be used as a reference when you are faced with a situation that requires any type of decision.

Step A: Clearly state the decision to be made.

____

Step B: List the possible choices or alternatives involved in your decision.

1. ____
2. ____
3. ____

Step C: Consider the short- and long-term consequences (advantages and disadvantages) of each choice. (Is it safe, healthy, legal, and respectful of yourself and others? Does it reflect your personal values?)

Alternative 1

Advantages: ____

Disadvantages: ____

Alternative 2

Advantages: ____

Disadvantages: ____

Alternative 3

Advantages: ____

Disadvantages: ____

Step D: Make a decision, and list your reasons for your choice.

____

____

____

Step E: Evaluate your decision. (Why do you feel that this is the best choice?)

____

____

____

Suggestions for Possible Group Scenarios

1. Dan is in seventh grade and is the shortest kid in his class—including all of the girls. A couple of kids have recently started to make fun of him, calling him names like "stumpy" and "shorty." At first he tried to ignore them, but the name-calling has gotten worse, and he is getting more upset and angry every day.

2. Tanya is thirteen and started her period when she was ten. She is also more "developed" than most of the girls in her class. Some of the boys stare at her breasts, with some making crude comments. This makes her feel uncomfortable. She wishes they would stop.

3. Ricardo is of average height and has gone through some of the changes that come at puberty. Unfortunately, one of those changes has been a problem with acne, which he is self-conscious about. One day he woke up with a large pimple on his chin. It was all red and inflamed. At lunch, Mike, one of the kids he regularly eats lunch with, said, "Ricardo, if you eat that greasy burger and fries, that zit on your chin is gonna explode." Some of the other kids laughed, but Maria, whom Ricardo has a crush on, stood up for him, saying, "That wasn't very nice to say. Just about all teenagers have problems with their complexion from time to time. Why don't you just keep your comments to yourself?"

   Ricardo did not know what to do, or what to say to Mike or Maria.

4. Chris is a freshman in high school. Chris has secretly been dating Pat for three months. Chris's friends and family would probably not like the fact that Chris is dating Pat. Pat has recently been pressuring Chris to go further physically and sexually than Chris is comfortable with. Chris likes Pat, but does not feel ready for a sexual relationship. Chris doesn't want to be alone and feels that any relationship is better than no relationship.

5. Beth is hesitant to change clothes for her eighth-grade physical education class. She has not gone through many of the changes at puberty that other girls have experienced, and she is uncomfortable changing in front of them in the locker room. They all seem to have larger breasts and a more mature figure. During the basketball unit, one of the more developed girls looked over to Beth as she was changing and said, "I guess *you* don't need a sports bra." Some girls started to laugh. Because of this, Beth cut her next physical education class. When approached by Mrs. Roberts, her physical education teacher, she lied and said that she had "cramps" and went to the nurse's office. She does not want to fail the class, but does not want to be made fun of, either.

(continued)

Suggestions for Possible Group Scenarios (*continued*)

6. Sean has a presentation to give to his health class on the importance of good nutrition, hygiene, and exercise during adolescence. He has worked hard and feels prepared for his presentation. He is concerned, though, because his voice has been changing and he does not know what will happen during his presentation. Sean's voice is getting deeper, but it occasionally cracks. When it happens, he gets embarrassed and turns bright red.

   The presentation is not optional and is worth 25 percent of his grade. He cannot decide what would be worse—getting a lower grade by not doing the oral presentation or embarrassing himself in front of everyone.

7. Mai Lu is in sixth grade. Many of the other girls in her class have gotten their period, but she has not. The girls saw a film about menstruation in health class, but Mai Lu is still nervous about getting her first period. She has questions like: "How will I know when it will come? What should I do to prepare for it? What kinds of menstrual hygiene products should I use?"

   She and her mother have always been close, but they have never talked about this issue. Her family is very conservative, and she does not want her mom to think that she is thinking about sexual things. She knows that she will probably get her first period soon, yet is worried that she will not know what to do and be totally embarrassed, especially if it happens in school.

8. Coach Roberts, Domingo's seventh-grade health instructor, was talking about puberty and hormones. He said, "That's what causes guys to be attracted to girls and girls to be attracted to guys." That confused Domingo because he really doesn't feel attracted to girls *or* guys. He is concerned that there may be something wrong with him, like a hormone problem.

   He doesn't really know Coach Roberts that well and might feel embarrassed telling him how he feels. He has an older brother, Alberto, who is in high school. There is also his school counselor, Mrs. Morales, who helped him last year when some kids were bullying him in school. He wants to talk to someone, but doesn't know whom to go to.

LESSON 7: PUBERTY GRAB BAG

Level: Middle school

Time: 40 minutes, plus time for presenting and discussing the public service announcement homework assignment in a follow-up session

National Health Education Standards

1. Core Concepts
3. Accessing Information
7. Self-Management

National Sexuality Education Standards: Performance Indicators

- Explain the physical, social and emotional changes that occur during puberty and adolescence.
- Identify medically-accurate information and resources about puberty and personal hygiene.
- Explain ways to manage the physical and emotional changes associated with puberty.

Rationale

Puberty is a time of rapid growth and body changes. Many of these changes require teens to become more aware of personal hygiene habits. The grab bag activity serves as a stimulus for discussions about changes in males and females as well as the new responsibilities accompanying these changes. After creating public service announcements related to the changes at puberty for homework, students will share their positive messages advocating healthy coping skills.

Materials and Preparation

Front board

Paper bags

The following items, each of which is to be placed in a paper bag:

- Commercial deodorant (stick, roll-on, or spray)
- Sports cup or jock strap
- Sports bra
- Lotion of SPF 30 or higher
- Breast self-exam (BSE) model
- Testicular self-exam (TSE) model
- Bar of facial soap and washcloth
- Toothbrush, toothpaste, and floss
- Bottle of shampoo
- Any other age-appropriate items or pictures of items

Pamphlets, brochures, or texts with information about puberty

Computers or personal mobile devices with Internet access (if available)

Copies of "Student Project: Public Service Announcement" homework

Procedure

1. To begin the class, ask students to list in their notebook common concerns preteens and teens have about their bodies, including those dealing with physical appearance. Because students' bodies are going through adolescent growth and other changes, ask them also to list common health habits young people should be following.
2. Ask students to volunteer to share items from the list they have compiled in their notebook. Write these items on the board, noting the awareness the students have about taking care of their bodies.
3. Then inform students that to further ensure that they understand healthy habits pertaining to puberty, they will become "health experts." For this, students will be placed in groups, with three to four students per group. Each group will be given a "puberty grab bag." Students will be asked to discuss a health habit represented by the object or objects in their group's paper bag, and to answer the following questions:
   a. What item or items are in the bag? Explain this as fully as you can, including giving any directions for its use.
   b. What health habit is represented by this object or objects?
   c. Why is this health habit of importance?
4. Remind the class to answer all three questions using available resources. To do this, students may use personal mobile devices, including cell phones, or computers with Internet access.
5. After groups have finalized their answers, ask for student volunteers to begin a class discussion. It is recommended to start with volunteers because not all students will feel comfortable with the given topic. After some students volunteer, others will feel more comfortable explaining their group's item or items. If no one volunteers, start with the more basic items (for example, a toothbrush).
6. If a group does not give important information, add it to the group's response.
7. Students may note that they started using some of the items, such as toothbrushes, earlier in their lives. Explain that these items were still placed in paper bags because some people need reminders or were never taught their proper use. For example, a child might have been given deodorant without anyone's having explained how and where it should be applied.
8. End the lesson by having students answer the processing questions.
9. Give students the "Student Project: Public Service Announcement" homework. This assignment serves as a culminating activity for the unit on puberty and adolescent development. Students can work individually or with a partner, as approved by you. Spending a few minutes of classroom time on the project is helpful in getting students started, but this is primarily a take-home assignment, with most of the work done outside of class. Students will be allocated three days to complete their projects. Students are responsible for briefly presenting their public service announcement to the class on the assigned date.

Processing

1. What surprised you during today's lesson? Explain.
2. How often are commonsense habits not common sense? Explain.
3. What habit do you wish a person had taught you more about?
4. If you had a child, what habit or habits would you make sure you taught him or her? At what age?
5. Because there are so many body changes accompanying puberty, you may sometimes have concerns about your body image (the image you have of yourself and your physical appearance) and self-concept (the mental image or picture you have of yourself).

   Discuss how each of the following may influence your body image and your self-concept:

   a. **Peers.** (*Possible responses:* They may have a negative effect by making fun of you, or a positive effect by complimenting you.)
   b. **Family.** (*Possible responses:* They may build up your self-concept by reminding you that you are loved for who you are, and by offering support when you have questions or concerns about the changes you are experiencing. They may also have a negative effect by putting you down, embarrassing you, or comparing you with siblings or peers.)
   c. **The media and society.** (*Possible responses:* The media may make it easier to get information that portrays an unrealistic view of what the "ideal" male or female should look like. Comparing yourself to the models in magazines and on TV may lead to a poor self-image and, in severe cases, an eating disorder.)

Assessment

- Groups correctly describe grab bag items and explain how they relate to pubertal changes.
- Students complete the additional homework assignment.

Names: ______________________________

Student Project: Public Service Announcement

Puberty: What's Happening?

Directions: You are responsible for creating a public service announcement (PSA) related to puberty and adolescent development. You may work individually or with a partner. Please use the following criteria when creating your PSA:

- Your PSA should cover common changes occurring in boys and girls during puberty, why some changes may be stressful or confusing, and how to best deal with those changes in a healthy way.
- When read out loud, your PSA should be from **one to two minutes long.**
- A minimum of five changes experienced at puberty should be mentioned in your PSA.
- The PSA should inform your peers where they can get accurate information and help in dealing with these changes. Mention at least one **person,** in school or at home, to whom they can go to for help and advice. You should also reference at least one **Internet resource** from which reliable information about puberty can be obtained. Explain why each of these is an appropriate resource.
- Be prepared to share your PSA project with the class on the day it is due.

LESSON 8: UP CLOSE AND PERSONAL

Level: Middle school

Time: 40 minutes

National Health Education Standards

1. Core Concepts
4. Interpersonal Communication

National Sexuality Education Standards: Performance Indicators

- Describe the physical, social, cognitive and emotional changes of adolescence.
- Explain ways to manage the physical and emotional changes associated with puberty.
- Demonstrate communication skills that foster healthy relationships.

Rationale

This Up Close and Personal (UCP) lesson encourages students to engage in an open, honest discussion by using sentence stems. The objective of this lesson is to integrate the affective (emotional) and cognitive (informational) domains related to the changes at puberty. Students will communicate personal opinions, feelings, and values related to puberty and sexual health. This will occur in an atmosphere of mutual trust and respect for each member of the class.

Note: It is unlikely that you will get through all sentence stems in one class session. You can decide which statements would be most appropriate for your students. Choices may be based on background information discussed in previous lessons, students' developmental level, restrictions you may have concerning what topics *can* and *cannot* be discussed, and your own comfort level in facilitating discussion.

Because UCP lessons deal mainly with the affective or emotional domain, they have a greater potential for personal disclosure on the part of students. You should be aware of and prepared to handle this. Sometimes it simply involves reminding the class that what is said in class stays in class. At other times, it may involve discussing issues with students privately to offer advice, resources, and support.

Materials and Preparation

Small lamp (optional)

Up Close and Personal sheet with several UCP sentence stems. (*Note:* Prior to teaching this activity, you should familiarize yourself with "Facilitating a UCP Session," which can be found at the end of the lesson.)

Procedure*

1. Ask students to form a circle with their chairs. Turning off the overhead lights and using a lamp may make the environment more conducive to an informal discussion.

---

*Unfinished sentences have been a useful learning tool for many years. The specific format used in this lesson has been adapted from the book *Up Close and Personal: Effective Learning for Students and Teachers* (Raleigh, NC: Lulu Press, 2007), by teacher, colleague, and friend Robert Winchester. Robert can be contacted at trustinbob@aol.com.

2. Introduce the activity in the following manner:

   Today we are going to do an activity called Up Close and Personal. It is simple to do, but for it to go smoothly, there are some rules to follow.

   First, understand this is not group therapy. Instead it is an opportunity for you to talk about how you feel about yourself, relationships, likes, dislikes, things that have come up in class, memories, and life in general. Although I will be facilitating the activity, I will also be sitting in the circle and participating along with everyone else.

   The activity is in the following format: I will read an unfinished sentence. Each of you will think about how you would finish this same unfinished sentence. Someone in the circle will then raise his or her hand and state his or her completed sentence. He or she will point to his or her right or left to determine which way around the circle we will proceed.

   When going around the circle, there should be no talking by anyone else. If something is said that you want to respond to or comment on, you must wait until we have gone all the way around the circle. If you cannot think of anything to say, or choose not to respond when it is your turn, you may simply say, "Pass" or "Come back to me." Everyone, including the teacher, is allowed to pass.

   When we have gone around the entire circle, I will ask anyone who passed if he or she would like to respond at this time. I will also ask for any questions or comments about anything that was said when going around the circle. At this point, there can be open discussion.

   Please note that during this activity, no names should be mentioned at any time. Instead, say something like, "I know someone who . . ."

   In addition, as with other lessons, what is said in class stays in class. However, please do not share anything that is too personal, that makes you feel uncomfortable, or that you wish to keep to yourself.

3. Once the rules have been explained and agreed on, read the first sentence stem aloud. After allowing a few moments for reflection, ask a student volunteer to start by stating his completed sentence. That student will then point to his left or right to note in which direction the remaining students will be given a chance to complete the sentence. Students then give their responses until everyone around the circle has spoken or passed.

4. At times, a student may simply not be ready to respond to a particular question. When this happens, remind her to pass, noting that she can answer after everyone else has spoken. It is also not unusual for many students to have the same response to a question or statement. "Repeats" reinforce the important concept that although all people are unique, they often share many of the same thoughts, feelings, and values.

5. After all students have responded, open up the discussion by asking if anyone has any questions or comments about anything that was said. Encourage students to talk in more detail about why they completed the sentence the way they did. Students may also ask others in the circle, including the teacher, to expand on their answer. Students may do so, or they may choose to pass.

6. Continue the circle discussion for as long as it is viable, constantly monitoring and enforcing the rules. When the discussion on a given sentence has run its course, move on to the next unfinished sentence.
7. Share the processing statements.
8. All UCP sessions should end with some brief closure in the form of another unfinished sentence. Examples include the following: "Today I learned . . ." "I learned that I . . ." "Right now I feel . . ." and "Something I want to say to one of my classmates is . . ."
9. Conclude the day's activity by summarizing what occurred in the session, making appropriate connections to the subject matter and curriculum. Then thank the class and say, "This ends our Up Close and Personal class for today."

Processing

1. If anyone has any concerns or questions about what was discussed during our UCP session today, he or she can speak to me privately after class or can bring it up for discussion during our next class session.
2. There are many people, including teachers, coaches, counselors, or school psychologists, who can assist you with any personal issues that you may want to share with them. Keep in mind that these individuals, as mandated reporters, *must* report any verbalization or indication that you may want to hurt yourself or hurt others, or revelations of abuse of any kind, to the appropriate authorities for follow-up and counseling services.

Assessment

- Students actively participate in the UCP activity. Even though some students may decide to pass on one or more questions, as long as they are actively listening and following the ground rules, they are "actively participating."

Facilitating a UCP Session

- Facilitation is a skill that you can improve with practice.
- Silence is not a negative phenomenon. Silence often indicates that higher-level thinking is taking place.
- Going over ground rules at the beginning of each session is a needed and helpful technique to prevent inappropriate behavior.
- Unacceptable behavior should be stopped the moment it is recognized. To do this, pause the activity and point out the offense to the individual. For example, say, "What was just said is a put-down (or personal name), and it is not allowed in the circle discussion. Please do not do it again," or "Please do not talk to your neighbor when you should be listening to the one person who is supposed to be talking."
- If a student persists in breaking the activity's rules, talk to him one-on-one after class. Let the student know that if his behavior continues, he may not be able to participate in the future. This almost always stops the offensive behavior.
- Remind students of the information teachers *must* report if shared:
  1. If they are going to hurt themselves
  2. If they are going to hurt others
  3. If they are being abused

Possible UCP Sentence Stems: Changes at Puberty

1. Right now I feel . . .
2. When I hear the word "puberty" . . .
3. I think the biggest change for girls or guys during puberty is . . .
4. One thing I have learned about puberty that I did not think was true is . . .
5. One thing I have learned about puberty and females is . . .
6. One thing I have learned about puberty and males is . . .
7. One way to cope with the physical and emotional changes of puberty is . . .
8. When it comes to puberty, one thing guys or girls may worry about is . . .
9. One good thing about puberty is . . .
10. The best thing about being a guy or girl is . . .
11. One adult I feel comfortable talking to about puberty is . . .
12. People who have gone through puberty may be able to reproduce and have a baby. One reason why I might not want to have a baby at this point in my life is . . .
13. One thing I learned today is . . .

LESSON 9: HOME-SCHOOL CONNECTION

TALKING ABOUT PUBERTY AND GROWING UP

Level: Middle school

Time: Varies

National Health Education Standards

1. Core Concepts
2. Analyzing Influences

National Sexuality Education Standards: Performance Indicators

- Describe the physical, social, cognitive and emotional changes of adolescence.
- Analyze how peers, media, family, society and culture influence self-concept and body image.
- Identify parents or other trusted adults of whom they can ask questions about puberty and adolescent health issues.

Rationale

Parents or guardians are the primary sexuality educators of their children. The role of the school is to supplement family teaching by providing students with accurate information, as well as to engage them in discussions in which they can explore their attitudes and develop and practice interpersonal skills. It is the responsibility of parents or guardians to communicate family values and beliefs. The main purpose of the Home-School Connection activities is to provide teens and their parents or guardians with the opportunity to privately spend time discussing human sexuality issues at home.

After completing the assignment, parents or guardians are requested to sign on the bottom. All responses from teens and parents or guardians on the Home-School Connection activity will be kept confidential. It will not be turned in to the teacher or graded. On the due date, students will be asked to *voluntarily* share any interesting comments or insights they learned or observed by participating in the assignment. Students *and* parents or guardians can choose to pass on any discussion they wish to keep private.

After completing the assignment, parents or guardians are requested to sign on the bottom. All responses from teens and parents or guardians on the Home-School Connection activity will be kept confidential. It will not be turned in to the teacher or graded. On the due date, students will be asked to *voluntarily* share any interesting comments or insights they learned or observed by participating in the assignment. Students *and* parents or guardians can choose to pass on any discussion they wish to keep private.

With family input and support, the overall goal is to encourage teens to become well-informed, caring, respectful, and responsible adults.

Materials and Preparation

Copies of "Parent or Guardian Interview: Talking About Puberty and Growing Up" worksheet

Procedure

1. Explain to the class that they are going to have an assignment to complete with one or more parents or guardians.
2. Distribute a copy of the "Parent or Guardian Interview: Talking About Puberty and Growing Up" worksheet to each student. Students will be interviewing one or more parents or guardians and writing down their responses on the worksheet.
3. Assign a due date for the assignment.
4. On the day the assignment is due, check that students have completed it by noting whether or not it was signed at the bottom. Do not collect or grade it.
5. Ask for volunteers to share some results of the discussion they had with the adult or adults they interviewed. Then ask the processing questions.
6. To conclude the lesson, have students participate in a "class whip," with each student making a brief statement related to knowledge gained or values expressed during the interview process (for example, "I learned . . ." "I feel (or felt) . . ." or "I was surprised . . .").

Processing

1. Which family members did you choose to speak to?
2. What was it like talking to family members about this topic? Were you comfortable with this discussion? Were your parents or guardians? Why is it sometimes difficult talking to parents, guardians, or other adults about issues related to human sexuality?
3. What were some of the messages your parents or guardians received about puberty? How many of your parents or guardians did not really talk to *their* parents or guardians about puberty? Did they give a reason for why this conversation never took place?
4. Did your parents or guardians talk about puberty in a health or other class when they were in school? If so, what do they remember about that experience?
5. What did your parents or guardians say have been some of the positive changes in the "world of teens" today? Do they feel that some of the changes have *not* been positive? What are some of the things they experienced or enjoyed doing when they were teenagers?
6. How did you feel about the messages or advice that your parents or guardians shared with you?
7. Did anything surprising come up during the conversation?
8. What did you learn from doing this assignment?
9. What did you learn from our class discussion? Did the parents or guardians of your classmates offer some of the same messages?

Assessment

- Students indicate that communication occurred with at least one family member by bringing to class an assignment signed by one or more parents or guardians.
- Students participate in the follow-up discussion pertaining to the assignment.
- Students participate in the class whip.

Parent or Guardian Interview: Talking about Puberty and Growing Up

We have been talking about the physical, mental, and emotional changes at puberty in health education class. Keeping the lines of communication open between parents or guardians and teens is always important, but it is especially important during this time of life, when young people start to transition from children into sexually mature adults. It is sometimes difficult or embarrassing to talk about this topic with parents or guardians. Yet the good news is that every adult went through and can relate to these changes—even your parents or guardians!

Directions: Find a parent or guardian who will answer the following questions about his or her own thoughts, feelings, and recollections about that time in his or her life. Write down his or her answer to each question in the space provided. At the end of the interview, you are required to write a reaction statement based on the answers of the person you interviewed. Your reaction statement should include what you learned, how his or her experiences were similar to or different from yours, and how comfortable you were doing this exercise. To get credit for the assignment, you and the person you interviewed should both sign at the bottom of the assignment after talking. This is simply to ensure that you have completed the assignment. It will not be turned in to the teacher or graded. All teen and adult comments on the Home-School Connection activity will be kept confidential.

If you interview a second adult, you will receive five extra credit points.

Note: The person you interview has the right to "pass" on any question he or she chooses not to answer.

Name of person interviewed: ____

Relationship to student: ____

1. About how old were you when you started to go through changes at puberty? What were some of the first signs that you were starting to mature?

   ____

   ____

   ____

2. When you started to go through puberty, were you able to talk to your parents (or guardians) about any questions or concerns? If so, were they comfortable discussing these concerns with you? Were *you* comfortable with the conversation? If you did not have this conversation, why do you think this was the case?

   ____

   ____

   ____

Parent or Guardian Interview: Talking about Puberty and Growing Up (*continued*)

3. Do you remember discussing this topic in school? If so, was this in a health class, or with the school nurse or another faculty member? What did your peers teach you? Were these discussions helpful? Comfortable? Embarrassing? Explain.

____

____

____

____

4. What did you enjoy when you were my age (sports, activities, TV, music, and so on)?

____

____

5. Since you were a teenager, the world has changed, especially in regard to technology (computers, cell phones, the Internet, and social networking sites). What do you feel have been some positive changes in the "world of teens" today? Do you have any concerns about the changes that have taken place since you were a teen?

____

____

____

____

____

6. What **advice** can you give about the changes at puberty and becoming a responsible, sexually mature young man or young woman?

____

____

____

____

____

Parent or Guardian Interview: Talking about Puberty and Growing Up (*continued*)

My Reaction Statement

Parent or guardian signature(s): ______________________

Student signature: ______________________

Identity

3

In every society, gender norms and gender roles influence people's lives, including their sexual lives. Greater equality and more flexible gender roles give all of us more opportunities to develop to our full potential as human beings. Young people can help promote gender and social equality by

- Not using degrading language or telling demeaning or sexist jokes
- Speaking out against discrimination and gender-based violence
- Supporting and reaching out to those who are being harassed because of their beliefs, appearance, race, nationality, or sexual orientation.
- Reporting harassment to a teacher, counselor, administrator, or other trusted adult

Within this chapter's lessons, effective communication is imperative. Students have the right to their opinions and values, yet need to be respectful of others when sharing them. To create a classroom of respect, the following rubric can be displayed on a classroom wall to remind students of what respectful and disrespectful forms of communication look like. The chart can also be used for assigning participation points during group discussions.

	ASSERTIVE COMMUNICATION (FULL POINTS)	PASSIVE COMMUNICATION (HALF POINTS)	AGGRESSIVE COMMUNICATION (NO POINTS)
Words	• "I" statements • Comments referring to behaviors, not to specific people	• Such statements as "Um . . ." "I don't know," and "What he said"	• "You" statements • Profanity • Put-downs
Tone (how words are said)	• Audible statements • Tone that is kept under control	• Statements that sound like questions • Speech that is too quiet to hear easily • Mumbling	• Raised voice • Condescending tone
Body language	• Good, firm posture • Pleasant facial expression	• No eye contact • Arms folded across chest	• Leaning forward • Tense muscles • Scowl on face • Rolling of eyes

LESSON 1: IDENTITY BINGO

Level: Middle school, High school

Time: 40–50 minutes

National Health Education Standards

1. Core Concepts
4. Interpersonal Communication

National Sexuality Education Standards: Performance Indicators

- Differentiate between gender identity, gender expression and sexual orientation.
- Differentiate between biological sex, sexual orientation, and gender identity and expression.
- Distinguish between sexual orientation, sexual behavior and sexual identity.
- Communicate respectfully with and about people of all gender identities, gender expressions and sexual orientations.

Rationale

Terms used within sexual identity lessons are often misunderstood and misused. This lesson reviews the appropriate terms and their definitions so that students will come to understand what terminology is appropriate when discussing sexual identity.

Materials and Preparation

Copies of "Identity Bingo" worksheet

Slips of paper, each with one term and one definition written (see examples provided at the end of this lesson). These should then be folded.

Container to hold the terms and definitions

Procedure

1. Begin the lesson by explaining that people need to understand appropriate terminology to discuss sexual identity. To do this, a game dealing with the class's knowledge of terms related to gender and sexual identity will be played.

   Note: Because the topic of gender roles and sexual orientation may make some students uncomfortable, plan ways to diffuse potential disagreements and maintain open and respectful discussion. As always, students have the right to their opinions. Students also have the right to "pass" on any uncomfortable questions. Discussion must be focused on the concept of tolerance and acceptance of differences among all people.

2. Inform the students that they will be playing a game of "identity bingo" using sexual identity terminology. The objective of the game is to obtain one of the traditional bingo wins. To do this, the teacher will read definitions of the listed terms one at a time. Each student is to determine what term best fits the definition and, if that term is in a box, mark the box with an *X*. A bingo win can be any of the following:

   - Five boxes in a row horizontally
   - Five boxes in a row vertically

- Five boxes in a row diagonally
- Four corners
- The full board

3. Distribute copies of the "Identity Bingo" worksheet. Allow approximately five minutes for students to randomly fill in *all* the boxes with the terms below the bingo board. The middle box with the term "Identity Bingo" is a free space. Additional terms are included. Make sure to check that students have filled in all of the boxes.
4. Place the term and definition cards in a container. After students have filled in all of their boxes, begin the game by picking one card out of the container and reading the definition to the class. Students then mark an *X* on the square containing the word they believe matches the definition.
5. When a student attains a bingo win, she should yell out, "Bingo!" The student will then verify her win by reading the terms on her sheet. You should also verify the win by comparing those terms with the definitions read aloud.
6. Once a particular win has occurred, such as the four corners, this option is no longer in play. Students will then focus on other ways to win (a vertical, horizontal, or diagonal row, or the entire board).
7. The game continues until all various bingo wins have occurred. You can give incentives to winners, including extra credit or a homework pass.
8. To reinforce the use of proper terminology, ask students the processing questions.
9. Conclude the lesson with a discussion on the following statement: "Almost everything males can do, females can do. Almost everything females can do, males can do." Obviously, there are some things, like giving birth, that would be exceptions to this statement. In general, though, student discussion should generate critical thinking related to equality of the sexes and acceptance and tolerance of all people.

Processing

1. What terms were you familiar with?
2. Where have you heard these terms?
3. How often are these terms used in an appropriate manner?
4. For which terms did you think you knew the meaning, only to discover you had the incorrect definition?
5. What new terms did you learn today?
6. Why do you think we are going over these terms?

Assessment

- Students complete the bingo game, recognizing each term's proper use and definition.
- Students actively participate in the bingo game and discussion (refer to the communication rubric).

Name: ____________________

Identity Bingo

Identity Bingo Game Board

		Identity Bingo		

List of Terms

Female	Heterosexual	Stereotypes	Sexual orientation	Transgender
Male	Homosexual	Gender identity	Lesbian	Respect
Gender	Bisexual	Gender roles	Tolerance	Advocacy
Nature	Transsexual	Feminine	Heterosexism	Coming out
Nurture	Questioning	Masculine	Homophobia	Gay
GLBTQ	Transvestite			

Definitions of Identity Terms

Advocacy—displaying support for and encouragement of something.

Bisexual—a person who is emotionally, physically, or sexually attracted to members of both sexes.

Coming out—a term used when a person informs others that he or she is gay.

Female—a person who is physically a girl or woman.

Feminine—having qualities or traits traditionally associated with females.

Gay—a homosexual person. This term is usually used to describe men but may be used to describe women as well. Once thought of as a negative term, it is now preferred by many homosexual people because, in their ongoing struggle for rights, it has come to be associated with a positive and proud sense of identity.

Gender—the behavioral or emotional traits typically associated with being male or female.

Gender identity—a person's inner sense of being male or female, resulting from a combination of genetic and environmental influences.

Gender roles—the characteristics, responsibilities, and expectations held by society about how men and women are supposed to behave simply because they are male or female.

GLBTQ—an acronym that stands for "gay, lesbian, bisexual, transgender, or questioning."

Heterosexism—discrimination by heterosexual individuals against gays and lesbians.

Heterosexual—a person who is attracted to a person of the opposite sex.

Homophobia—the fear or hatred of someone who identifies as gay, lesbian, bisexual, or transgender.

Definitions of Identity Terms (*continued*)

Homosexual—a person who is attracted to a person of the same sex.

Lesbian—a female who is predominantly or exclusively attracted to other females.

Male—a person who is physically a boy or male.

Masculine—having qualities or traits traditionally associated with males.

Nature—physical or biological factors influencing behaviors and personal traits.

Nurture—environmental factors influencing behaviors and personal traits.

Questioning—a term referring to a person who is questioning his or her gender identity, sexual identity, or sexual orientation. People who experience this may be unsure of their sexuality or may still be exploring their sexual feelings. This is most common among teens and young adults.

Respect—consideration, appreciation, or both for another or oneself.

Sexual orientation—the direction of a person's sexual interest toward members of the same sex, the opposite sex, or both sexes.

Stereotypes—generalized beliefs about a particular group or class or people.

Tolerance—the ability to respect the beliefs of others even though they may be different from one's own.

Transgender—a term used to describe a person who is born male or female but identifies with a gender identity that is different from the sex at birth.

Transsexual—a person who has had a sex-change operation.

Transvestite—a person who dresses like and assumes the role of a member of the opposite sex.

LESSON 2: "WHO ARE YOU?" NATURE VERSUS NURTURE

Level: Middle school, High school

Time: 40–50 minutes

National Health Education Standard

2. Analyzing Influences

National Sexuality Education Standards: Performance Indicators

- Analyze external influences that have an impact on one's attitudes about gender, sexual orientation and gender identity.
- Analyze the influence of peers, media, family, society, religion and culture on the expression of gender, sexual orientation and identity.

Rationale

This lesson introduces the concept of misperceptions about sexual identity, including the belief that people can "choose" to be different from who they naturally are. Although some behaviors and traits are influenced by environmental factors, others are inherent or natural to the individual. This lesson attempts to demonstrate that there are both external *and* internal influences on sexual identity, yet sexual orientation is not a choice.

Note: The last processing question allows students to discuss the myths behind homosexuality. The belief that people can be taught to be gay—or taught not to be gay—may be stated by a student. There is no research to support this myth. Many people who "come out" as teens or adults often explain how they knew as a child that they were attracted to people of their same sex, yet did not tell anyone because of societal norms and the fear of being ostracized.

Materials and Preparation

Copies of "Who Are You? (Nature Versus Nurture)" worksheet

Front board

Procedure

1. Begin by explaining that the lesson will focus on the personal traits and characteristics of students in the class. Hand out the "Who Are You? (Nature Versus Nurture)" worksheet and ask students to complete it.
2. After students have completed the worksheet, ask them to share answers of their choice. To do this, you can go through the questions one by one and ask for answers from three or four different students for each. You can also foster discussion about how much they enjoyed noting their personal traits and characteristics (people usually enjoy talking about themselves). Similarities and differences within the class should also be noted.

3. Refer to the "Nature Versus Nurture" part of the worksheet's title. Ask students to explain and discuss what the terms "nature" and "nurture" mean. Overall, students should comprehend that

   - Internal traits or characteristics are natural or inherent (nature).
   - Students were taught to have certain traits or characteristics (nurture).

   Students can brainstorm examples of environmental influences—for example, messages in music, TV commercials, and peers—with you or a student writing a list on the front board.

4. After students understand the difference between nature and nurture, ask them to refer to their worksheet again. This time they are to discuss whether each answer is caused by nature or nurture. If it is caused by nature, students have checked under the "Nature" column. If it is caused by nurture, students should have checked under the "Nurture" column. Allow students time to discuss their answers.

   Note: Students may not agree on certain answers. For example, students may say that they enjoy a particular type of music because of their friends. However, other students may disagree because they instinctively enjoyed that type of music as soon as they heard it.

5. Bring closure to the lesson by having students answer the processing questions. You can also ask students to answer the last two processing questions in their notebook or journal for further reflection, either in class or at home.

Processing

1. What does the phrase "nature versus nurture" refer to?
2. What traits or characteristics occur naturally in people?
3. What traits or characteristics occur because of the influence from outside sources?
4. What are examples of external influences?
5. How does "nature versus nurture" affect whom a person is attracted to?
6. How does "nature versus nurture" affect sexual identity and sexual orientation?

Assessment

- Students provide answers on the worksheet, indicating whether each answer is caused by nature or nurture.
- Students brainstorm a list of external influences.
- Students complete additional notebook or journal entries.

Name: ______________________________

Who Are You? (Nature Versus Nurture)

Directions: Write down your answers to the following questions. Then note if you believe your answer is something that comes naturally to a person (nature) or is learned (nurture) by making a check mark in either the "Nature" column or the "Nurture" column, respectively.

	My Answer	Nature	Nurture
1. What is your favorite color?			
2. What hand do you usually write with?			
3. What is your favorite sport?			
4. Are you able to roll your tongue?			
5. What is your favorite TV show?			
6. Which of your toes on your left foot is the longest?			
7. Are you able to touch the tip of your nose with your tongue?			
8. What is your favorite store?			
9. Where do you usually hang out with friends?			
10. What, if any, foods are you allergic to?			
11. What is your favorite type of music?			
12. What musical talent do you have?			
13. What toy did you play with the most growing up?			
14. What political issue concerns you the most?			
15. Do you wear any type of glasses or contact lens?			
16. What subject do you excel at in school?			

LESSON 3: MESSAGES ABOUT GENDER ROLES AND SEXUAL STEREOTYPES

Level: Middle school, High school

Time: 40 minutes

National Health Education Standards

1. Core Concepts
2. Analyzing Influences
4. Interpersonal Communication

National Sexuality Education Standards: Performance Indicators

- Differentiate between gender identity, gender expression and sexual orientation.
- Explain the range of gender roles.
- Analyze the influence of peers, media, family, society, religion and culture on the expression of gender, sexual orientation and identity.
- Communicate respectfully with and about people of all gender identities, gender expressions and sexual orientations.

Rationale

Too often, people watch movies or TV programs or play video games without recognizing the gender roles supported in them. The purpose of this lesson is to increase awareness of gender messages in the media.

Materials and Preparation

Front board or poster paper and markers to create the table of gender roles

Video media source most students have seen, shown using a computer and LCD projector or Smart Board

Scrap paper for exit card responses (optional)

Copies of "Messages in the Media" homework

Procedure

1. To begin the class, ask students to define the term "gender roles." A sample definition is "the characteristics, responsibilities, and expectations held by society about how men and women are supposed to behave simply because they are male or female."
2. After students understand the proper definition of "gender roles," ask them to answer the following questions in their notebook:
    a. What are two traditional gender roles shown in the media for females? What are two shown for males?
    b. What are gender roles shown in the media that are not traditional for females? For males?

c. What is a gender role you wish were shown more often in the media for either females or males?

As students are writing down their responses, create a table on the board (or poster paper), with one side for females and the other for males, that looks something like this:

Traditional Roles for Females	**Traditional Roles for Males**
Nontraditional Roles for Females	**Nontraditional Roles for Males**

3. Ask students to give their answers for the roles they have seen for one gender. Students should also note if each role would be considered traditional or nontraditional. As this is done, you or a student should write the answers in the appropriate box of the table. Then have students share their responses for the other gender.
4. Students should then share the role they would like to see portrayed in media sources. Ask, "Is this a traditional or nontraditional role?" for each additional item being noted on the table.
5. Next, inform the class that they are to create a similar table in their notebook. Explain that a video clip from a popular movie (for example, *Pocahontas*) or TV show (for example, *G. I. Joe*) will be shown, and that students are to fill in their table with the gender roles portrayed in the clip. (You could also show a set of commercials, or use some other media source.)
6. Show the clip, and monitor the students as they take notes on the gender roles on their table. This should take approximately ten minutes.
7. After showing the clip, ask students to discuss the traditional and nontraditional roles they saw. In addition, students may point out any symbolism pertaining to gender. For example, a student may note specific colors of clothing the females and males wore. This discussion can first occur with a partner or in a small group, and then be shared with the whole class.
8. Ask students the processing questions. Students can answer the last two questions on an exit card or in their journal.
9. Another way to conclude the lesson is to ask students to read and respond to a quote on female and male roles. Examples of these can be found online.
10. Ask students to analyze the messages in one media source they have seen or heard by completing the "Messages in the Media" homework.

Processing

1. What are obvious and not-so-obvious messages about gender roles shown in movies? In TV shows? In video games?
2. Are the roles of males and females shown in the media more traditional or nontraditional? Explain.
3. Who creates the messages we see?
4. How do these messages affect our society?
5. How have these messages affected you?

Assessment

- Students complete the class and individual tables.
- Students demonstrate assertive and respectful communication in class discussions (refer to the communication rubric).
- Students write answers on an exit card or in their journal.
- Students complete the "Messages in the Media" homework.

Name: ______________________________

Messages in the Media

Directions: Before our next class, you are going to continue to analyze messages you see or hear from another appropriate media source. This media source can be a song you often listen to, a TV show you watch, or a set of commercials shown during your favorite show.

If you are stuck, choose one of the following to analyze:

- *Free to Be . . . You and Me* video clips "Billy Wants a Doll" or "Atlanta"
- "If I Were a Boy" by Beyoncé
- "Girls Just Want to Have Fun" by Cyndi Lauper
- "Boys Don't Cry" by The Cure
- "Guys Do It All the Time" by Mindy McReady
- "I'm Just a Girl" by No Doubt

After watching or listening, answer the following questions:

1. What is your initial reaction when you see or hear the messages in your media source? Why do you think this is?

____

____

____

____

2. What are your feelings toward the messages seen or heard in your example?

____

____

____

____

3. How appropriate are the messages? Explain.

____

____

____

____

4. If you had a daughter or son who saw or heard these messages, how would you feel about that?

____

____

____

____

5. What would you say to your daughter or son about these messages?

____

____

____

____

LESSON 4: "ONCE UPON A TIME"

Level: Middle school, High school

Time: 40 minutes

National Health Education Standards

1. Core Concepts
2. Analyzing Influences
4. Interpersonal Communication

National Sexuality Education Standards: Performance Indicators

- Differentiate between gender identity, gender expression and sexual orientation.
- Differentiate between biological sex, sexual orientation, and gender identity and expression.
- Analyze external influences that have an impact on one's attitudes about gender, sexual orientation and gender identity.
- Communicate respectfully with and about people of all gender identities, gender expressions and sexual orientations.

Rationale

From birth, people receive messages about how males and females are expected to behave. Although some messages are changing, boys and girls may be treated differently and be given separate tasks, reinforcing stereotypes and restrictive gender roles. The objective of this lesson is to introduce the concepts of gender roles and perceptions, particularly those characteristics that society considers masculine or feminine. Because students are to be grouped by sex, they should feel more comfortable in brainstorming differences between the sexes; such a division also helps avoid potential interference and comments from members of the opposite sex. After exchanging lists and discussing the actual physical differences and stereotypes at play, students will gain a better understanding of how gender role stereotypes can be restrictive and harmful for both males and females.

Materials and Preparation

Copies of "Definitions of Identity Terms," as a handout, from Lesson 1 in this chapter (optional)

Two sheets of newsprint titled "Differences Between Males and Females," along with two markers

Front board, with the following table displayed:

Differences Between Males and Females

MALES	FEMALES
1. Males have a penis. (Biology)	1. Females have a vagina. (Biology)
2. Males are more aggressive. (Stereotype)	2. Females are more emotional. (Stereotype)
3.	3.

Scrap paper for exit card responses

Procedure

1. Without any introduction of the topic of the day, read the following story, "Once Upon a Time," aloud. Ask students to listen carefully to solve the riddle:

   Once upon a time, a nurse was getting married. It was a beautiful, sunny day in June, and the bride and groom's friends and family had gathered for the happy occasion. The bride looked beautiful in her white dress, and the groom, a retired Marine, looked very handsome in his tuxedo.

   Later at the reception, a "fast" song started playing. Uncle Harry, who was a real character, ran over to the dance floor and started dancing. He was twirling and jumping around, then tried to spin on his back like a break dancer.

   All of a sudden, Uncle Harry stopped dancing, grabbed his chest, and collapsed right there on the dance floor from an apparent heart attack.

   The bride, who was standing nearby, did nothing to help. Why?

2. At the end of the story, ask the class, "Why didn't the bride do anything to help Uncle Harry?"
3. After students state incorrect guesses ("She was in shock," "She didn't want to get her dress dirty," "She was going to be left a lot of money in his will"), go back and read the first sentence of the story slowly while emphasizing the word "nurse." If no one still gets it, reveal the answer: "The *groom* was the nurse!" Explain to the students that the groom was trained as a medic when he was in the Marines. When he got out of the military, he decided to stay involved in the medical field. He did not want to spend a lot of time and money training to be a doctor, and nursing seemed to be a career he would enjoy while still being able to put his military training to work.
4. Say, "The story did not state that the bride was the nurse, but many people assume this. Why? Could she have been a doctor? A teacher? A construction worker?"
5. If desired, distribute the "Definitions of Identity Terms" from Lesson 1 as a handout. Discuss each of the terms related to gender roles and sexual identity.
6. Once students have a better understanding of the terms, break the class up into two groups, one consisting of all females and the other consisting of all males. Ask the groups to form a circle with their chairs at opposite ends of the room, as far away from the other group as possible. Explain that students are going to work together quietly in their group to brainstorm a list of how males and females are different.

7. Give each group a piece of newsprint and a marker. Assign one student from each group to be a group recorder who is in charge of writing items on the list, and another as the group's spokesperson to share their list at the completion of the brainstorm.
8. Have recorders copy down on their newsprint the table begun on the board.
9. Explain to the groups that their gender roles, either masculine or feminine, are determined by biological differences and society's stereotypes. Their group task is to brainstorm as many differences between males and females as they can come up with in fifteen minutes. The girls' group will only work on the "Males" column. The boys' group will only work on the "Females" column. If time permits, the groups can begin to complete the other column.
10. To get them started, you might ask each group to come up with a biological difference to list as the first item, and a stereotyped view of males or females to list as the second. From there, they can list any combination of physical differences and stereotypes. For example, for the first item, the boys might say, "Females have a vagina." The girls might state, "Males have a penis." Examples of stereotypes might be "Females are more emotional" and "Males are more aggressive."
11. Explain that each group's list should include as many physical differences as they can think of, but also should include many of society's stereotypes related to males or females. They can also consider how boys and girls may be treated differently from the time they are born. Other things to consider might be differences in personalities, interests, clothing, roles in the family, typical jobs, relationships, dating, sexual activity, sports, and so on. Remind students that stereotypes need not apply to all males or all females. For this activity, if a group believes that a difference is more often related to one gender than the other, it is okay to list it—even if members of the other group may not agree. The point of this activity is to have an open, honest interchange of ideas, even if some of the items on the list may be controversial.
12. While groups are compiling their respective lists, go back and forth to note how each one is progressing. You can give some general ideas to each of the groups, like "How is a mother different from a father?" "Are sisters and brothers treated differently?" "Does one gender express feelings more openly than the other?" "Are there any body parts you have left out?" Encourage each of the groups to come up with a minimum of twenty to thirty differences in the fifteen-minute period.
13. When the time is up, the group spokespeople will take turns reading statements from their list. When a spokesperson mentions an item from her group's list, the recorder in the other group should list it on his group's newsprint.
14. As each item is read aloud and recorded, groups have an opportunity to explain whether it is a physical difference or a stereotype. In some cases, there may be disagreement between the groups. You should allow some of these discussions and debates to take place, but should insist that students not use abusive language or make any derogatory remarks. Giving students a chance to state their viewpoint in an assertive manner lets them practice expressing their opinions respectfully. The main point of the activity is to separate the biological differences from society's stereotypes, and that many of these stereotypical views of males and females can be hurtful and insulting. This lesson is designed to increase awareness of this point and, therefore, decrease the use of stereotypes in everyday life.

15. When the lists have been exchanged, have the class look at how many items were based on biological differences and how many were stereotypes. Generally, there will be many more stereotypes than actual biological differences.
16. To conclude the lesson, ask the processing questions. Question 3 may be used for an exit card. In addition, students can discuss these "out the door" statements:
    a. "Men can be responsible, caring, gentle, loving, tender, and compassionate human beings. Spread the word!"
    b. "Women can be assertive, gentle, independent, loving, adventurous, strong, and compassionate human beings. Spread the word!"

Processing

1. What is one thing you learned today about the physical differences between males and females that you did not know before?
2. What did you notice about gender stereotypes?
3. In your opinion, are stereotypes healthy or unhealthy? Explain your answer.
4. In addition to sexual stereotypes, people are often stereotyped by their race, age, ethnic background, body shape and proportions, appearance, and so on. What are some examples of stereotypes for each of these? What are some examples to show how these stereotypes are hurtful or harmful?

Assessment

- Groups complete their chart.
- Students are assertive when speaking (refer to the communication rubric).
- Students complete an exit card for processing question 3.

LESSON 5: GENDER STEREOTYPES AND POPULARITY

Level: Middle school, High school

Time: 50–60 minutes

National Health Education Standards

1. Core Concepts
2. Analyzing Influences

National Sexuality Education Standards: Performance Indicators

- Explain the range of gender roles.
- Analyze the influence of peers, media, family, society, religion and culture on the expression of gender, sexual orientation and identity.
- Differentiate between gender identity, gender expression and sexual orientation.
- Differentiate between biological sex, sexual orientation, and gender identity and expression.

Rationale

Every day, teens are bombarded with media messages about what it means to be popular. Often, these media messages portray negative stereotypes that are not health enhancing. As young adults attempt to define who they are, they are often confused about what roles they should play, especially in regard to their sexuality. This lesson first allows students to discuss common stereotypes found within cliques of males and females. Then, after reflecting on the small group and class discussions, they are asked to create personal definitions for themselves.

Materials and Preparation

Video clip taken from a DVD or the Internet, shown using a computer and LCD projector or Smart Board

Large poster paper and markers for each group of students

Scrap paper for prompt responses

Materials for students to create collages or type performance projects

Procedure

ACTIVITY 1: WHAT IS A CLIQUE?

1. Begin the class by having students watch a short video clip on common groups formed in high school, if one is available. One example is the scene from the movie *Mean Girls* in which characters describe the different cliques in their school. After showing the video clip, ask students to define the term "clique."

2. If a video clip is not available, ask students to define the term "clique" and explain how common cliques are in today's society. Extend the discussion further by inquiring if the group someone is "in" defines who that person is.
3. Separate the class into groups of five or six students each. Groups can be single sex or mixed. Distribute the large poster paper and markers to each group. Explain that groups will have ten minutes to discuss traits ascribed to "popular" teenage males and females. Make sure to emphasize the point that names of actual students *should not* be mentioned.

   Specifically, students should answer the following questions:

   a. What common words and phrases come to mind when you think of a high school female who is "popular"?
   b. What common words and phrases come to mind when you think of a high school male who is "popular"?

   Students can include illustrated examples of popularity stereotypes on their poster as well as written ones.
4. As the groups work on their respective posters, walk around the room to ensure that students are on task and are being respectful.
5. After ten minutes have passed, ask each group to tape their poster up on a wall. Allow the class a few minutes to walk to each poster, noting similarities and differences between groups' answers. Then have students return to their seat.
6. Begin a discussion by asking what common themes appear for one sex. Then ask about the opposite sex. Continue to discuss where these ideas come from, and then ask the processing questions.
7. Conclude this part of the lesson by asking students to respond to the following prompt on a piece of scrap paper: "How fair are these popularity stereotypes? Explain your answer."

ACTIVITY 2: PERFORMANCE PROJECT

1. After students have discussed common themes portrayed for males and females, ask students to complete one of the following projects, which require students to come up with their own definition of who they are:

   a. Create a collage displaying how you define yourself as a female or a male.
   b. Describe in writing who you are as a male or a female. This can include how you think, feel, and act. The description should be at least one full typed page or two handwritten pages (with no spaces between lines).

   Note: Students may at first be confused by the second option, but after some contemplation they should be able to provide a description.

2. If they choose to do so, students can share their writing or collage during the next class. (Students may also complete the project at home.) Here is a possible grading rubric for your reference:

Performance Project Rubric (10 Points Total)

	4–5 POINTS	2–3 POINTS	0–1 POINT(S)
Proper terminology	All terms relating to identity were used correctly.	Some terms relating to identity were used correctly.	Most or all terms relating to identity were used incorrectly.
Personal description	The student fully explained or showed his or her definition of being a male or a female.	Some thought was apparent in the final product, although it seemed rushed, brief, or both.	No personal reflection was apparent. Work was done quickly or not given any thought.

Processing

1. How easy was it for your group to create a list of popularity stereotypes associated with each sex? Why do you think it was like this?
2. Where do these popularity stereotypes come from? Be specific.
3. Do you remember any particular time when you were told you could not do or be something because of a gender stereotype? Explain.
4. What happens if you are a male with female popularity traits? A female with male popularity traits?
5. How can we make sure we do not allow stereotypes to affect relationships with others?

Assessment

- Groups complete their poster.
- Students participate in the class discussion.
- Students answer the prompt question.
- Students each create a performance project.

LESSON 6: SUGAR AND SPICE AND EVERYTHING NICE

GENDER ROLES AND SEXUAL STEREOTYPES

Level: Middle school, High school

Time: 40 minutes

National Health Education Standards

1. Core Concepts
2. Analyzing Influences
4. Interpersonal Communication

National Sexuality Education Standards: Performance Indicators

- Explain the range of gender roles.
- Differentiate between biological sex, sexual orientation, and gender identity and expression.
- Analyze the influence of peers, media, family, society, religion and culture on the expression of gender, sexual orientation and identity.
- Communicate respectfully with and about people of all gender identities, gender expressions and sexual orientations.

Rationale

Often, members of both sexes will have stereotyped views of what it would be like to be someone of the opposite sex.

Analyzing the influences of friends, family, the media, and culture on beliefs about what is typically masculine or feminine behavior encourages critical thinking in students. It allows them to explore myths, attitudes, and feelings about their own and the opposite sex. The purpose of this lesson is to allow students to compare and contrast the biological and sociocultural aspects of human sexuality. In addition, common stereotypes related to sexual identity and gender roles will be discussed.

Note: Students tend to make broad generalizations related to typical masculine and feminine roles, some of which may provoke a retaliatory response from students of the opposite sex. Your job is not to be a referee, but rather to reinforce the fact that although males and females are different in many ways, these differences are based much more on external influences than on biology.

Materials and Preparation

Copies of "Gender Roles People Search" worksheet

Copies of "Twenty-Four Hours as a Member of the Opposite Sex" homework

Procedure

1. Begin the class with the following story:

    A woman walked into the kitchen to find her husband stalking around with a fly swatter.

    "What are you doing?" she asked.

    "Hunting flies," he responded.

    " Oh . . . killing any?" she asked.

    "Yep, three males, two females," he replied.

    Intrigued, she asked, "How can you tell?"

    He responded, "Three were on a beer can, two were on the phone."

    Allow students to discuss this "joke." Ask, "Did this joke offend anyone in class? Might this joke offend someone? Why?" (This joke may offend someone because it contains examples of sexual stereotypes.)

2. Have a class discussion to define and give examples of stereotypes. Examples may include labeling or generalizing about someone based on race, religion, sex, nationality, age, or clothing.
3. Explain that the class will explore some statements related to stereotyping people based on their gender. At this point, distribute the "Gender Roles People Search" worksheet and read the instructions aloud as students follow along on the page.
4. Allow five minutes for students to gather names. At the end of five minutes, have students return to their seat.
5. Facilitate the discussion by starting with the first statement. Ask if anyone found a female who does not "like to shop or talk on the phone." There are usually at least one or two girls in a class who do not fit this stereotyped image of females. Ask any of these girls *why* they do not particularly like to do these things. Does this mean that they are abnormal or weird? Stress the point that even though society expects females to like these things, not all females do. Stereotyping people is more common than people think and is perfectly normal. Then ask if there are any boys in the class who like to shop and talk on the phone. If there are some boys who like these things, does it mean there is something wrong with them? Are they strange? Feminine? Obviously, again, this is perfectly normal.
6. Go through the remaining statements from the worksheet. Your role is to encourage open, honest communication and to insist that students communicate respectfully with each other. The interaction between members of the class should not develop into a "war of the sexes." Express to students that there is no right way to think, feel, or act. The discussion should not be about which is the better or a "winning" sex, and instead should focus on gender-related information in an unbiased way.
7. Ask the processing questions.
8. To bring closure to the lesson, explain that although some of the differences between the sexes are biological, many more are based on society's stereotyped views. State:

    From birth, boys and girls are expected to act in certain ways. Friends, family, the media, society, and culture influence how boys and girls think they should behave.

Many people believe that society's strict views of male and female roles have changed over the last fifty years, especially with the rise of the Women's Liberation Movement in the 1960s. However, society's views of what is typically masculine or feminine are still a part of everyday life.

Gender stereotypes can have a negative impact on someone's professional and personal relationships. In addition, making fun of people for not acting the way society expects them to act is disrespectful and hurtful.

Note: The most important outcome of this people search and follow-up discussion is making students aware that male and female stereotyping can discourage males and females from reaching their true potential as human beings.

9. Distribute copes of the "Twenty-Four Hours as a Member of the Opposite Sex" homework. During the next class, ask volunteers to share how their lives would be different and how they would be the same if they were members of the opposite sex. Here is a possible rubric for grading the homework assignment:

"Twenty-Four Hours as a Member of the Opposite Sex" Homework Rubric (10 Points Total)

	5 POINTS	2–3 POINTS	0–1 POINT(S)
Proper terminology	All terms relating to identity were used correctly.	Most terms relating to identity were used correctly.	Some terms were used incorrectly, or no terms were used.
Personal description	The student fully explained what a school day would be like as a member of the opposite sex.	Some thought was apparent in the student's explanation, although it seemed rushed, brief, or both.	No or very little personal reflection was apparent. Work was done quickly or not given any thought.

Processing

1. How often do people assign others' gender roles?
2. What roles are placed on you that you agree to?
3. What roles are placed on you that you do not agree to?
4. How do gender roles differ depending on where you live?
5. How do gender roles differ depending on your age? Depending on where you live?

Assessment

- Students participate in the people search and follow-up discussion.
- Students show assertive communication (refer to the communication rubric).
- Students successfully complete the homework assignment.

Name: ______________________________

Gender Roles People Search

Directions: To complete this activity, you must search for students in your class who match one or more of the characteristics listed here. When you find someone, have him or her **print** his or her name on the appropriate line. No person may print his or her name on more than **two** lines on any individual's paper. You may sign your name on **one** of the lines of your own sheet. Your objective is to obtain as many names as possible in the five-minute time limit.

Find someone . . .

1. Who is a female and does not like to shop or talk on the phone:

____

2. Who is a female and rarely wears makeup or jewelry:

____

3. Who has a "best friend" of the opposite sex:

____

4. Whose mother is a full-time wife, mother, and homemaker:

____

5. Who is male and enjoys texting and talking on the phone:

____

6. Who has been treated by a male nurse:

____

7. Who had a male teacher in kindergarten or first grade:

____

8. Who knows a female who works on a construction crew:

____

9. Who is a female and is very competitive:

____

10. Who is not very interested in sports:

____

11. Who has changed a dirty diaper:

____

12. Who thinks a female would make a good U.S. president:

____

13. Who has cried in the last week:

____

14. Who thinks women can do just about everything men can do:

____

15. Who thinks men can do just about everything women can do:

____

Twenty-Four Hours as a Member of the Opposite Sex

Directions: Imagine that when you wake up tomorrow, you will have magically transformed into a member of the opposite sex. This means that if you are a male today, you will be a female tomorrow. If you are a female, you will be a male. This will only be a temporary change; the following morning when you wake up, you will be back to your original self.

Your assignment is to write a composition (minimum of two hundred words) about what you imagine one day at school as someone of the opposite sex would be like. Include some of the following in your composition:

- When do you wake up?
- How long does it take to get ready for school?
- What do you wear?
- What is it like on the bus, in your classes throughout the day, in the halls, at lunch, and after school?
- Whom do you talk to?
- What do you talk about?
- Are your relationships with your family, teachers, and friends different?
- Do you like the same types of music? Food? Social activities?
- How do you feel about your body? Your self-image?
- Are you looked at differently? Treated differently? Do you like this, or not?
- What is the best part of the day?
- What is the worst part of the day?
- How do you feel by the end of the day?
- What stereotypes about the opposite sex do you experience?

Be creative with your composition and use your imagination!

LESSON 7: IMPLICIT ASSOCIATION TEST

Level: High school

Time: 40–50 minutes

National Health Education Standard

2. Analyzing Influences

National Sexuality Education Standards: Performance Indicator

- Analyze the influence of peers, media, family, society, religion and culture on the expression of gender, sexual orientation and identity.

Rationale

From birth, people receive messages about how males and females are expected to behave. This lesson allows students to think "outside the box" about preconceived thoughts or concepts pertaining to gender and gender roles. Students will question whether their thoughts are intrinsic or caused by outside sources. To do this, each student will go online and complete two Implicit Association Tests (IATs) pertaining to gender. These IATs were designed by researchers associated with Harvard University.

The Implicit Association Test allows an individual to answer simple questions about how words are associated with other words or pictures. How quickly one responds to an association, as well as how many correct responses are given, are evaluated to show if the test taker prefers a particular pattern of thought. For example, a test might determine how likely an individual is to categorize females in traditional female roles.

After taking the test, a summarizing statement is given. This one statement, although brief, allows individuals to consider their automatic preference and/or association concerning the given topic. This test compares the result to the results from past participants and allows test takers to question their own preferences or prejudices in regard to other people.

This assignment can be completed as homework. However, processing what the assessment is about requires an in-depth discussion in a classroom setting. (*Note:* Although students may complete this assignment at home, the directions are written as if the completion will occur in class.)

Materials and Preparation

Smart Board or TV screen for demonstrating the test

Copies of "The Implicit Association Test" worksheet

Computers with Internet access, one for each student

Procedure

1. Introduce the lesson by asking students to respond to the following quote:

> Women have one great advantage over men. It is commonly thought that if they marry they have done enough, and need career no further. If a man marries, on the other hand, public opinion is all against him if he takes this view.
>
> **Rose Macaulay, a novelist found at http://goodquotes.org/opinion-quotes.html**

2. Allow students to think about this quote and discuss whether thoughts like this exist in today's society.
3. After a brief discussion, introduce the day's activity by going over the Implicit Association Test. If you are able to do so, display the website on a Smart Board or TV screen. It is important to explain what "implicit" and "association" refer to. This online "test" can seem confusing, but if you demonstrate its use and foster class discussion around the test's significance, students will come to understand its purpose.
4. Distribute the "The Implicit Association Test" worksheet to all students. You or a student should then read the information about the test aloud.
5. To give students a better understanding of how the IAT works, consider doing one of the assigned tests in front of the class, going page by page. Through your modeling of the activity, students will better comprehend the day's task.
6. Allow students to read the directions and ask questions before anyone begins the test.
7. Students will then log onto the computer and complete the IATs for:
    a. Gender and science
    b. Gender and career
8. Students can print out the final page or write down the responses for each of their IATs. As students are waiting for others to finish, they can journal about their results and whether or not they agree with them. Others will journal at home.
9. For closure, ask the processing questions to allow the students to process their final responses.

Processing

1. What were your results from the Gender-Science IAT?
2. What were your results form the Gender-Career IAT?
3. How do you feel about your results? Are they accurate? Explain.
4. Where do you believe your responses came from? Are they intrinsic, or were you taught them?
5. Do you think a test like the IAT can accurately predict if certain thought patterns exist? Explain your answer.

Assessment

- Students complete two IATs and answer questions from the worksheet.
- Students analyze their IAT results in a journal entry.

Name: ______________________________

The Implicit Association Test

In the late 1990s the Implicit Association Test (IAT) was presented as a social psychological tool to measure an individual's automatic association of ideas. In other words, it measures how certain thoughts occur by reflex (involuntarily) because of one's memory. Although this concept can be difficult to understand, after completing one of the Implicit Association Tests, a person may be better able to assess if he or she has underlying beliefs about a particular topic.

For today, you will be given the opportunity to explore the IAT by taking two tests specifically geared toward gender: the Gender-Career IAT and the Gender- Science IAT.

Note: Your final assessment on each IAT will not include a lot of information. Instead, it will show you a preference for gender and science or gender and career, depending on the test. It will also show the results from others who have taken the IAT before you. Although brief, this summary can be enlightening for people who wish to better understand thought patterns they were not previously aware of.

Directions: To take the tests, please follow these steps:

1. Go to https://implicit.harvard.edu.
2. On the page titled "Project Implicit," click on "Go" in the "Project Implicit Social Attitudes" box. You will be signing on as a guest and only need to note your country of origin.
3. Read the page titled "Preliminary Information." If you choose not to proceed, tell your teacher. If you do want to continue, read over the whole page and then click "I wish to proceed."
4. On the page "Take a Test," click on one of the following:
   a. Gender-Science IAT
   b. Gender-Career IAT
5. Read over all of the directions carefully. Click on the "Click Here to Begin," then "Continue."
6. On the next page(s), complete the questions about yourself to the best of your ability. These questions are for the purpose of the website's research. Your name, address, and phone number will not be requested. Then click to the next page.
7. The next page will display terms that will be used for your IAT. Read the information carefully. You will need to keep your fingers on the E and I buttons on the keyboard while taking the test. Start the test by pressing either the E or the I button for the noted term or picture. You will repeat this procedure about four to six times.
8. After you have completed pressing the E and I buttons, allow the computer to calculate your results. Press on the space bar to go on to the next page. Additional questions will be shown. Answer these, then press "Continue." On the next page, your result will be shown. Remember—this result will be brief, yet it can be telling. Write on the back of this worksheet what your result was, then answer the additional questions.
9. Below your result, additional questions are asked. Answer these, and then proceed to the next page. The next page will show you how other respondents have replied. Note this on your worksheet.
10. At the bottom of this page, click on "Additional Demonstration Tasks" to complete the other IAT.

Responses to the Implicit Association Tests

Gender-Career IAT

1. After completing this test, what "preference" or final note was provided from the website about your answers?

2. Summarize the bar chart showing the results of all Gender-Career IAT respondents.

3. How did your result compare to the results of other test takers?

4. How accurate do you feel the IAT was for you? Explain your answer.

Responses to the Implicit Association Tests (*continued*)

Gender-Science IAT

1. After completing this test, what "preference" or final note was provided from the website about your answers?

2. Summarize the bar chart showing the results of all Gender-Science IAT respondents.

3. How did your result compare to the results of other test takers?

4. How accurate do you feel the IAT was for you? Explain your answer.

LESSON 8: ADVOCACY AND GENDER IDENTITY

Level: Middle school, High school

Time: 40–50 minutes

National Health Education Standards

3. Accessing Information
4. Interpersonal Communication
8. Advocacy

National Sexuality Education Standards: Performance Indicators

- Communicate respectfully with and about people of all gender identities, gender expressions and sexual orientations.
- Demonstrate communication skills that foster healthy relationships.
- Access accurate information about gender identity, gender expression and sexual orientation.
- Develop a plan to promote dignity and respect for all people in the school community.
- Advocate for school policies and programs that promote dignity and respect for all.

Rationale

Policies in regard to expected respectful behaviors exist at the school, district, community, state, and federal levels, yet often people are not aware of these policies or how they are written. To enhance students' understanding of such policies, this lesson allows students to analyze and critique a current policy and apply it to sexual orientation, gender identity, and gender expression. In addition, students will be given the opportunity to rework the policy to further advocate dignity and respect for all students.

Note: Students may desire to take this lesson further by advocating for policy changes at the school or district level. This can include students' presenting suggestions to administrators, board members, or both at appropriate times.

Materials and Preparation

Current school or district policy relating to dignity for students and community members (such as a bullying or harassment prevention policy), displayed at the front of the classroom. Such a policy may be found in the student handbook or the district calendar or website.

Teacher copy of "Sexual Orientation, Gender Identity, and Gender Expression Scenarios," with Scenarios A through H cut into separate parts.

Appropriate resources to find information about school, district, community, county, state, or national policies (such as local legislation for university policies about harassment or bullying).

Procedure

1. Begin the class by having a student volunteer read aloud the chosen policy displayed at the front. Ask students if they recognize where it is from; some students may not be aware that the school or district even has such a policy. Ask, "What is the point of having a policy that people are not aware of?"
2. Create groups of four to five students. After students are seated with their respective groups, explain that each group is going to be given a different scenario related to the policy previously reviewed.
3. Distribute one of the eight scenarios to each group and allow time for a group discussion to occur. Groups should process the appropriateness of the behavior in their assigned situation.
4. After five minutes have passed, ask a representative from each group to read the group's situation. Ask another group member to explain the group's perceptions. Students from other groups can ask additional questions and give their perspective; you should ensure statements are appropriate.
5. After all of the groups' scenarios have been discussed, allow another five minutes for groups to create recommendations to strengthen the policy given earlier in a way that shows dignity and respect for all students, no matter what their gender expression, gender identity, or sexual orientation may be. Also, if available, provide students with correct information relating to the topic, in the form of either reliable websites or informational pamphlets, for example.
6. When time is up, ask one group member who did not speak earlier from each group to explain any improvements to the policy. Groups may have similar suggestions.
7. Conclude the activity by having students write in their journal about the featured school or district policy and the provided scenarios.
8. For an optional assignment, have students write a letter to a person in a leadership position who is able to make changes to the featured policy. This letter should be developed with respectful and appropriate language.

Processing

1. How does the school or district policy protect heterosexual students? Gay or lesbian students? Bisexual students?
2. Why do you think this policy was created?
3. Who is able to create or strengthen policies pertaining to gender identity, gender expression, or sexual orientation?

Assessment

- Students demonstrate assertive communication within their group and in the class discussion (refer to the communication rubric).
- Students respond correctly to their assigned scenario, according to the school or district policy, indicating whether the behavior is appropriate and what can be done within the school or district if it is not.
- Students each complete an individual journal entry.
- Students complete the optional letter writing assignment.

Sexual Orientation, Gender Identity, and Gender Expression Scenarios

Scenario A

Chuck and Larry are high school seniors. They have been dating for three months, and many students at school are aware that they are a couple. While walking by a classroom, another student yells aloud, "Hey, homos!"

Is this behavior shown by the student acceptable?

Explain your answer.

Scenario B

Bob and Debby have been dating for six months. One afternoon, they are seen making out in the lunchroom. A teacher walks by and sarcastically says, "Get a room, you two," and continues on his way.

Is this behavior shown by the teacher acceptable?

Explain your answer.

Scenario C

Erica is a fourth grader who loves to play sports. After school, she tells the recreation director she wants to join the football team. He explains that she cannot because "football is not meant for girls."

Is this behavior shown by the recreation director acceptable?

Explain your answer.

Scenario D

Stephen is in the third grade. Since the first grade, he has told everyone he really is a girl and wants to wear skirts and dresses to school and to be called Stephanie. His principal has told his mother that this is not allowed.

Is this behavior shown by the principal acceptable?

Explain your answer.

Sexual Orientation, Gender Identity, and Gender Expression Scenarios (*continued*)

Scenario E

Miguel is in the seventh grade and is experiencing the vocal changes of puberty. His voice squeaks when he speaks, going from low to high pitches, especially when he is nervous. While making a presentation in science class, his voice made squeaking sounds. The girls sitting on the side of the room giggled every time this happened, and started calling him "Michelle" after class.

Is the behavior shown by the girls acceptable?

Explain your answer.

Scenario F

Ms. Johnson, a high school physical education teacher, is rumored to be a lesbian. Some parents have requested that their daughters not have her as their teacher. They feel that she is not an appropriate role model and fear that her sexual orientation may encourage their daughters to "turn gay." The guidance counselor changed the girls' schedules to appease the parents.

Is the behavior shown by the parents acceptable?

Is the behavior shown by the guidance counselor acceptable?

Explain your answers.

Scenario G

Veronica loves wearing makeup and, as she likes to say, dress like a "girly girl." She often wears short skirts and shirts showing her cleavage. The principal decided to suspend her because she has already been told to wear appropriate clothing to cover her breasts and thighs.

Is the behavior shown by the principal acceptable?

Explain your answer.

Scenario H

The senior prom is approaching. The principal announces that only heterosexual couples can buy tickets to the event, knowing that there are some students who are gay and in a dating relationship.

Is the behavior shown by the principal acceptable?

Explain your answer.

LESSON 9: UP CLOSE AND PERSONAL

Level: Middle school, High school

Time: 40–50 minutes

National Health Education Standards

1. Core Concepts
2. Analyzing Influences
4. Interpersonal Communication

National Sexuality Education Standards: Performance Indicators

- Communicate respectfully with and about people of all gender identities, gender expressions and sexual orientations.
- Demonstrate communication skills that foster healthy relationships.
- Explain the range of gender roles.
- Analyze the influence of peers, media, family, society, religion and culture on the expression of gender, sexual orientation and identity.

Rationale

A variety of positive and negative influences within society affect our health. This Up Close and Personal (UCP) session will stimulate discussion about some of the internal and external factors that influence attitudes and behaviors among youth. In addition, students will practice effective communication skills while clarifying their personal beliefs, values, and perceived norms about gender and identity.

Because UCP lessons deal mainly with the affective or emotional domain, they have a greater potential for personal disclosure on the part of students. You should be aware of and prepared to handle this. Sometimes it simply involves reminding the class that what is said in class stays in class. At other times, it may involve discussing issues with students privately to offer advice, resources, and support.

Note: A student's "coming out" is confidential, and teachers are not required to share this with school authorities under mandated reporting laws. It is important, however, to ensure that no harassment of any kind results from such a revelation. Encouraging students to work together to promote dignity and respect for all people, regardless of race, religion, sex, ethnicity, or sexual orientation, should be the overriding theme of all class discussions.

Materials and Preparation

Small lamp (optional)

Up Close and Personal sheet with several UCP sentence stems. (*Note:* Prior to teaching this activity, you should familiarize yourself with "Facilitating a UCP Session," which can be found at the end of the lesson.)

Procedure*

1. Ask students to form a circle with their chairs. Turning off the overhead lights and using a lamp may make the environment more conducive to an informal discussion.
2. Introduce the activity in the following manner:

   Today we are going to do an activity called Up Close and Personal. It is simple to do, but for it to go smoothly, there are some rules to follow.

   First, understand this is not group therapy. Instead it is an opportunity for you to talk about how you feel about yourself, relationships, likes, dislikes, things that have come up in class, memories, and life in general. Although I will be facilitating the activity, I will also be sitting in the circle and participating along with everyone else.

   The activity is in the following format: I will read an unfinished sentence. Each of you will think about how you would finish this same unfinished sentence. Someone in the circle will then raise his or her hand and state his or her completed sentence. He or she will point to his or her right or left to determine which way around the circle we will proceed.

   When going around the circle, there should be no talking by anyone else. If something is said that you want to respond to or comment on, you must wait until we have gone all the way around the circle. If you cannot think of anything to say, or choose not to respond when it is your turn, you may simply say, "Pass" or "Come back to me." Everyone, including the teacher, is allowed to pass.

   When we have gone around the entire circle, I will ask anyone who passed if he or she would like to respond at this time. I will also ask for any questions or comments about anything that was said when going around the circle. At this point, there can be open discussion.

   Please note that during this activity, no names should be mentioned at any time. Instead, say something like, "I know someone who . . ."

   In addition, as with other lessons, what is said in class stays in class. However, please do not share anything that is too personal, that makes you feel uncomfortable, or that you wish to keep to yourself.
3. Once the rules have been explained and agreed on, read the first sentence stem aloud. After allowing a few moments for reflection, ask a student volunteer to start by stating his completed sentence. That student will then point to his left or right to note in which direction the remaining students will be given a chance to complete the sentence. Students then give their responses until everyone around the circle has spoken or passed.
4. At times, a student may simply not be ready to respond to a particular question. When this happens, remind her to pass, noting that she can answer after everyone else has spoken. It is also not unusual for many students to have the same response to a question or statement. "Repeats" reinforce the important concept that although all people are unique, they often share many of the same thoughts, feelings, and values.

---

*Unfinished sentences have been a useful learning tool for many years. The specific format used in this lesson has been adapted from the book *Up Close and Personal: Effective Learning for Students and Teachers* (Raleigh, NC: Lulu Press, 2007), by teacher, colleague, and friend Robert Winchester. Robert can be contacted at trustinbob@aol.com.

5. After all students have responded, open up the discussion by asking if anyone has any questions or comments about anything that was said. Encourage students to talk in more detail about why they completed the sentence the way they did. Students may also ask others in the circle, including the teacher, to expand on their answer. Students may do so, or they may choose to pass.
6. Continue the circle discussion for as long as it is viable, constantly monitoring and enforcing the rules. When the discussion on a given sentence has run its course, move on to the next unfinished sentence.
7. Share the processing statements.
8. All UCP sessions should end with some brief closure in the form of another unfinished sentence. Examples include the following: "Today I learned . . ." "I learned that I . . ." "Right now I feel . . ." and "Something I want to say to one of my classmates is . . ."
9. Conclude the day's activity by summarizing what occurred in the session, making appropriate connections to the subject matter and curriculum. Then thank the class and say, "This ends our Up Close and Personal class for today."
10. Specific to this particular UCP session, assign homework in which students must write a reflection paper (of at least two to three paragraphs). A good prompt might be, "Based on what I learned about gender and identity during today's UCP discussion, one thing I will consider changing about my attitudes, my future behavior, or both is . . ."

    This assignment allows students to reflect on and develop changes in attitudes and behaviors over time. When shared with the class in a subsequent lesson, it further allows the student, the class, and the teacher to observe changes in knowledge, attitudes, and values.

Processing

1. If anyone has any concerns or questions about what was discussed during our UCP session today, he or she can speak to me privately after class or can bring it up for discussion during our next class session.
2. There are many people, including teachers, coaches, counselors, or school psychologists, who can assist you with any personal issues that you may want to share with them. Keep in mind that these individuals, as mandated reporters, *must* report any verbalization or indication that you may want to hurt yourself or hurt others, or revelations of abuse of any kind, to the appropriate authorities for follow-up and counseling services.

Assessment

- Students actively participate in the UCP activity. Even though some students may decide to pass on one or more questions, as long as they are actively listening and following the ground rules, they are "actively participating."
- Students complete the homework assignment and share their response in a future class session.

Facilitating a UCP Session

- Facilitation is a skill that you can improve with practice.
- Silence is not a negative phenomenon. Silence often indicates that higher-level thinking is taking place.
- Going over ground rules at the beginning of each session is a needed and helpful technique to prevent inappropriate behavior.
- Unacceptable behavior should be stopped the moment it is recognized. To do this, pause the activity and point out the offense to the individual. For example, say, "What was just said is a put-down (or personal name), and it is not allowed in the circle discussion. Please do not do it again," or "Please do not talk to your neighbor when you should be listening to the one person who is supposed to be talking."
- If a student persists in breaking the activity's rules, talk to him one-on-one after class. Let the student know that if his behavior continues, he may not be able to participate in the future. This almost always stops the offensive behavior.
- Remind students of the information teachers *must* report if shared:
    1. If they are going to hurt themselves
    2. If they are going to hurt others
    3. If they are being abused

Possible UCP Sentence Stems: Gender and Identity

1. On a scale of one to ten, one being horrible and ten being wonderful, right now I am about a . . .
2. When I hear the word "heterosexual," the first thing I think about is . . .
3. One message I have received from parents (or guardians) or peers about gender roles and sexual orientation is . . .
4. Messages I have received from the media (movies, TV, music, advertising, and the Internet) about gender roles and sexual orientation are . . .
5. When it comes to being tolerant of people who are "different," most teenagers at this school . . .
6. If I thought a friend were being harassed because of his or her sexual orientation, I would . . .
7. Messages in the media tell us that men should . . .
8. Messages in the media tell us that women should . . .
9. If my best friend told me he or she was gay, I . . .
10. One stereotype that I have heard about males or females who are gay or lesbian is . . .
11. "People do not 'choose' their sexual orientation." My opinion about this statement is . . .
12. Something in my background or upbringing that has influenced my attitude about sexual orientation is . . .
13. Something I learned today is . . .

LESSON 10: HOME-SCHOOL CONNECTION

TALKING ABOUT GENDER IDENTITY

Level: Middle school

Time: Varies

National Health Education Standards

1. Core Concepts
2. Analyzing Influences
4. Interpersonal Communication

National Sexuality Education Standards: Performance Indicators

- Explain the range of gender roles.
- Communicate respectfully with and about people of all gender identities, gender expressions and sexual orientations.
- Analyze external influences that have an impact on one's attitudes about gender, sexual orientation and gender identity.

Rationale

Gender identity refers to a person's internal sense of being female, male, or a combination of both. Gender roles refer to the way society expects people to behave based on their biological sex. The role of the school is to supplement the teaching of parents or guardians by providing students with accurate information, and by engaging them in developing and practicing interpersonal skills. It is the parents' or guardians' responsibility to communicate family values and beliefs.

The first part of this Home-School Connection activity asks parents or guardians to share their beliefs and attitudes about when someone "becomes a man" or "becomes a woman." Different cultures and societies may have very different views on this subject. Having discussions about gender identity can often be difficult for both children and adults. It is important to realize, however, that a person's biological sex and gender identity play important roles in determining that individual's thoughts, feelings, attitudes, and behavior.

The second part of the assignment deals with how adults can promote tolerance for children and teens who do not fit the norm of their gender. By having discussions about people who are "different," parents or guardians can instill in their children the universal value of promoting dignity and respect for all people, regardless of their race, religion, ethnicity, or sexual orientation.

After completing the assignment, parents or guardians are requested to sign on the bottom. All responses from teens and parents or guardians on the Home-School Connection activity will be kept confidential. It will not be turned in to the teacher or graded. On the due date, students will be asked to *voluntarily* share any interesting comments or insights they learned or observed by participating in the assignment. Students *and* parents or guardians can choose to pass on any discussion they wish to keep private.

With family input and support, the overall goal is to encourage teens to become well-informed, caring, respectful, and responsible adults.

Materials and Preparation

Copies of "Talking about Gender Identity" worksheet

Procedure

1. Explain to the class that they are going to have an assignment to complete with one or more parents or guardians.
2. Distribute the worksheet and assign a due date.
3. On the day the assignment is due, check if students have completed the assignment by noting if the sheet was signed on the bottom. The assignment should not be collected or graded.
4. Go through the processing questions, asking for student volunteers to share the results of the discussion they had with the adult or adults they interviewed. All student comments are voluntary.
5. Conclude the lesson by asking students to participate in a "class whip." For this, each student will quickly share one brief statement related to the activity. Examples include "I learned . . ." "I feel (or felt) . . ." or "I was surprised . . ."

Processing

1. Which family members did you choose to speak with?
2. How did you feel talking to family members about this topic? Were you comfortable with this discussion? Were your parents or guardians?
3. Is it easy or difficult to talk to family members about issues related to gender identity and sexual orientation? Explain.
4. What were some of the messages you received about when a male "becomes a man" and a female "becomes a woman"?
5. What advice did you receive about how schools, parents or guardians, and other adults can reduce bullying or harassment and ensure that all students are treated with dignity and respect?
6. How did you feel about the messages that your parents or guardians shared with you?
7. Did anything surprising come up during the conversation?
8. What did you learn from doing this assignment?
9. What did you learn from our follow-up class discussion?

Assessment

- Students bring to class the completed and signed assignment.
- Students participate in the follow-up discussion related to the assignment.
- Students participate in the class whip.

Talking about Gender Identity

Parents or guardians, through their expressed thoughts, personal values, and actions, are the primary sexuality educators of their children. The role of the school is to supplement family teaching by providing students with accurate information and life skills. Therefore, both families and schools can encourage teens to become well-informed, caring, respectful, and responsible adults.

Directions: After discussing and filling out the questions that follow, please sign the bottom of the worksheet. This is simply to verify that your child has completed the assignment. It will not be turned in to the teacher or graded. All comments from teens and parents or guardians on this Home-School Connection activity will be kept confidential.

With these guidelines in mind, please take a few minutes to discuss the following assignment with your child. Thank you in advance for your participation.

1. In different cultures, there are celebrations and events noting when a young person is no longer considered a child and, instead, "becomes a woman" or "becomes a man." In our culture . . .
   a. What do you think signifies the transformation when a female "becomes a woman"?

   ____

   ____

   ____

   b. What do you think signifies the transformation when a male "becomes a man"?

   ____

   ____

   ____

2. Imagine a young person who does not fit the "norms" of his or her gender. How can parents or guardians, teachers, counselors, administrators, and religious leaders help prevent teasing or bullying and ensure that this child is shown dignity and respect?

____

____

____

____

____

Parent or guardian signature(s): ______________________________

Student signature: ______________________________________

Pregnancy and Reproduction

4

The United States continues to have one of the highest teen pregnancy rates in the industrialized world, despite a steady decline in rates since the 1990s. Providing teens with the information, skills, and motivation to make informed decisions about sexuality can help them avoid or reduce sexual risk taking, thereby lowering the risk of an unplanned pregnancy.

The lessons in Chapter Four include information about how pregnancy happens. Many of the activities also introduce or reinforce decision-making and other life skills that can help students avoid an unplanned pregnancy. Lesson topics and performance indicators include

- Defining sexual intercourse and its relationship to human reproduction
- Describing the signs of pregnancy, and prenatal practices that can contribute to or threaten a healthy pregnancy
- Assessing the skills and resources needed to become an effective parent
- Being aware of social norms and accessing valid, reliable information
- Explaining the health benefits, risks, and effectiveness of various methods of birth control, including abstinence, condoms, and emergency contraception

ADDITIONAL LESSONS IN THIS CHAPTER

For teens and young adults, decisions about whether or when to engage in sexual behaviors can have major short- and long-term consequences. Communication and decision-making skills can be learned and improved with practice. Teens can benefit from learning the sequential steps in a decision-making model. They can also learn and practice effective communication strategies, such as active listening; using refusal skills; and distinguishing between passive, aggressive, and assertive behaviors. Several of the activities in this chapter provide opportunities for students to practice and apply communication and decision-making skills related to their sexual health.

LESSON 1: PREGNANCY AND BIRTH 101

Level: Middle school

Time: 40 minutes

National Health Education Standard

1. Core Concepts

National Sexuality Education Standards: Performance Indicators

- Define sexual intercourse and its relationship to human reproduction.
- Identify prenatal practices that can contribute to a healthy pregnancy.

Rationale

Decisions about having children are based on personal values, cultural beliefs, and other factors.

Middle school children are especially curious about reproduction and the birth process, often because of a lack of accurate information about "where babies come from." Children need to be taught that men and women have different organs that enable them to have a child, as well as specific cells in their bodies (sperm and egg cells) that enable them to reproduce.

Through a guided visualization activity titled "The Story of Fertilization and Birth" in the first part of the lesson, students will be actively involved in a visual simulation of what occurs during conception and embryonic development. In the second part of the lesson, students will complete a worksheet on how life begins in addition to a crossword puzzle to assess functional knowledge.

Materials and Preparation

Seven cards large enough for the entire class to see, labeled using markers with the following words:

Sperm/X Chromosome	Sperm/Y Chromosome	Egg/X Chromosome	Ovary	Fallopian Tube	Uterus	Vagina

Anatomically correct models or labeled drawings of male and female reproductive systems. (*Note:* When explaining the process of fertilization, prenatal development, and birth, it is helpful to have drawings or models of the male and female reproductive systems. These drawings can be downloaded from many sites on the Internet and distributed to students. Another helpful model is the "Birth Atlas," which can be purchased through many health education catalogs.)

Teacher copy of "The Story of Fertilization and Birth"

Copies of "How Life Begins" worksheet

Copies of "Pregnancy and Birth Crossword Puzzle" homework

Procedure

ACTIVITY 1: "WHERE DID I COME FROM?"

1. Ask the class if they ever talked with their parents or guardians about where babies come from, and what their parents or guardians said. Responses may vary, depending on when they had "the talk" with their parents or guardians, ranging from "The stork brought you" or "You grew in Mommy's tummy" to very scientific, detailed information about sex and the process of fertilization and reproduction.
2. Explain that sometimes parents or guardians do not talk with their children about where babies come from. This may be because the topic never comes up, because of feelings of embarrassment, or because they just do not know what to say and how to say it.
3. Allow students to discuss the dilemma facing children who have never had "the talk" with a parent or guardian, and where these children might otherwise learn about sex and how babies are made. Sources may include peers, health class, the media, and books. Tell students that sometimes this information is accurate, and sometimes it is not.
4. Explain that in today's lesson, students will review terms related to male and female reproductive anatomy as well as the process of human reproduction and birth.
5. Ask seven volunteers to help with a demonstration: two students for the sperm cells; one student for the egg cell; and four students for the other reproductive organs. Hand them their corresponding cards.
6. Display a basic diagram of the female reproductive system. This can be either a drawing of yours, a poster, or an image found online and displayed on a Smart Board. The ovaries, fallopian tubes, uterus, and vagina should be labeled.
7. Ask the class, "Who knows what happens during sex?" Some giggles and perhaps embarrassment should be expected, but there will be some students who volunteer an answer. Ask students to use proper terminology when answering. Most students should have had some health or science instruction in elementary school, but this may not always be the case. A sample answer could be: "When a man and a woman have sexual intercourse, the male's penis is inserted into the female's vagina and deposits sperm. This discharge is called an ejaculation."
8. Have the student volunteers stand at the front of the room. The student with the card labeled "Egg/X Chromosome" should stand near the ovary in the diagram of the female reproductive system. Explain that you will read "The Story of Fertilization and Birth," during which the students holding the different cards are to move to demonstrate what occurs during the various steps of the fertilization process. Begin reading.

9. When you have finished the story, thank the volunteers. Ask the class if there are any questions. Have a Question Box available in the classroom in case students have a question they would like to ask anonymously.

   Note: This topic generally elicits many questions from middle school students, some of which may be embarrassing for them to ask openly in class. The Question Box (first described in Chapter One, Lesson 5) should be made available so students can anonymously ask questions at any time.

ACTIVITY 2: HOW LIFE BEGINS

1. Hand out the "How Life Begins" worksheet. Allow students to work in pairs or small groups to complete the worksheet, using the word bank provided to assist them in filling in the blanks.
2. Give students eight to ten minutes to complete the worksheet. Review the information by going around the room and having students each take a turn reading a completed sentence from their worksheet, while checking for accuracy.
3. When the worksheet has been completed and discussed, and after you have asked the processing questions, hand out the "Pregnancy and Birth Crossword Puzzle" homework. Students should complete the puzzle at home and bring it with them for the next class session, at which point their answers will be checked. Here is the answer key for your reference:

   Across

   2. Cervix
   5. Cesarean
   6. Identical
   9. Placenta
   12. Fraternal
   13. Zygote

   Down

   1. Fetus
   3. Gynecologist
   4. Umbilical
   7. Embryo
   8. Uterus
   10. Prenatal
   11. Amnion

4. As an optional summative activity to assess students' learning, you can develop and administer a posttest on information related to reproductive anatomy and physiology, prenatal development, and the birth process.

Processing

1. How comfortable did you feel during today's lesson? Explain why you felt this way.
2. How much information did you know already? Where did you learn this?
3. Why is this information important to review?
4. After hearing this information, what advice would you give to a future mother or father?

Assessment

- Students actively participate in the first activity, "Where Did I Come From?"
- Students correctly complete the "How Life Begins" worksheet.
- Students correctly complete the crossword puzzle homework assignment.
- Students complete a summative assessment (optional).

The Story of Fertilization and Birth

Once a girl reaches puberty, she starts to release specific chemicals called hormones. Those hormones cause the changes in her body during puberty. One of the most important changes takes place inside her body. This change occurs when the ovaries release mature egg cells, or ova. (Have the student with the "Ovary" card stand near the diagram of the female reproductive system, alongside the drawing of the ovary). A female egg cell is barely visible to the naked eye and is about the size of a poppy seed. Once a female begins her monthly menstrual cycle, the ovum starts to travel down the fallopian tube. (At this point, have the student with the "Fallopian Tube" card stand near the diagram of the female reproductive system, adjacent to one of the fallopian tubes.)

As you can see from the diagram, there are two ovaries and two fallopian tubes. The ovaries generally alternate, releasing one egg cell each month. (At this point, have the student with the "Egg" card move from the ovary to the fallopian tube.)

Meanwhile, there are also changes occurring in the male's body. Two glands, called the testes, begin to produce sperm. Sperm cells are much smaller than egg cells, and can only be seen under powerful microscopes. Before ejaculation, sperm mix with a white fluid that helps them move and keeps them viable. This fluid is called semen. During sexual intercourse, a male releases sperm into the female's vagina. On average, three hundred million sperm are released each time a male has an ejaculation, or discharge.

Almost every cell in the body contains forty-six chromosomes, which determine all the genetic traits that make us unique. The only exceptions are the sperm and egg cells. Instead of forty-six chromosomes, they only have twenty-three. All female egg cells have an X chromosome. About half of the sperm cells a male produces have an X chromosome. (At this point, have the student with the "Sperm" card containing the X chromosome stand next to the student with the "Egg" card, in close proximity to the area of the female reproductive system diagram where one of the fallopian tubes has been labeled.)

If a sperm with an X chromosome makes its way through the vagina, up into the uterus, and through the fallopian tube, it can combine with the egg in a process called fertilization. The new cell will then contain forty-six chromosomes. It also has two X chromosomes. This means the fertilized egg will develop into a baby girl. (Have the student carrying the "Sperm" card with the X chromosome leave and stand on the side of the room.) If, however, a sperm carrying a Y chromosome fertilizes the egg (have the student with the "Sperm" card carrying the Y chromosome join the egg cell in the fallopian tube), the fertilized egg will now have an XY combination of sex chromosomes, and develop into a baby boy. Because about half of the sperm carry the X chromosome and about half carry the Y chromosome, the odds of having a baby boy or girl are about fifty-fifty.

Occasionally, two eggs will be released from the ovaries. Fraternal twins are formed when two different eggs are fertilized by two different sperm. These two separate babies have no more in common than brothers and sisters born at different times. They may be two boys, two girls, or a boy and a girl, depending on whether the egg was fertilized by a sperm carrying an X chromosome (an XX combination, or a female) or a Y chromosome (an XY combination, or a male).

The Story of Fertilization and Birth (*continued*)

Identical twins occur when a single egg is fertilized by a single sperm and splits into two identical halves. Two separate zygotes are formed and are always the same sex. If a sperm carrying an X chromosome fertilizes the egg, they will be identical twin girls. If a sperm carrying a Y chromosome fertilizes the egg, they will be identical twin boys.

Once the egg is fertilized, it is called a zygote. It travels from the fallopian tube to the wall of the uterus. (Have the student with the "Uterus" card stand in front of the diagram.) The egg attaches itself to the lining of the uterus and begins to grow. After a few weeks, the egg cell starts changing shape, and is now called an embryo. Other structures start to develop, including the placenta on the uterine lining to help supply nutrients and oxygen to the growing embryo through a tube filled with blood vessels called the umbilical cord. A sac of fluid called the amnion or amniotic sac forms, surrounding and protecting the embryo. From about the eighth week until birth, the developing cells are referred to as a fetus. The average length of time from fertilization to birth is about forty weeks, or around nine months.

A pregnant woman must take extra care to maintain good health with exercise, healthy foods. If possible, she should avoid smoking, drinking alcohol, and taking drugs not recommended by her doctor, because these substances may be harmful to the developing baby. Throughout the nine months of her pregnancy, a pregnant woman should also make frequent visits to her gynecologist. This is referred to as prenatal (or "before birth") care. A gynecologist is a doctor who specializes in reproductive health care for women. Most gynecologists are also trained obstetricians. An obstetrician specializes in the delivery of babies.

When the baby is ready to be born, special hormones in the woman's body start to make the uterus contract. These contractions start to push the baby down to the lower end of the uterus and into the vagina, which is also called the birth canal. (At this point, have the student with the "Vagina" card come to the front of the room.) These contractions are like strong cramps through which the mother's body is working to help push the baby out of her body. A term used to explain these contractions is "labor."

The length of time a woman is in labor varies, but it is usually several hours. As the contractions get stronger, the baby is pushed farther down the birth canal. Finally, with one last contraction, the baby is pushed out of the mother's body and is born.

Sometimes babies are born by an operation called a cesarean section. This is a surgical procedure in which a doctor makes an incision through a woman's abdomen and uterus to deliver the baby.

Once the baby starts to breathe for himself or herself, the umbilical cord is clamped and cut. Neither the mother nor the baby feels this. After a few minutes, the placenta starts to dislodge from the wall of the uterus, and is pushed out of the body along with the other end of the umbilical cord. This is called the afterbirth.

Finally, the baby is given some medical tests to ensure he or she is healthy. After a few minutes, the baby is wrapped in a blanket and can be placed into the mother's arms. This ends the story of how a new life comes into the world.

Name: ______________________________

How Life Begins

Directions: Fill in the blanks on the worksheet by using words from the list that follows.

Drugs	Ovary	Canal	Labor	Cesarean
Sperm	Prenatal	Fraternal	Umbilical	Fallopian tube
Gynecologist	Blood	Genes	Diet	Vagina
Identical	Alcohol	Boy	Girl	Obstetrician
Smoke	Ovum	Fetus	Hours	Uterus
Zygote	Placenta	Embryo	Cells	Forty-six

The body is made up of millions of ________________. Almost all of these contain ________________ chromosomes, or the hereditary material that determines your appearance and just about everything else making **you**! Your mother's egg cell, or ________________, contributed twenty-three of these. Your father's ________________ cell also contributed twenty-three of these.

During sexual intercourse, sperm from the male are deposited into the ________________ of the female. If a woman has released an egg from her ________________, the sperm can fertilize it in the ________________.

The fertilized egg starts dividing into a ball of cells called a(n) ________________. This ball of cells travels down the fallopian tube and attaches to the wall of the ________________. From the second to around the eighth week, the ball of cells starts to change shape. It is now called a(n) ________________. From the eighth week until birth, the developing baby is referred to as a ________________. If a sperm with an X chromosome fertilizes the egg, which always has an X chromosome, the developing baby will be a(n) ________________. If a sperm with a Y chromosome fertilizes the egg, the XY combination will produce a baby ________________. Occasionally, two eggs will be released and fertilized by two different sperm. The two babies are born and are

Name: ______________________________

How Life Begins (*continued*)

called _______________ twins. They can be two boys, two girls, or one girl and one boy. _______________ twins form when one egg is fertilized by one sperm and, shortly after fertilization, the egg splits into two equal parts. Because the twins have the same chromosomes and _______________, they will look exactly alike.

While growing in the uterus, the baby gets food and oxygen through the _______________ cord. This cord is connected to the _______________, a special organ attached to the wall of the uterus, absorbing nutrients from the mother's body. Although the mother is feeding the baby and giving oxygen through these two structures, the mother's _______________ never mixes with the baby's _______________ (repeat word).

After about nine months, the uterus will start to contract and push the baby out through the vagina, also referred to as the birth _______________. These contractions are referred to as _______________ and can last for several __________. Sometimes, for various reasons, a baby is not born through the vagina. Doctors then have to perform a special kind of surgery to remove the baby from the uterus. This is called a _______________ section.

When a woman is pregnant, she has to take very good care of herself. Everything she puts into her body can affect her developing baby. She should go for regular checkups to her _______________, a doctor specializing in taking care of women, especially when they are pregnant. Most of the time this doctor also delivers the baby. This special type of doctor is called a(n) _______________.

A pregnant woman should not _______________ or drink _______________. She should not use any other _______________ unless it is under the supervision of her doctor. She should also eat a balanced _______________. _______________ care is very important if a woman wants to have a healthy baby.

Name: ______________________________

Pregnancy and Birth Crossword Puzzle

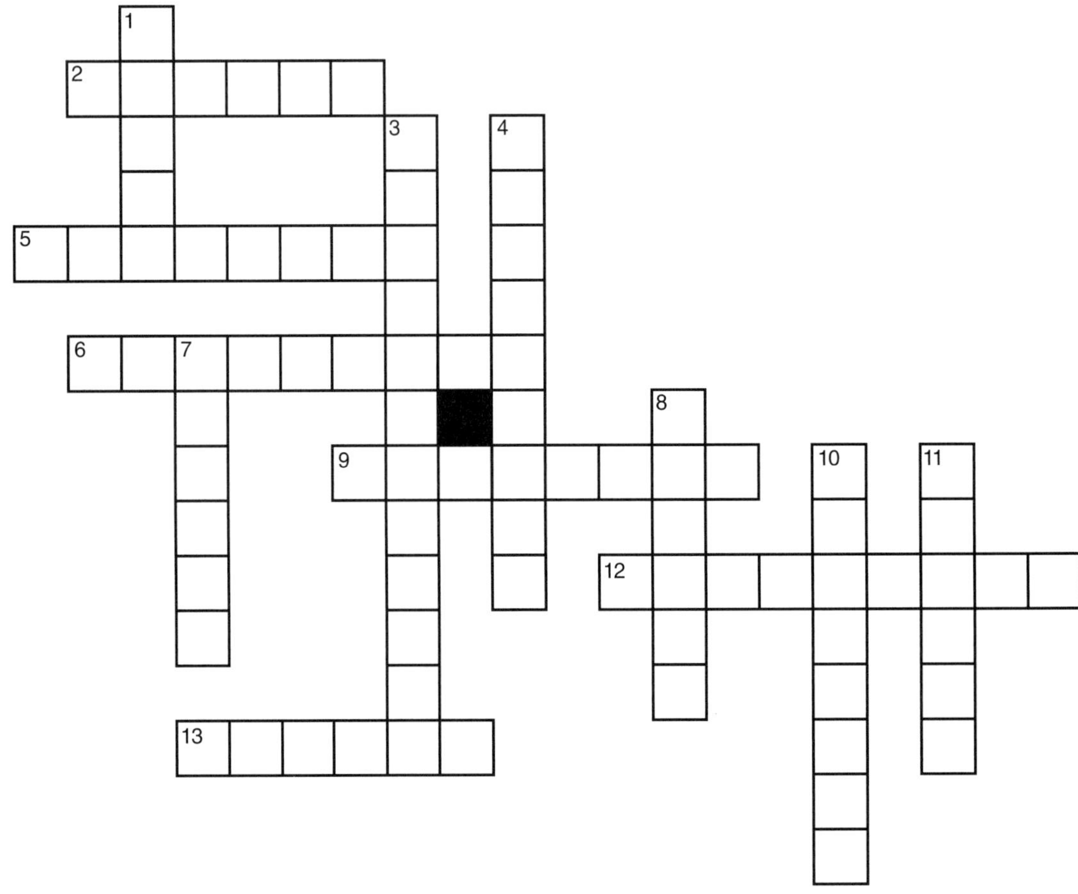

Across

2. Lower end of the uterus
5. ________________ section (surgical delivery of a baby through the abdominal and uterine walls)
6. Twins formed from a combination of one egg and one sperm that "splits" into two separate babies
9. Organ attached to the uterus to nourish the unborn baby
12. Twins formed from two eggs and two different sperm
13. Fertilized egg cell

Down

1. Developing baby from the eighth week until birth
3. Doctor who specializes in the reproductive needs of women
4. Cord serving as a supply line between the mother and the unborn child
7. Growing baby from the second to the eighth week
8. Pear-shaped female reproductive organ
10. Before birth
11. Protective sac of fluid surrounding the fetus

LESSON 2: THE ABSTINENCE PILL

Level: Middle school, High school

Time: 30 minutes

National Health Education Standards

1. Core Concepts
4. Interpersonal Communication

National Sexuality Education Standards: Performance Indicators

- Compare and contrast the advantages and disadvantages of abstinence and other contraceptive methods, including condoms.
- Demonstrate the use of effective communication skills to support one's decision to abstain from sexual behaviors.

Rationale

Young teenagers are generally not mature enough for a sexual relationship that includes intercourse. Sexual abstinence means not engaging in any sexual behavior that could result in a pregnancy or STI, including HIV. In this activity, students will brainstorm the advantages and disadvantages of abstinence. They will then discuss and debate the following statement: "Vows of abstinence break far more often than condoms." Finally, you will reveal what an imaginary "abstinence pill" would look like, including instructions for its use.

Materials and Preparation

Front board

Large, clear, cylindrical container to simulate a prescription bottle

Prescription bottle label (sample included at the end of this lesson). You can modify the label in any appropriate and creative way. Consider the dosage, the frequency of use, the doctor's name, the "have it with you at all times" statement, side effects, and the need to not mix it with alcohol or other drugs.

Plastic egg or other container simulating a pill to be placed into the prescription bottle

Small piece of paper inside the pill that reads "no"

Copies of "Abstinence and Communication Skills: Nat and Brenda" homework

Procedure

1. Begin the lesson by asking students to define the word "abstinence." After some discussion, have students copy a definition into their notebook (as it is displayed on the front board). Although there is much debate about what sexual abstinence actually is, a generally accepted definition might be as follows:

   Sexual abstinence—choosing not to participate in any type of sexual activity, including vaginal, anal, or oral sex.

2. Write the following quote on the board: "Vows of abstinence break far more often than condoms."
3. To encourage students to discuss the quote, ask the following questions:
    a. How effective or realistic is it to discuss abstinence with adolescents?
    b. Should abstinence be a mandatory part of a sexual health unit?
    c. How many of you have discussed abstinence with a parent or guardian? With friends? In school? In religious instruction? What messages have you heard about abstinence?
    d. What kinds of things do people abstain from? (Food, voting, alcohol, drugs, sex . . .)
    e. Why do they abstain? (To protect health, to avoid making a decision, to avoid negative consequences, because of religious beliefs . . .)
4. Next, inform the class that they will brainstorm the advantages and disadvantages of abstinence.
5. On the front board (or newsprint), write the word "abstinence" in large letters. Draw a line down the center of the paper. To complete the left side of the chart, have students brainstorm the *advantages* of abstinence. To complete the right side, ask the class to brainstorm the *disadvantages* of abstinence.

    Some suggested answers are as follows:

ADVANTAGES	DISADVANTAGES
Abstinence lessens chances of pregnancy. It may be in line with family or personal values. It is a good way to get to know your boyfriend or girlfriend without the complications of sex. It allows you to focus on school, sports, or other interests.	Abstinence may be viewed as unnatural or unrealistic in the eyes of some teens and young adults. You may feel confused about media messages portraying sex as the norm.

6. Conclude this brainstorm with a class discussion. Stress that although sexual feelings are normal and natural, most young teenagers are not mature enough for a sexual relationship that includes intercourse. There are many ways that teenagers in romantic relationships can express their feelings without engaging in sexual intercourse. Delaying sex until they are older and more mature is the most responsible, healthy choice.
7. Show the model of the abstinence pill. State, "It is difficult to talk about something you cannot see, so I decided to invent an abstinence pill. Let me read the directions on the label." Then begin to read the text on the label, allowing students time to process what you are reading.

8. Open up the bottle and take out the pill. Say, "As you can see, for a lot of people, this abstinence pill is going to be difficult to swallow." Allow students to make any comments.
9. Now open up the pill, take out the only ingredient (the small piece of paper), and read the word "no."
10. Ask students the processing questions. Make sure to stress to students that abstinence does not have to mean a lack of love, intimacy, romance, sensuality, or fun.
11. Distribute copies of the "Abstinence and Communication Skills: Nat and Brenda" homework. Assign and explain the homework assignment due at the next session.

Processing

1. What are your thoughts on the abstinence pill?
2. When would people decide to "go off" the abstinence pill? At a certain age? When they find the right partner? When they get married? When they find another method that works for them?
3. How easy is it for someone to say "no" to a person he or she cares about or is attracted to?
4. How might a relationship be affected if one of the partners continues to put pressure on the other to have unwanted sex?
5. What are some ways a person can express physical attraction to or feelings for another person without having sex?

Assessment

- Students participate in the discussion of the quote and the advantages and disadvantages of abstinence.
- Students complete the homework assignment.

Sample Abstinence Pill Label

Abstinence Pill

Rx (Number One Way to Protect Yourself)

Dosage: One pill, as often as needed. Make sure you have it with you at all times, especially when on a date, at a club, or whenever the "urge to merge" hits you.

Side effects: Occasionally may make you feel "left out." Positive side effects include enhanced self-image and not having to worry about pregnancy or STIs. It is estimated that 50 percent of high school students take the abstinence pill with very few negative side effects.

Caution: Do not mix with alcohol or other drugs.

Dr. Al Waysbesafe 1-888-555-SAFE

For refill or other medication questions, call 1-888-555-SAFE.

Name: ______________________________

Abstinence and Communication Skills: Nat and Brenda

Scenario: Nat and Brenda are freshmen in high school. They are at Brenda's house, and her parents are gone for the evening. Brenda is pressuring Nat to have sex. Nat is a virgin and made a pledge at an assembly program in middle school that he will remain abstinent until marriage.

Directions: Write a **conversation** between Brenda and Nat. In that dialogue, Nat should give at least two reasons why abstaining from sex is a healthy choice for him. He should also use at least two refusal or assertive communication skills to effectively get his message across to Brenda. Brenda will start the conversation.

Brenda: Nat, I think we are ready to take our physical relationship to the next level.

Nat: ____

____

____

Brenda: ____

____

____

Nat: ____

____

____

Brenda: ____

____

____

Nat: ____

____

____

Brenda: ____

____

____

Nat: ____

____

____

LESSON 3: PARENTING PEOPLE SEARCH IDEAL PARENTS

Level: High school

Time: 40 minutes

National Health Education Standard

2. Analyzing Influences

National Sexuality Education Standards: Performance Indicator

- Analyze factors that influence decisions about whether and when to become a parent.

Rationale

Raising children is an enormous responsibility, and being a teenage parent can be extremely difficult. Although there is no such thing as an "ideal parent," effective parents share many common traits and qualities. In this session, students will conduct a parenting people search and discuss these traits and qualities. Students will then list and rank healthy parenting indicators by identifying conditions necessary to promote a child's health, safety, and positive development.

Materials and Preparation

Copies of "Parenting People Search" worksheet

Copies of "Qualities of Ideal Parents" worksheet

Front board

Procedure

ACTIVITY 1: PARENTING PEOPLE SEARCH

1. Explain that the goal of the day's lesson is to discuss what it means to be a good parent.
2. Distribute the "Parenting People Search" worksheet to all students. Read the directions to make sure that students understand the rules of the game. Inform the class that when the first person to fill all twelve boxes yells "Bingo," the game is over and students should return to their seat.
3. Begin the game. After four minutes, if no one has completed all twelve boxes, say "Time is up," and ask students to return to their seat.
4. Ask the person who yelled "Bingo" to come to the front of the room. If no one filled all twelve boxes, ask for someone who got eleven signed names to stand at the front of the room. (If there is a tie, have both students come to the front of the room and alternate reviewing their sheet.)
5. Ask the student at the front of the room to name the person who signed each box, starting with the top box on the left-hand side. The person who signed the first box should be able to answer the question or give his opinion related to that question, and so on.

6. Continue going through each of the boxes, asking students who have signed their names in the various boxes to provide their answer and opinion. Often this will spark a response from additional students and a brief discussion by other class members, who may state a different opinion or add information. You should encourage and facilitate such discussion.
7. When all boxes have been discussed, exclaim that the person whose sheet was read is the winner! A small prize, like extra credit points or a homework pass, may be offered.

ACTIVITY 2: QUALITIES OF IDEAL PARENTS

1. Distribute the "Qualities of Ideal Parents" worksheet and read the directions. Allow five minutes for students to complete their individual rankings.
2. Pair off students. Ask students to share and discuss their top five answers on their list with their partner. They should try to come to some agreement on two items they both consider to be very important.
3. Reconvene as a large group. Ask pairs of students to share their top two qualities. Make a list on the front board of the items mentioned, noting which are given most often.
4. Ask the processing questions.
5. Bring closure to the lesson by stating that parenting is one of the most important jobs people can have in their lives. Being an effective parent requires a lot of skill and patience.
6. At the conclusion of the lesson, allow a few minutes to have students write a reflection statement of at least a few paragraphs based on the day's discussion. Instruct them to analyze two important factors that would influence someone's decision about whether and when to become a parent. As students complete this, you can walk around the room and, without reading them, make sure that entries have been made in student journals. If time allows, students can also volunteer to read their reflection statement aloud to the class, or they can choose to keep their journal entry private.

Processing

1. Why are your "top" qualities important?
2. How can the qualities listed on the worksheet improve the health and well-being of children?
3. How many of you think you might want to be a parent someday? Why or why not?
4. What type of parent will you be?

Assessment

- Students participate in the parenting people search and discussion.
- Students complete the "Qualities of Ideal Parents" worksheet and participate in the follow-up discussion.
- Students each write a reflection in their journal.

Name: ______________________________

Parenting People Search

Directions: You are going to get to know more about the people in this room by completing a people search. You have four minutes to walk around the room with this paper and a pen or pencil to find others who "fit" with the statements in the boxes. When you find someone, have that person **print** his or her name in that box. No person may sign your sheet more than twice. You are allowed to sign one box on your own sheet. Your objective is to get all boxes filled in with a name. If you get all twelve boxes filled in before the four minutes are up, yell "Bingo!"

Note: Do not sign your name if you cannot honestly answer the question!

Find Someone Who . . .

1. Knows one thing a pregnant woman should **not** do	7. Was brought to a babysitter or to day care so both parents or guardians could work
2. Would consider adopting a child	8. Has watched at least one episode of *Teen Mom* or *16 and Pregnant*
3. Thinks his or her parents have done a good job raising him or her	9. Knows what to do if a baby swallows poison
4. Has changed a messy diaper	10. Thinks most teenagers are not mature enough to be good parents
5. Lives with only one parent or guardian	11. Thinks teens should have a curfew for school nights, weekends, and special occasions
6. Thinks he or she knows approximately what percentage of teen marriages end in divorce	12. Thinks he or she will be a good parent someday

Name: ______________________________

Qualities of Ideal Parents

Directions: Following is a sample list of characteristics and qualities of the "ideal parent." Look over the list and choose five you feel are most important. When you have your five qualities, list them in order of importance on the lines that follow. (Rank them from 1 to 5, with 1 being most important.) If there are some important qualities or characteristics you feel are missing, add them to your list.

Ideal parents . . .

- Are easy to talk to (talking *to* you, not *at* you)
- Are understanding, yet firm
- Encourage you to do your best, but do not put too much pressure on you
- Are involved in your life, but do not try to control your life
- Are loving and caring
- Are good role models
- Provide you with necessities (food, shelter, "brand-new red sports car"!!)
- Are not too strict, but not too easy either
- Are not too nosy and respect your privacy
- Build up your self-image
- Are patient
- Have a sense of humor and are fun to be with
- Do not "baby" you or embarrass you in front of your friends
- Do not compare you to siblings, relatives, and friends
- Are pretty cool (not "totally out of it")
- Are not afraid to say "no" sometimes
- Do not assume things or jump to conclusions
- Are willing to compromise
- Are always there for you and give you a sense of security
- Spend time with you
- Other: ______________________________
- Other: ______________________________

My List of Characteristics of Ideal Parents

1. ______________________________
2. ______________________________
3. ______________________________
4. ______________________________
5. ______________________________

LESSON 4: ARE YOU PREPARED FOR PARENTHOOD?

Level: Middle school, High school

Time: 45 minutes

National Health Education Standard

2. Analyzing Influences

National Sexuality Education Standards: Performance Indicator

- Analyze factors that influence decisions about whether and when to become a parent.

Rationale

Each year in the United States, a number of teenagers become parents. Many of them are unprepared when it comes to having the important skills necessary to be a responsible parent. This lesson will identify and discuss the qualities of effective parenting and define the terms "parent," "parenting," and "family." Concepts to be raised include the physical, mental, emotional, and social needs of a child. Students will also analyze how having a baby as a teen can affect present and future goals.

Materials and Preparation

Front board, with the following written down:

GROUP 1	GROUP 2	GROUP 3	GROUP 4
Daily Routine and Free Time	Friends and Social Life	Finances	Education and Career
Male + Changes – Changes *Female* + Changes – Changes	*Male* + Changes – Changes *Female* + Changes – Changes	*Male* + Changes – Changes *Female* + Changes – Changes	*Male* + Changes – Changes *Female* + Changes – Changes

Four sheets of newsprint and four markers

Masking tape

Copies of "Parenting" worksheet

Fourteen index cards, each with a parental responsibility written in large print. Examples include responsibilities from the following four categories:

Physical: Nutritious food, medical care, clothing, shelter, protection

Mental: Solving problems, making decisions, stimulating thinking, providing education

Emotional: Love, empathy, values, traditions, self-respect

Social: Having a caring provider for basic needs, having someone spending time with him or her

Box or other type of container labeled "Parenting Contract," placed at the front of the room, to hold the parental responsibility cards

Procedure

ACTIVITY 1: PARENTHOOD—HOW IT CAN CHANGE YOUR LIFE

1. Divide the class into four mixed-sex groups. Give each group a sheet of newsprint and a marker, and assign them each a number from 1 through 4. Have the groups each write one of the four columns from the board on the newsprint, based on their group number.
2. Instruct the groups to make lists of how having a baby as a teenager would affect a person's life. Specifically, they are to write how this would affect the male and female and their (1) daily routine and free time; (2) friends and social life; (3) finances; or (4) education and career (depending on their group number). For example, having a baby would limit the amount of time a female teenager can spend with her friends.

   One person should be designated as the recorder, and another person should be the spokesperson for the group. Allow approximately six to eight minutes for groups to complete their chart.
3. When lists are completed, have the spokesperson for Group 1 come to the front of the room and tape the completed newsprint to the front board for the class to see. The spokesperson should review all the ways having a baby would affect the daily routines and free time of a typical male teenager and female teenager.
4. Follow the same procedure with Groups 2, 3, and 4, allowing each to discuss their given topic.
5. Conclude this activity by asking processing questions 1 through 9.

ACTIVITY 2: PARENTING CONTRACT

1. Distribute the "Parenting" worksheet and lead a discussion on the definitions of the provided terms. After student input, the following definitions should be written on the board, and students should copy them down on their worksheet:

   Parent—a father or mother of a child; may or may not be biologically related

   Parenting—meeting a child's PHYSICAL, MENTAL, EMOTIONAL, and SOCIAL needs

   Family—a group of two or more persons who are related by birth, marriage, or adoption, and may or may not live together

2. Discuss the qualities of a strong family, as outlined on the worksheet. Discussion should center on students' comparing the characteristics of the ideal family with those of their own family.
3. At this point, explain to students that they are going to discuss what the physical, mental, emotional, and social needs of children actually are by playing a brief matching game. Write down the following four column headings on the board in large letters: "Physical Needs," "Mental Needs," "Emotional Needs," and "Social Needs."
4. Explain that it is easy to become a mother or father, but that unfortunately it is *not* so easy to be a good parent. Although they do not need a license or have to sign a contract, by having children, parents take on very big responsibilities when they bring their baby home from the hospital. Explain the next activity:

   What I have at the front of the room is a box labeled "Parenting Contract." Inside the box are many of the responsibilities involved in being a responsible parent written on cards. What I would like is for volunteers to come up, pull out one of the cards with a parental responsibility written on it, and decide whether it meets a child's *physical needs, mental needs, emotional needs,* or *social needs.* You will then use a piece of masking tape to place that card under one of the columns. If the class agrees, all students should write that term under the appropriate column on their worksheet.

5. After all cards have been assigned to the appropriate category, ask processing questions 10 through 13.

Processing

1. If you were a teen parent, would you miss your free time and privacy?
2. Would you be willing to cut back on your social life to spend more time helping take care of a baby?
3. Do you think you could afford to support a child?
4. What kinds of expenses are involved in having and providing for a new baby? Where would you get the money? Would it be difficult to manage a child and a job at the same time?
5. How would having a child change your plans for your education or your plans for the future? Do you think you would try to continue to finish high school? What about any plans you may have had for college?

6. How would your parents or guardians feel about your being a new parent? Supportive or not? Would they be willing to give their time or money to help you out?
7. What are some differences in how having a baby would have an impact on a teenage girl's life or a teenage boy's life? Is one sex affected more than the other?
8. There have been documentaries and reality shows on TV depicting the lives of teens in this situation. What are some common problems these girls (and couples) face?
9. How many of you think you would like to be a parent someday? Do any of you feel you are ready to be a parent at this point in your life? Why or why not?
10. Where have you seen examples of teenage parents?
11. Do the messages in songs, in movies, on the Internet, or on TV influence teens? Explain.
12. What types of families are on TV? Single-parent families? Same-sex couples with children? Extended families?
13. Name some TV shows centering on families. Are these families typical? Realistic? Do they portray positive or negative role models?

Assessment

- Groups complete their respective charts.
- Students participate in the parenting contract activity, correctly identifying and categorizing a child's needs.

Name: ______________________________

Parenting

Definitions

Parent: ____

____

Parenting: ____

____

Family: ____

____

Qualities of a Strong Family

- **Commitment.** Members are committed to one another, promote each other's welfare, and work to make each other happy.

- **Appreciation.** Family members make one another feel good about themselves. They find good qualities in one another and express appreciation for them.

- **Good communication.** All family members spend time talking and listening to each other.

- **Enjoyment of time spent with each other.** Family members spend quality time together.

- **Strong value system.** Family members believe in something, and those beliefs are understood and supported by all family members.

- **Ability to deal with crisis and stress in a positive manner.** Strong families are good at solving problems; they unite in a crisis—it does not divide them.

People who become parents must fulfill a large number of responsibilities. A responsibility is a duty or an obligation that is expected of you. If parents were to sign a "contract," it would require them to meet the physical, mental, emotional, and social needs of their children, as outlined on the following "Parenting Contract."

Parenting Contract

"If I become a parent someday, I agree to provide the following for my child(ren)":

Physical Needs	Mental Needs	Emotional Needs	Social Needs

LESSON 5: THE PREGNANCY GAME

Level: Middle school, High school

Time: 45 minutes

National Health Education Standards

1. Core Concepts
3. Accessing Information
4. Interpersonal Communication

National Sexuality Education Standards: Performance Indicators

- Compare and contrast the advantages and disadvantages of abstinence and other contraceptive methods, including condoms.
- Define emergency contraception and describe its mechanism of action.
- Identify medically-accurate information about contraceptive methods, including emergency contraception and condoms.

Rationale

In this activity, students will be involved in a simulation exercise in which they imagine what it would be like to get pregnant or to get someone else pregnant while still in high school. Follow-up discussion will focus on analyzing the internal and external influences on decisions about pregnancy options.

Note: Discussion about preventing teen pregnancy is certainly appropriate in a human sexuality class. It is important to keep in mind, however, that there may be some students who have previously dealt or are currently dealing with this very issue. Every effort should be made to be sensitive, and you must remind the class about general rules for classroom discussion. No put-downs, listening respectfully to everyone's opinions, and the right to "pass" are especially important, and should be strictly enforced. Students should also be reminded that there are many resources available in the school and community to confidentially assist them with any concerns or issues they may have in regard to this topic.

Materials and Preparation

Front board or newsprint and markers

Two different colors of wrapped candies (for example, Andes candies, or Hershey's Kisses with and without almonds) in a ratio of four to one. In a class of twenty-five, for example, you will need twenty green (chocolate mint) and five red (chocolate cherry) Andes candies or twenty plain Hershey's Kisses wrapped in silver and five Hershey's Kisses with almonds wrapped in gold. (*Note:* Be cautious about students with allergies.)

Paper bag, to be filled with candy

Six index cards with questions for discussion, numbered 1 through 6

Copies of "Creating a Persuasive Essay" homework

Procedure

1. Begin the class by writing "Unplanned Teen Pregnancy" on the front board (or newsprint).
2. Instruct students to think about words or phrases that come to mind when they hear this term. Ask student volunteers to share with the class some of the words or phrases they associate with the term. Compile this list on the board.
3. Ask students how many of the items on the list have a *negative* connotation. Then ask about *positive* connotations. Typically there will be many more negative terms or phrases in response to the term "unplanned teen pregnancy" than there are positive. If a term has a negative connotation, place a minus sign next to it on the board. If a term has a positive connotation, place a plus sign next to it.
4. Summarize by saying that for most teens an unplanned pregnancy means a time of confusion, fear, and mixed emotions on the part of both partners involved.
5. Inform the class that to come to understand this point better, they will play the Pregnancy Game. Reinforce the idea that the most common reason teens give for not using contraception is "they did not plan on having sex." Then say something like the following: "In this bag are candies wrapped in two different colors of wrappers. One in five is red. If you pick a green candy, it means you are not pregnant or did not get anyone pregnant. But if you pick a red candy, you are pregnant, or, if you are a male, got a female pregnant."
6. Make sure students do not peek into the bag when they reach in to pick a candy. When all students have picked, have those students who "got pregnant" or "got someone pregnant" bring their chair to the front of the room and sit in a line as if on a panel.
7. At this point, distribute the index cards randomly to members of the class. Explain that those students who are up at the front of the room are to imagine that they have actually gotten pregnant or gotten someone pregnant at this point in their lives. They are to answer the questions based on their own personal goals, attitudes, and values. For some of the questions, students can "make up" answers, responding as if they were a pregnant teen or the partner of a pregnant teen. The "audience" is to ask the questions written on the cards.
8. Have the person with the first question read the card aloud. Ask people on the panel to answer as best they can, imagining this situation has actually happened to them. They may pass if they choose to.
9. After all panelists have expressed their opinion on the first question, open up discussion to the entire class. Then proceed to the next question. When all panelists have been asked all of the questions, thank the panel and have them return to their seat.
10. Ask students to raise their hand if they know of a teenager who either became pregnant or got someone pregnant. Ask for volunteers who are willing to share, without revealing names, what that individual decided to do and how it worked out. Stress the point that entering into a sexual relationship brings with it lots of responsibilities. Too often, teens enter into sexual relationships before they have really thought about

the possible consequences of their actions. Abstinence, or delaying having sex until an older age, is a responsible decision for most teens. Having sex is not a sign of maturity. Understanding the possible consequences of having sex and taking precautions to make sex safer *is* a sign of maturity.

11. Conclude by asking the processing questions and assigning the "Creating a Persuasive Essay" homework.

Processing

1. How realistic was today's activity?
2. "We weren't planning on having sex. One thing led to another, and it just kind of happened." This is a common explanation teens give when they are faced with an unplanned pregnancy. How can partners communicate more effectively about contraception, including abstinence and condoms?
3. How comfortable would you be talking to a parent or guardian about contraception? How comfortable do you think your parents or guardians would be discussing this topic?
4. What local resources are available in your community for teens to access medically-accurate sources of pregnancy-related information, counseling, and support?

Assessment

- Students participate in the Pregnancy Game simulation and discussion.
- Students complete the "Creating a Persuasive Essay" homework assignment.

Possible Questions for Index Cards

Index Card 1

How did each of you feel when you picked the candy that meant you were pregnant or had gotten someone pregnant? What thought or emotion came to your mind first?

Index Card 2

How long had you been going out with the mother or father? Did you use protection? Why or why not?

Index Card 3

If this really happened to you, whom would you tell? (No one? The male involved, if you are a female? A best friend? Your parents or guardians? A counselor? Someone else?) If you told your parents or guardians, how would they take the news? Are there any girls who would not tell the boy involved? Why or why not?

Index Card 4

Would you be happy that this happened to you? Do you think that some teenagers are happy when they find out they are pregnant or their girlfriend is pregnant?

Index Card 5

The three options available to most teenagers in this situation are

1. Have the baby and keep it
2. Have the baby and give it up for adoption
3. Have an abortion

What internal factors (personal experiences, values) or external factors (peers, family, religion, the media) might play a significant role when you are choosing among your options? How can teenagers best make this decision?

Index Card 6

Emergency contraception prevents pregnancy after having unprotected sex. The most common form of emergency contraception is called Plan B, which consists of two pills containing a synthetic hormone, progestin. These are taken within five days of unprotected intercourse, but it is best to take them as soon as possible. They work by keeping a woman's ovaries from releasing an egg for longer than usual. If there is no egg to join with the sperm, pregnancy cannot occur. Federal law says that emergency contraception can be bought over the counter.

How do you feel about emergency contraception? Is it something you would consider? Why or why not?

Creating a Persuasive Essay

Directions: "Teen pregnancy is a serious problem in the United States." Please respond to this statement according to the following guidelines:

1. You will have one week to write a persuasive essay in response to the provided statement. The target audience for your essay will be high school students.
2. You must research your topic. To back up your rationale for your argument, you should use the trusted sites listed after these directions to access accurate, up-to-date information related to teen pregnancy. A minimum of ten facts or statistics should be gathered, and you should cite the websites from which you obtained them.
3. Your essay should have an introduction, body, and conclusion.
4. The introduction should clearly state the problem and explain why it is worth discussing.
5. In the body of your essay, you should use the facts gathered from the websites to make your argument. Statistical data, facts, and real-life examples will help make your essay convincing.
6. You must highlight at least two ways teens can eliminate or reduce the risk of becoming teen parents.
7. In your conclusion, please restate your main thesis and the strongest point or points made in your essay.
8. Your essay will be evaluated on how well you access information and how it was used to present a convincing argument to your peers.

Reliable Internet Resources

www.cdc.gov/HealthyYouth/yrbs/index.htm
www.advocatesforyouth.org
www.SEICUS.org
www.thenationalcampaign.org
www.guttmacher.org

LESSON 6: EIGHT WEEKS

Level: Middle school, High school

Time: 40–50 minutes

National Health Education Standards

1. Core Concepts
2. Analyzing Influences
5. Decision-Making

National Sexuality Education Standards: Performance Indicators

- Analyze factors that influence decisions about whether and when to become a parent.
- Apply a decision-making model to various sexual health decisions.

Rationale

Thousands of teenagers are faced each year with a decision about an unplanned pregnancy. The couple involved must make an informed choice while considering their state laws and options, as well as their personal feelings and values.

By reading the provided scenario, teenage males and females will gain a better understanding of how an unplanned pregnancy would affect their lives. Students will practice working through the decision-making model in relation to the scenario, noting that the different possible choices have various consequences involved. At the end of the lesson, students should be able to verbalize their final decision about what they believe the couple in this particular scenario should do.

Materials and Preparation

Copies of "Eight Weeks" handout

Copies of "Decision-Making Model" worksheet

Procedure

1. Introduce the lesson by asking the class how many have seen the TV shows *Teen Mom* or *16 and Pregnant*. Ask the class what messages these shows provide. Do they glamorize teen pregnancies, or do they have the opposite effect?
2. After some discussion, distribute the "Eight Weeks" handout to each student. Ask students to read the scenario quietly by themselves.
3. When students have finished reading the scenario, hand out the "Decision-Making Model" worksheet. Briefly review the steps on the worksheet as a class.
4. Students should then fill in their worksheet, completing the steps in the decision-making process for the situation described in the scenario. Allow approximately eight to ten minutes for this task.

5. When students each have completed their worksheet, ask for volunteers to share what they felt the best decision would be. Encourage a wide range of thoughts and feelings. Be cognizant of the fact that the "pro-choice versus pro-life" debate is a delicate issue. Students have the right to their individual opinions, and each should be respected. Also, students who wish to keep their decisions to themselves should not have to share them.

   Note: Students who are not involved in verbalizing their personal opinions can still participate by actively listening to the class discussion.
6. Conclude the activity by asking the processing questions.

Processing

1. How easily did you come up with your final decision?
2. What factors helped you make a final decision?
3. What factors did not help you make a final decision?
4. If a friend confided in you that he or she were in this situation, what would you say or do?

Assessment

- Students complete the "Decision-Making Model" worksheet.
- Students participate in the follow-up discussion about their personal opinions and values in regard to pregnancy options.

Eight Weeks

Directions: Read the following scenario. After reading the story, answer the questions on the "Decision-Making Model" worksheet as best as you can, using the decision-making process to decide on what you believe each of the main characters in the story should do.

In the back of her mind, seventeen-year-old Christy Richards knew what the test result was going to be, but she was hoping it was a false alarm. When she saw the doctor at the clinic, she found out for sure . . . she was eight weeks' pregnant!

Her first indication was that she had missed her period. This did not necessarily mean anything—a lot of teenage girls are irregular and occasionally miss a period—but not her. She had always been like clockwork, ever since the seventh grade. Every twenty-eight days she would get it. She knew when it was coming, how long she would have it . . . she even thought she knew when she ovulated. Every month around the middle of her cycle, she just felt different. She could not explain how, but she did.

She knew abstinence was the only 100 percent safe way to avoid pregnancy and STIs. She thought she would remain a virgin at least until she graduated from high school. But then she met Jim. They started out as friends, then started dating and getting more serious. They never planned on having sex. But, well, you know how it is. Her parents were gone for the evening . . . Jim came over to watch TV . . . they started making out on the couch. . . One thing led to another, and it just happened!

Eight weeks ago. The longest eight weeks of her life. Because "it just happened," they did not use a condom. She was a little worried at first, but figured that because they had only done it once, the odds were in her favor. Looking back on it now, though, she felt stupid. They both had taken health class in school and learned that the "guess" method was not reliable. She even remembered her health teacher trying to emphasize that there are "at least three hundred million sperm all looking for that one egg!"

She worried some more when she was late with her period that month. When it never came, she started to think about it all the time. Oh, how she wished she could take back that night. Since that night eight weeks ago, whenever she and Jim were alone, she pretended everything was okay. They would kiss and make out and stuff, but she would stop things before they went too far. Jim was starting to get frustrated and felt that if they really liked each other and were responsible, sex would make their relationship stronger. He told her he would use a condom, but she would remind him that condoms did not always work and she did not want to take a chance. He also said that they had already had sex once . . . so "What was the big deal?"

(continued)

Eight Weeks (*continued*)

Now Christy has to deal with a situation that she thought only happened to "other people." Now she *is* one of those "other people" and is worried sick about it.

She remembers when her married twenty-four-year-old sister, Carmen, found out she and her husband were going to be parents. Carmen was so happy! She could not wait to tell everyone. Society seems to be pleased with and proud of young married women who get pregnant, yet seems to turn its back on unmarried pregnant girls. Views may have liberalized somewhat since Christy's parents were teenagers. There are even shows on TV about pregnant teens and teen moms. But for Christy, being seventeen and pregnant is certainly not going to make her mom and dad happy.

Christy has been so worried lately, she has not been much fun to be around. She and Jim have been arguing a lot over the last few weeks. She did not want to say anything to him until she was sure. And now she cannot hide her resentment toward him—she is angry that he did not take any precautions against getting her pregnant.

She remembers that night so clearly now. Why didn't she stop him? Why didn't she say "no"? They were just fooling around, having fun. Well, life is not much fun for her right now. She has got to make a decision—a decision that will affect the rest of her life.

She decided to confide in her sister, Carmen. The first question Carmen asked was: "How do you feel about Jim right now?" When Christy told her of her resentment, Carmen said Jim would probably feel the same way toward *her*! "It takes two, you know," she said.

After talking with Carmen, Christy drove over to Jim's house to tell him that she is pregnant. Jim was not too happy about the news. He stormed around the living room, saying, "You gotta be kidding!" But of course she was not. The test she took at the clinic only confirmed the home pregnancy test she'd taken a week earlier. No doubt about it—she is eight weeks' pregnant.

Name: ______________________________

Decision-Making Model

Directions: Work through the steps in the decision-making process that follows. Put yourself in this couple's position, and answer based on your attitudes, beliefs, and values. If you are comfortable doing so, you will be encouraged (but not required) to share your final decision with classmates and to justify it.

Step A: State the decision to be made.

____

Step B: List possible options.

1. ____

2. ____

3. ____

Step C: List one positive and one negative consequence for each option.

Option 1	Option 2	Option 3
+	+	+
–	–	–

(*continued*)

Name: ______________________

Decision-Making Model (*continued*)

Step D: Gather information.

1. If I were in this situation, I would seek advice from ______________________

   because ______________________

   ____

2. The state and local laws I need to be aware of are ______________________

   ____

3. Being in this situation would effect on my short- and long-term goals by

   ____

   ____

4. My family, religious, and personal values are ______________________

   ____

   ____

Step E: Based on the information just gathered, make a decision.

1. If I were in this situation, I would decide to ______________________

   because ______________________

2. The two biggest factors in my decision are

   a. ______________________

   ____

   ____

   b. ______________________

   ____

   ____

LESSON 7: SEX—WHAT ARE TEENS *REALLY* DOING?

ASSESSING CURRENT STUDENT KNOWLEDGE, BELIEFS, AND ATTITUDES ABOUT TEENS AND SEX

Level: Middle school

Time: 40 minutes

National Health Education Standards

1. Core Concepts
3. Accessing Information

National Sexuality Education Standards: Performance Indicators

- Define sexual abstinence as it relates to pregnancy prevention.
- Identify medically-accurate resources about pregnancy prevention and reproductive health care.

Rationale

Current research suggests that when students believe *most* or *almost all* of their peers are engaging in a *risky* behavior, they are more likely to engage in the behavior themselves. Conversely, when students believe that they are in the majority with respect to positive health beliefs, attitudes, and behaviors, they will continue to act in those health-enhancing ways.

Very often, however, adolescents overestimate the norm (for example, "All teenagers are having sex") or underestimate the norm ("Just about all teens use condoms when they have sex"). The reality is that only about half of high school students have had sex, and only about 60 percent used a condom during their last act of intercourse.

In this lesson, students will predict and evaluate data from the most recent Youth Risk Behavior Survey (YRBS) from the Centers for Disease Control and Prevention (CDC). They will first complete a questionnaire in pairs or triads without seeing the actual data. Then each group of students will use the Internet to access information to fact-check their responses.

Materials and Preparation

Copies of "Sex: What Are Teens *Really* Doing?" worksheet

Several computers or student personal mobile devices with Internet access

Procedure

1. Put students in pairs or triads, depending on the size of the class and the number of available computers (or personal mobile devices).
2. Hand out the "Sex: What Are Teens *Really* Doing?" worksheet.

Note: The answers to this particular questionnaire have not been given because statistics change all the time. The main objective of the activity is for students to guess what the answers are and then to find out the correct answers *themselves* by accessing the YRBS website. The YRBS is administered every two years. You should visit the YRBS website regularly to update and create new questions relevant to your student population.

3. Explain that the pairs or triads will have approximately five minutes to predict what the correct answers are to the eight-question survey. Students are *not* to use any Internet-enabled device to assist them in answering the questions. They should discuss the questions with their partner or partners, but should record their own answers on their individual worksheet.
4. When the time is up, tell students that they can now use the Internet to check for the correct answers to the survey. Explain that the questions on this worksheet are based on the results of the latest Youth Risk Behavior Survey, conducted every two years by the CDC. The survey's data consist of actual anonymous and random responses from teenagers all over the country.
5. Instruct students to turn on the computer and go on the Internet. Students will still be working in the pairs or triads that were formed earlier.
6. Direct students to the YRBS website, www.cdc.gov/nccdphp/dash/yrbs, and give the following directions for navigating it:
   a. On the left side of the home page, click on "Sexual Risk Behavior."
   b. On the next page, click on "Data and Statistics." You will be researching national statistics (U.S. data).
   c. On the next page, under "Select Sexual Risk Behavior," scroll down to "Ever had sexual intercourse." By navigating through this page, the correct answers to the first five questions should be found.
   d. Click on the "back" button. Go to the drop-down menu. By scrolling down the various menu items, the correct answers for the remaining statements should be found.
7. As students are researching their answers, circulate throughout the room to assist them. Allow approximately ten minutes for pairs or triads to access the information and self-correct their own answers.
8. After they have found all eight answers, ask students to count the number of answers they answered correctly and put that number at the top of their worksheet.
9. Facilitate a class discussion by asking the processing questions.
10. As an additional follow-up assignment, students may choose from any of the individual or group projects listed here. Instructors may develop their own rubrics to assess student work.

Individual and Group Projects

- Individually or in groups, students can create a product (a poster, game, video, or brochure) or give a presentation (a PowerPoint, public service announcement, demonstration, puppet show, or role-play) to encourage students to engage in healthy behaviors. Results from the YRBS should be incorporated into the product or presentation.
- Small groups of students can create products or performances related to the results of the YRBS statistics on teens and sexual health. Each product or performance

should incorporate facts and statistics and demonstrate one or more health skills—for example: (1) students can illustrate goal-setting skills by developing a plan to attain a personal goal, and they can then identify ways in which an unplanned pregnancy can have an impact on short- and long-term goals; (2) students can address communication and refusal skills, including being able to assertively say "no" to unwanted sex; and (3) students can show advocacy by writing letters to administrators, board of education members, and legislators, advocating for more instruction in health class related to comprehensive human sexuality education.

Processing

1. Many teens tend to overestimate the percentages of students who engage in sexual behaviors. Why do you think this is so?
2. On which specific questions did you overestimate the amount of sexual activity teens were involved in?
3. Why do you think it is common for teens to believe a higher percentage of students engage in sex or risky sexual behaviors than is actually the case? (Answers may include peer influences; the idea that "everybody is doing it"; media messages that make it seem like everyone is drinking, smoking, and having unprotected sex; and thinking it is cool to do.)
4. What are some of the internal or external influences affecting the decisions you make about your sexual health? (Answers may include self-esteem; goals for the future; the fear of getting pregnant or getting someone pregnant; the fear of an STI; individual values; peers; parents or guardians; the media; siblings; religion; and other adults, such as teachers, coaches, and counselors.)
5. Of the influences just listed, which do you believe have the greatest influence on your age group? Why?
6. Do you think parents or guardians can influence teenagers to make healthy choices and behaviors? How? What advice have you gotten from your parents or guardians related to any of these issues? Is it easy to talk to them about these issues? Why or why not?
7. What generalizations, if any, can you make about the results of the Youth Risk Behavior Survey?
8. The statistics in this activity were taken from the *national* Youth Risk Behavior Survey. Each state has its own individual results. How do you think your state's results compare with the national statistics?

Assessment

- Students each complete their worksheet and correct their answers.
- Students participate in the follow-up discussion on teen behavior.
- Students demonstrate evidence of accessing a reliable source of information by navigating the YRBS website appropriately.
- Students complete an individual or group project (product or performance).

Name: ______________________________

Sex: What Are Teens *Really* Doing?*

Directions: Working with a partner or in triads, discuss the following eight statements. For each statement, take your best guess at what you feel is the correct answer by circling "True" or "False." You will have five minutes to complete the survey. You do not have to agree with your partner or partners, but you should discuss the possible answers.

Survey Questions

1. Among all races and ethnicities, 59 percent of high school students in grades nine through twelve have had sexual intercourse.

My Answer		**Actual Answer**	
True	False	True	False

2. Among all races and ethnicities, more high school males have had sex than high school females.

My Answer		**Actual Answer**	
True	False	True	False

3. Among all races and ethnicities, the percentage of high school students who have had sexual intercourse **increases** as students move from ninth grade to twelfth grade.

My Answer		**Actual Answer**	
True	False	True	False

4. Among all races and ethnicities, 86 percent of high school senior males have had sex.

My Answer		**Actual Answer**	
True	False	True	False

Note: All statistics are based on nationwide results.

Name: ____________________________

Sex: What Are Teens *Really* Doing? (*continued*)

5. Among all races and ethnicities, the percentage of twelfth-grade females who have ever had sex is 50 percent lower than that of twelfth-grade males.

My Answer		**Actual Answer**	
True	False	True	False

6. Among students who are sexually active, 11 percent drank alcohol or used drugs before their last act of sexual intercourse.

My Answer		**Actual Answer**	
True	False	True	False

7. Among high school females who are currently sexually active, over half reported that they used birth control pills to prevent pregnancy before their last act of sexual intercourse.

My Answer		**Actual Answer**	
True	False	True	False

8. Among high school students who are currently sexually active, 20 percent did not use a condom to prevent pregnancy during their last act of sexual intercourse.

My Answer		**Actual Answer**	
True	False	True	False

LESSON 8: ABSTINENCE TILL MATURE CREATING YOUR OWN ATM POSTER

Level: Middle school, High school

Time: Two 40-minute sessions

National Health Education Standards

1. Core Concepts
2. Analyzing Influences

National Sexuality Education Standards: Performance Indicators

- Define sexual abstinence as it relates to pregnancy prevention.
- Compare and contrast the advantages and disadvantages of abstinence and other contraceptive methods, including condoms.
- Analyze influences that may have an impact on deciding whether or when to engage in sexual behaviors.

Rationale

Delaying sexual intercourse until they are older and more responsible is the healthiest choice for teens, especially younger teens. This activity is designed to afford students the opportunity to create a personal poster related to abstinence and delaying sexual activity. Students will use computer graphics to create their poster. In making their "Abstinence Till Mature" posters, students will have a chance to analyze internal and external influences that may affect their decision making in regard to sexual activity.

Materials and Preparation

Copies of "Creating Your Personal ATM Poster: Abstinence Till Mature" handout

Copies of "Poster Rubric" handout

Teacher copy of "ATM Poster (Sample)" to be shown to the class

Computers with a writing or publishing program. (*Note:* Alternately, access to old magazines, scissors, glue, markers, or other materials is needed if students are creating posters in the traditional manner.)

Printers to print out students' completed posters

Card stock, one piece for each student, to print out individual posters

Procedure

ACTIVITY 1: DAY 1—WORKING IN THE MEDIA CENTER

1. Ask students to brainstorm personal reasons to choose abstinence, and to record these in their notebook. Remind students to think of the physical, mental, emotional, social, and spiritual benefits of choosing abstinence. Ask each to generate a list of at least ten items.
2. Ask students to volunteer any reasons for remaining abstinent. Remind the class that this choice is a valid option for young people. Delaying sexual activity until they are older, more mature, and more responsible for their own health decisions is a healthy choice.

3. Explain that for the rest of the class time, students will each create a poster that reflects their personal beliefs, attitudes, and values related to delaying sexual activity. This poster will be labeled their "personal ATM (abstinence till mature) poster." Tell them that they will have one day to create this poster using a computer, but that they can also work on it at home if they have the technology. Posters will be shared and evaluated based on a distributed rubric.
4. Distribute the student handout and go over the assignment and the assessment criteria. Allow students to ask questions. Be sure to explain the rubric fully, including the doubling of points for some sections.

   Note: A sample ATM poster has been included in this lesson as a model to show to students. This model uses text alone. Based on the rubric given to students, student posters should include clip art, graphics, and possibly personal drawings if they are to receive the maximum grade.
5. Students should spend the rest of the class creating their respective ATM posters. Remind them to be creative, including poems, slogans, or rhyming words. They should also incorporate some facts or statistics from credible sources to reinforce their message. Creative use of text, color, fonts, graphics, drawings, and clip art can also make the poster more visually appealing
6. While students are working at computers, assist students with the technology. Students who are more technologically advanced can also assist others with the assignment.
7. When students have each completed their poster, give them a piece of card stock to print it out. If they decide to continue working on their poster at home, make card stock available to them so they can print out their poster at home.

ACTIVITY 2: DAY 2—SHARING OF ATM POSTERS

1. Tell students that they will have a chance to share their ATM poster in this class.
2. Posters can be displayed on a bulletin board or hung up around the room. Alternately, students can sit in a circle and pass their poster to the person on their right. Everyone has thirty seconds to look at each poster, and then pass it again to the right until all posters have been read by every student. Students then have the opportunity to explain the messages in their poster to the class, with follow-up questions and discussion from classmates.
3. Finish the lesson by asking the processing questions.

Processing

1. What are some good reasons not to get involved in a sexual relationship as a teenager?
2. How do you think most teens feel about the concept of "abstinence till marriage"?
3. When do you believe you or your peers will be ready for a sexual relationship?

Assessment

- Students complete their ATM poster, including the required information.
- Students grade their own poster using the provided rubric.
- Students share and discuss their ATM poster with the class.

Creating Your Personal ATM Poster: Abstinence Till Mature

Directions: In class, we have been discussing the benefits of choosing abstinence as it relates to your physical, mental, emotional, social, and spiritual health. For some, the goal is to remain abstinent until marriage. For others, the goal is to delay sexual activity until they are more mature and responsible. As you look at your own personal list of the physical, mental, emotional, social, and spiritual benefits of abstinence, note the factors that are most important to you. Using your list, create an ATM poster to reflect your own beliefs, attitudes, and values on this topic.

- You will be using a software program to create your poster. If you need assistance with the technology, ask the teacher or peer to help you.
- You are encouraged to be creative and original by using text, clip art, pictures, color, and graphics to personalize your poster. When you have finished designing your ATM poster, you will be given a sheet of card stock to print out a copy of your poster.
- The only mandatory items that must appear somewhere on your poster are the letters "**ATM**" and your **signature**.
- Be prepared to share and discuss your poster with the class.
- Your ATM poster will be assessed on the qualities described on the rubric provided.

Performance Task Assessment

Poster Rubric (Exceptional = 4; Good = 3; Fair = 2; Poor = 1)

ELEMENT	POSSIBLE SCORE	POINTS EARNED
Message		
The message or recommendation of the poster is readily apparent. The theme encourages health-enhancing risk reduction behaviors. The poster is appropriate for the target audience. The abbreviation "ATM" is prominently displayed somewhere on the poster. **(2x)**	8	
Factual Information		
Information is accurate and up to date. Statistics have been cited and referenced. **(1x)**	4	
Drawings, Graphics, and Illustrations		
Graphics and drawings (including the use of color, different fonts and text sizes, clip art and other illustrations, and so on) add to the purpose and interest of the poster. **(2x)**	8	
Creativity		
The poster is original and highly creative. (For example, it may include acrostic or other poetry formats, slogans, jingles, or other text or visual illustrations that reflect creative thought.) **(2x)**	8	
Attractiveness		
The poster is attractive in terms of design, layout, and neatness. The poster gets the attention of the viewer. **(1x)**	4	
Oral Presentation		
The student communicates the main theme to the target audience. The student's voice and body language support the message when presenting to the class. **(1x)**	4	
Grammar		
There are no grammatical or spelling mistakes on the poster. The student's signature appears on the poster. **(1x)**	4	
Total	40	

TEACHER COPY: ATM Poster (Sample)

Rx - Religion
- Values
- Love
- Soul Mate
- Monogamous Partner
- *DO NOT MIX WITH ALCOHOL!!

Abstinence

Till

Mature

Think with your
HEAD
Not your
HORMONES

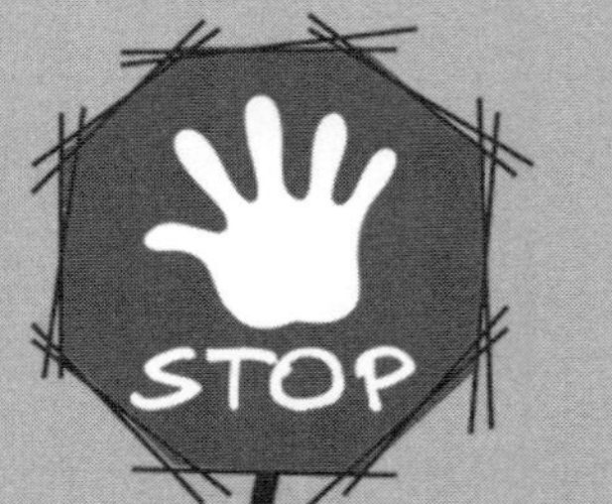

NO STI's, HIV, GUILT, WORRY OF PREGNANCY
RESPECT + RESPONSIBILITY = THE RIGHT TIME!!!!!!!!
WAIT FOR MS. RIGHT, NOT MS. "RIGHT NOW"

Signature ____________________

Phone: 555-I'll-WAIT
Fax: 555-NOT READY-YET
E-mail: NO GLOVE NO LOVE@WAITING.COM

LESSON 9: PARENT-TEEN CIRCLE SKITS

Level: High school

Time: 40 minutes

National Health Education Standards

2. Analyzing Influences
4. Interpersonal Communication
5. Decision-Making

National Sexuality Education Standards: Performance Indicators

- Analyze influences that may have an impact on deciding whether or when to engage in sexual behaviors.
- Demonstrate ways to communicate decisions about whether or when to engage in sexual behaviors.
- Assess the skills and resources needed to become a parent.

Rationale

Effective communication is an important part of all relationships. It is sometimes difficult, however, to communicate with parents or guardians about sexual issues. Learning to be assertive can be an important skill in improving relationships with parents or guardians, peers, and romantic partners. In this activity, students will practice communication techniques in the dual roles of parent and teen. Having students play the role of the parent often makes them more understanding of the responsibilities that parents or guardians feel when it comes to setting limits on their children's sexual activity.

Materials and Preparation

Copies of "Communicating about Sex: Assertive, Aggressive, and Passive Communication" handout

Copies of "Parent-Teen Communication: Circle Skits" worksheet

Procedure

1. Distribute the "Communicating about Sex: Assertive, Aggressive, and Passive Communication" handout. Review it with students, allowing for about ten minutes of practicing assertive, aggressive, and passive communication.
2. Have students rearrange their chairs in a large circle. Once they are in a circle, distribute the "Parent-Teen Communication: Circle Skits" worksheet.
3. Explain that the activity they are about to experience will require each student to alternate between thinking as a teenager and thinking as a parent. State: "The person on your right is your mother or father, and the person on your left is your teenage son or daughter."

4. Next, share the scenario:

   It is around 9:00 on a Saturday night. Your parents are going to a party and are not expected home until about 1:00 or 2:00 in the morning. You are their sixteen-year-old child who is currently home alone. Around 9:30, your partner shows up with a DVD, chips, and soda. So the two of you sit on the couch to watch the DVD and have the snacks. At one point, you begin to kiss your partner, and your partner kisses you back. Before you know it, you are both topless, making out on the living room couch.

   All of a sudden, the front door opens and one of your parents comes in, saying, "We were having trouble with the car, so we came back to take the other . . ." At this point, your parent realizes what is going on, and says . . .

5. All students should now assume the role of the mother or father in this story. On the top line of the "Parent-Teen Communication" worksheet, they should write in silence what they think their response to the situation would be.
6. After one minute has passed (most students should be finished writing what they think they would say as the parent in this situation), ask them to pass their paper to the person on their left. This person is their teenage son or daughter.
7. At the same time, they will also receive a paper from the person on their right, who is their mother or father.
8. Explain that all students in the circle are now in the role of the teenager. They should forget about what they wrote as the mother or father and concentrate on the paper in front of them. They should read what their mother or father wrote, and respond to this on the "Teen" line (without talking aloud). Allow one minute for students to respond in writing.
9. When they are finished, they will give their paper back to the person on their right, the parent, who will read what their son or daughter said and respond to it appropriately.
10. This back-and-forth will continue until all students have reached the bottom of the page. Make sure students know when they will be playing the role of the teen and parent for the last time. They should try to bring some resolution to the conversation.
11. When the entire page has been filled in, make sure all students have the paper they started with.
12. Ask volunteers to read their skit. For each skit, have students try to determine whether the parties involved were communicating *aggressively, assertively, passively,* or using a combination of communication styles.
13. Allow students to consider the challenges of being a parent or guardian by asking the processing questions.
14. End the class with a "class whip," having each student complete the following sentence stem: "One thing I think will be helpful when talking to my parents or guardians about sex is . . ."

Processing

1. If this really happened to you, how do you think a parent or guardian would react? Why?
2. Would it matter whether you were a daughter or a son? Why or why not?
3. Would it matter if it were a father or a mother who walked in on you? Why or why not?
4. Would it matter how old you were? How long you and your partner had been going out? Whether your partner was of the same or the opposite gender?
5. When do you think it is appropriate for a couple to start a sexual relationship? At what age or maturity level?
6. Now that you have had a chance to think about some of the situations and pressures parents or guardians have to face, are you better able to understand your parents' or guardians' point of view?

Assessment

- Students participate in the circle skits activity and follow-up discussion.
- Students participate in the class whip.

Communicating about Sex: Assertive, Aggressive, and Passive Communication

Communication is the key to becoming informed about sex and making the right decisions. Communication can start when you are very young and want to ask your parents or guardians or another trusted adult questions about sex. But communication should not stop there. You need to make sure your friends and the people you have relationships with always know your thoughts, feelings, and values. To do this you must communicate effectively.

Overall, there are three main ways to communicate:

A passive person does not make eye contact, her voice is soft and difficult to hear, and her body language or facial expressions may give you the impression that you could change her mind if you were to pressure her. Being passive often results in being taken advantage of.

An aggressive person uses a louder voice, and her body language is forceful or even threatening. She may stand close to the other person and "invade space." Her facial expressions are usually very serious or angry. She will often try to get what she wants by taking advantage of others.

An assertive person clearly and calmly states how she feels, why she feels that way, and what she wants or needs. She sticks up for herself, but in a way that does not take advantage of another person or put that person down.

There are three key elements of communication: eye contact, tone of voice, and body language. Based on the information just given, the statement "**I don't want to**" can be "said" by an individual in a variety of ways:

Passively: Not making eye contact and speaking very softly, he may say, "Well, . . . I don't . . . want . . . to."

Aggressively: Looking you straight in the eye, he may say in a loud, angry voice, "I don't want to!!!"

Assertively: Looking you in the eye, standing up straight, and with a moderate tone of voice, he may say, simply but convincingly, "I don't want to."

The benefits of being assertive are that you can honestly express how you feel without putting someone else down. Being assertive is almost always the best way to communicate because you are being respectful, and the other person knows exactly how you feel.

Being able to communicate assertively about sexual issues with parents or guardians, or with other adults, peers, and romantic partners, is an important skill that you can improve with practice.

Name: ______________________________

Parent-Teen Communication: Circle Skits

Parent: ____

____

____

____

Teen: ____

____

____

____

Parent: ____

____

____

____

Teen: ____

____

____

____

Parent: ____

____

____

____

Teen: ____

____

____

____

Parent (last comment): ____

____

____

____

Teen (last comment): ____

____

____

____

LESSON 10: SKILLS-BASED SEXUALITY SCENARIOS

Level: Middle school, High school

Time: 40 minutes

National Health Education Standards

1. Core Concepts
4. Interpersonal Communication
5. Decision-Making
6. Goal Setting

National Sexuality Education Standards: Performance Indicators

- Compare and contrast the advantages and disadvantages of abstinence and other contraceptive methods, including condoms.
- Demonstrate ways to communicate decisions about whether or when to engage in sexual behaviors.
- Apply a decision-making model to choices about contraception, including abstinence and condoms.
- Develop a plan to eliminate or reduce risk for STIs, including HIV.

Rationale

By learning and practicing health skills, such as communication and decision making, students can become healthy sexual beings.

In this activity, students will be given the opportunity to discuss scenarios dealing with a variety of sexual issues. To resolve the presented challenges, students will practice one or more of these important health skills.

Materials and Preparation

Teacher copy of "Skills-Based Scenarios: What Would You Do?," cut up into five cards. (*Note:* Suggested answers to the group scenarios for use in facilitating discussion are also included at the end of this lesson.)

Procedure

1. Divide the class into five groups. Assign a recorder and speaker for each group, or have groups determine who will fill those roles on their own.
2. Explain that a card with a scenario and questions written on it will be distributed to each group. After reading, groups are to answer the questions to resolve the scenario.
3. Hand out one scenario to each group. Allow ten minutes for the groups to read the scenario, brainstorm possible choices, and then write responses—fully answering the questions.

4. When groups have completed their work, ask one of the groups to volunteer to read their scenario and their completed response. After that group's response to the scenario has been given, open up the discussion to the entire class. During this class discussion students may offer comments or different opinions about how to handle the situation.
5. After the first group's scenario has been discussed, move on to one of the other groups and follow the same procedure.
6. Conclude the lesson by asking the processing questions.

Processing

1. Which of the situations are the most relevant to teenagers in our school?
2. What skill, of the ones presented, is the most important in your eyes?
3. What skill do you feel students need more practice with?

Assessment

- Students actively participate in the small and large group discussions.
- Group members offer complete responses to their scenario.

Skills-Based Scenarios: What Would You Do?

Card 1: Communication

Sexual Harassment

Tina is sixteen. She is upset and crying when she calls her friend Debbie on the phone. She confides that her basketball coach from her church team, who is in his twenties, has been making her feel uncomfortable. He has repeatedly asked her personal questions about her sex life, corners her when he is alone with her, and "jokes" that they should "go back to his place after practice" to "get to know each other better." She asks Debbie for advice on what she should do.

1. Define sexual harassment.
2. Based on your definition, explain why this situation is clearly a case of sexual harassment.
3. Write a conversation between Tina and Debbie, in which Debbie suggests two healthy options for dealing with the situation.

Card 2: Goal Setting

Avoiding Unplanned Pregnancy

Lee is a fifteen-year-old high school student. In health class, Lee has been learning about the difficulties encountered by teen couples having to deal with an unplanned pregnancy. Lee is a virgin and plans to delay starting a sexual relationship. Lee plans to go to college and feels that becoming a teen parent would interfere with those plans.

1. Write a plan to help prevent Lee (male or female) from being involved in an unplanned pregnancy. The plan should have a clear goal statement, specific steps to meet that goal, and the short- and long-term benefits of achieving the goal. The plan should
   a. State one short-term goal
   b. State one long-term goal
   c. Analyze possible external influences that may hinder Lee from reaching his or her goal
   d. Identify personal support systems and explain their importance to Lee in achieving his or her goal
2. Write a brief conversation Lee might have with a friend, parent, guardian, or other trusted adult who is supportive of this goal.

Skills-Based Scenarios: What Would You Do? (*continued*)

Card 3: Decision Making

Risk for HIV

Roberto is considering taking an HIV test. He has been sexually active with two girls, and is worried he may have been exposed to the virus. Roberto must make a decision about whether or not to get tested for HIV.

1. List and explain the steps in the decision-making process that specifically relates to Roberto's situation.
2. Write a conversation that Roberto might have with a doctor about being tested. In this conversation, Roberto should use assertive communication techniques to clearly get his message across to the doctor about his concerns related to being tested and his fears about the possible results of the test.

Card 4: Accessing Information

Contraception

Lori is the editor of her high school newspaper. She has heard many of her peers say they wished they had more information about the different forms of birth control. She decides to write an article describing four different forms of birth control that are commonly used by teens.

1. Write an outline of an article (an itemized list) for Lori, noting the four different forms of birth control commonly used by teens.
2. List at least three sources people can go to for reliable health information.

Card 5: Communication

Abstinence

Tiffany, a freshman, feels pressured to have sexual intercourse by her boyfriend, Tom, a junior. She wants to remain abstinent, but does not know how to discuss this with him without hurting his feelings or getting him angry.

1. Describe three reasons why postponing sex at her age is a healthy choice.
2. Describe three effective communication skills Tiffany can use to communicate her true feelings to Tom.
3. Write a conversation between Tiffany and Tom about remaining abstinent in which Tiffany uses assertive communication, including an "I message."

Skills-Based Scenarios: What Would You Do?

Possible Answers for Scenarios

Card 1: Communication

Content

The actions of Tina's coach constitute sexual harassment, which includes unwelcome comments, gestures, touching, or other verbal or nonverbal actions of a sexual nature.

Skill

- If comfortable doing so, as a first step Tina should give a clear "no" statement and exhibit multiple refusals if necessary.
- Debbie can suggest that Tina cannot remain silent, because things will only get worse. Tina should assertively tell the coach that his comments are unwelcome and a form of sexual harassment. If Tina is too intimidated to do this alone, Debbie can agree to go with her.
- Debbie can advise Tina to tell her parents, and they can then contact the coach or other authorities to make this behavior stop.

Card 2: Goal Setting

Content

1. Lee's short-term goal is to remain abstinent and eliminate the risk of an unplanned pregnancy.
2. Lee's long-term goal is to attend college. Having a child could affect this long-term goal due to parental responsibilities, financial problems, or lack of family support.
3. Possible external influences that may hinder Lee's goal may be peer pressure to have sex; media influences that encourage sexual activity; or being under the influence of alcohol or other drugs, which may increase the possibility of engaging in unprotected sex.
4. Support systems may be friends or family, counselors, teachers, or other trusted adults who would be supportive of Lee's goal.

Skill

Effective communication would involve any of the following:

- Employing active listening and response skills
- Using effective verbal (assertive) and nonverbal communication
- Demonstrating healthy ways to express needs, wants, and feelings

Card 3: Decision Making

Content

Things Roberto must consider in making his decision might include:

- Did he have unprotected sex?
- Did he have sex while under the influence of drugs or alcohol?
- Does he know the sexual backgrounds of his two partners? Are they promiscuous?
- Did either partner show signs or symptoms of illness? STIs?
- Did either partner share needles?

Skills-Based Scenarios: What Would You Do? (*continued*)

Skill

Steps in the decision-making process would be

1. Stating the decision
2. Listing possible alternatives
3. Noting the positive and negative consequences of each alternative
4. Gathering information and evaluating whether the decision supports his personal, family, or religious beliefs and values
5. Making a decision
6. Evaluating the results

Card 4: Accessing Information

Content

Four common methods of birth control used by teens and their effectiveness are as follows:

- Abstinence—100 percent effective
- Birth control pill—99 percent effective when used correctly
- Male condom—86 percent to 97 percent effective, depending on whether it is used correctly every time
- Withdrawal—very ineffective due to the presence of pre-ejaculate, with a high risk of failure

Skill

Accessing information involves

- Identifying specific sources (people with some form of expertise, such as a personal physician or a counselor; a clinic; Planned Parenthood; Internet sites ending in .gov, .edu, or .org; and so on)
- Evaluating the validity of each source

Card 5: Communication

Content

Reasons for Tiffany not to have sex include

- No risk of pregnancy
- No risk of STIs
- Improved self-esteem
- Alignment with religious or family values

Skill

- Possible assertive communication strategies are sharing clear, organized thoughts; using clear "no" statements; providing a reason; making repeated refusals if necessary, and ending the relationship.
- A possible example of an "I" message is: "**I feel** uncomfortable **when you** put pressure on me to have sex, **because** I care about you, but I'm just not ready to take that step. **I want you to** respect my decision to remain abstinent at this time."

LESSON 11: ASK THE "SEXPERTS"

Level: High school

Time: Two 40-minute sessions

National Health Education Standards

1. Core Concepts
3. Accessing Information
4. Interpersonal Communication

National Sexuality Education Standards: Performance Indicators

- Compare and contrast the advantages and disadvantages of abstinence and other contraceptive methods, including condoms.
- Access medically-accurate information about contraceptive methods, including emergency contraception and condoms.
- Demonstrate ways to communicate decisions about whether or when to engage in sexual behaviors.
- Compare and contrast behaviors, including abstinence, to determine the potential risk of STI/HIV transmission from each.
- Describe the signs, symptoms and potential impacts of STIs, including HIV.
- Access medically-accurate prevention information about STIs, including HIV.
- Demonstrate the use of effective communication skills to reduce or eliminate risk for STIs, including HIV.
- Describe characteristics of healthy and unhealthy romantic and/or sexual relationships.
- Demonstrate effective ways to communicate personal boundaries as they relate to intimacy and sexual behavior.
- Identify sources of support such as parents or other trusted adults whom they can go to if they are or someone they know is being bullied, harassed, abused or assaulted.

Rationale

To make good decisions about their sexual health, students need to be able to access valid sources of information. The most commonly used source of information for teens today is the Internet. Because unreliable information can also be found online, students must be able to distinguish between reliable and unreliable sources. In this lesson, to practice the skill of accessing medically accurate information, students will research answers to commonly asked questions about sexual health. They will then present their findings to the class as part of an "Ask the Sexperts" TV panel.

Materials and Preparation

Computers or personal mobile devices with Internet access, at school or at home. If Internet access is not available, or if sex-related sites are blocked in the school, students will have to meet as a group, split up their tasks, and do this assignment at home. The website used for this particular activity is www.sexetc.org.

Index cards

Overhead projector and blank transparency sheets or Smart Board

Miscellaneous materials to be used as visual aids in student presentations, such as models of male and female reproductive systems and condoms and other examples of contraception (if allowable and available)

Copies of "Oral Presentation Rubric" handout

Table and chairs or several extra student desks, to be placed in front of the classroom prior to the beginning of class on the second day

Microphone (real or simulated)

Procedure

ACTIVITY 1: DAY 1—GROUP WORK

1. Begin the class by explaining that the topic of sexual health seems to raise a lot of questions. Often sexuality education classes teach students about the "basics" of reproduction, yet may not answer some of the "real" questions students have. This activity will attempt to address this problem.
2. Briefly review how to judge the reliability of a website. Generally, websites that end in .gov (government agencies); .edu (educational institutions, like colleges and universities); and .org (community organizations, like the American Lung Association) tend to be reliable sources of information. Sites that end in .com may contain reliable information, but often represent commercial organizations that are trying to sell a product. Depending on the product a given organization is selling, the website may or may not be trustworthy.
3. Tell students that over the course of the next day, they will be researching information related to sexual health topics. One trusted site used by many health and sexuality educators as well as teenagers is www.sexetc.org. Sex, Etc. is monitored by Answer, a national organization dedicated to providing and promoting comprehensive human sexuality education for young people.

   Note: For more information about Answer, including contact information, visit http://answer.rutgers.edu.
4. Break students into five groups, and assign each group one of the following topics:
   a. Teen pregnancy
   b. Abuse and violence
   c. Love and relationships
   d. Sexually transmitted infections
   e. Birth control and safer sex

5. Explain the groups' "mission": students will have one research day to gather twelve questions asked on the Sex, Etc. website pertaining to their group's topic. This website offers many different questions, and students should choose the ones most relevant to their school and community. In addition to finding twelve questions (and their answers), students will require some sort of visual aid related to their topic. You may have to assist students in determining which visual aids are available and appropriate.

   Note: One class period is needed for online research. If the school blocks the Sex, Etc. website, group members should divide up research tasks and each log onto the site at home.

6. Have students log onto the Sex, Etc. website. Make sure they focus on their group's topic—they should only review the list of frequently asked questions sent in by teens from across the country.

   Note: Group members should decide which questions they feel are most interesting or relevant to their classmates. They should divvy up responsibility for answering the questions evenly. They must then look up the answer to each of the questions on the website. Each individual question should be written out on a separate index card. These cards will be distributed randomly to the "audience" for the actual "show" the following day.

   Note: Each group should find or create some type of visual aid related to the topic they are presenting. For example, the group dealing with teen pregnancy might use a model of the female reproductive system, which you could provide. The groups dealing with STIs and birth control and safer sex may have various forms of contraception available to demonstrate proper use. Groups for whom props or models are not appropriate or available should create an overhead transparency, poster, or PowerPoint slide, for example, addressing at least one of the questions they present. For example, the group dealing with love and relationships may create an overhead transparency or poster listing "signs of an unhealthy relationship." In some cases, you may have to assist in gathering props or making the other visual aids from student-created lists and pictures.

7. Distribute the "Oral Presentation Rubric" handout to all students and briefly review the assessment criteria.

ACTIVITY 2: DAY 2—SEXPERTS GROUP PANEL PRESENTATIONS

1. The table and chairs or extra desks should be set up in a row in front of the classroom for the presenting group. The rest of the class can be in rows or a semicircle.
2. Before class begins, ask the first presenting group to distribute their index cards to random audience members.
3. You should play the role of "host" introducing the panel and their area of expertise.
4. After introductions, ask if any of the audience members have a question for the panel. Once someone with an index card raises her hand, take the microphone to that member of the audience, and she will ask the question on the card. The appropriate member of the panel will answer the question. Often, the answer will generate further discussion, which you should moderate.

5. Continue with the questions from the audience until all have been answered. If the group did not use the visual aid to clarify questions, they should use it in summarizing their presentation.
6. Thank and dismiss the panel and move on to the next group. Follow the same procedure until all groups have completed their presentation.
7. After all presentations have been given, ask the processing questions to elicit more discussion on the topics at hand.

Processing

1. How useful was the Sex, Etc. website? Explain.
2. What questions did you find interesting? Why?
3. What questions surprised you? Why?
4. How comfortable would you feel if a peer approached you to ask you any of the mentioned questions? What would you say?

Assessment

- Groups complete their research and presentation (to be assessed by the instructor based on the rubric provided).
- Students participate in a group discussion of the processing questions.

Oral Presentation Rubric (12 Points Total)

CRITERION	EXEMPLARY 4	ACCOMPLISHED 3	DEVELOPING 2	BEGINNING 1
Content	❑ Content was accurate. ❑ Content was organized. ❑ Students showed full understanding of the topic.	❑ Content was mostly accurate. ❑ Content was mostly organized. ❑ Students showed good understanding of the topic.	❑ Content was partially accurate. ❑ Content was partially organized. ❑ Students showed fair understanding of the topic.	❑ Content was inaccurate. ❑ Content was not organized. ❑ Students did not understand the topic.
Verbal Skills of Group Members	❑ Students spoke clearly. ❑ Students projected their voice. ❑ Students shared responsibility for answers.	❑ Students spoke clearly most of the time. ❑ Students projected their voice most of the time. ❑ Students shared responsibility for answers.	❑ Students spoke somewhat clearly. ❑ Students projected their voice somewhat. ❑ One or two group members answered most questions.	❑ Students did not speak clearly. ❑ Students had weak voice projection. ❑ One group member answered questions.
Mechanics and Visual Aid	❑ Correct grammar was used. ❑ Spelling was correct. ❑ Graphics and pictures were attractive and supported the theme.	❑ Correct grammar was used most of the time. ❑ There were one to two spelling errors. ❑ Some graphics and pictures were supportive of the theme.	❑ Sometimes poor grammar was used. ❑ There were three to five spelling errors. ❑ Graphics and pictures were not supportive of the theme.	❑ Poor grammar was used. ❑ There were six or more spelling errors. ❑ Graphics and pictures detracted from the presentation or were not included.

LESSON 12: EASY, DIFFICULT, IMPOSSIBLE

ARE YOU REALLY READY FOR SEX?

Level: Middle school, High school

Time: 40 minutes

National Health Education Standards

1. Core Concepts
2. Analyzing Influences
4. Interpersonal Communication

National Sexuality Education Standards: Performance Indicators

- Explain the health benefits, risks and effectiveness rates of various methods of contraception, including abstinence and condoms.
- Compare and contrast the advantages and disadvantages of abstinence and other contraceptive methods, including condoms.
- Analyze influences that may have an impact on deciding whether or when to engage in sexual behaviors.
- Identify the laws related to reproductive and sexual health care services (i.e., contraception, pregnancy options, safe surrender policies, prenatal care).

Rationale

Values are the ideas, feelings, and beliefs that make up what is important to a person. Values play a major role in determining decisions and behaviors, including those related to sexuality. In this panel activity, students will be made aware of their values and compare their values with those of their peers. They will also analyze how health-related decisions are influenced by individual, family, and community values.

Note: It is useful for there to have been prior discussion of effective communication skills. Students should also have a basic understanding of the decision-making model.

Materials and Preparation

Front board

Four sets of three laminated cards. With text written in marker in large letters, one card in a set will read "Easy," the second card will read "Difficult," and the third card will read "Impossible."

Four extra chairs set up in front of the room

List of statements to be read to student volunteers. (*Note:* Twenty suggested values-based scenarios are included at the end of this lesson. You should choose those scenarios that are most relevant and developmentally appropriate for your students.)

Procedure

1. Begin the discussion by asking students what it means to be "responsible." Expand the discussion to focus on what it means to be "sexually responsible." Answers can be listed on the board. (Answers may include having knowledge of one's reproductive system and how it works, respecting yourself and others, avoiding physical or emotional harm, communicating feelings and values honestly, and taking precautions to avoid an unwanted pregnancy or STIs.)
2. Next, ask students to discuss what the word "relationship" means to them. Again, students' answers can be written on the board. (Answers may include sharing a close, personal feeling with someone, such as a friend, parent or guardian, or boyfriend or girlfriend; seeing one person on a regular basis or being "with" someone; and developing a sense of trust and intimacy with someone.)
3. Begin the panel activity: ask for four volunteers (two males and two females, if possible) to come to the front of the room and serve as a panel. Explain that a series of statements will be read aloud, and each member of the panel will think about the statement and then hold up one of three signs ("Easy," "Difficult," or "Impossible") to answer.

   Announce the following: "All the statements about to be read have something to do with either relationships, sexual behavior, risks and consequences, future decisions, or values. Some situations might be *easy* for you to deal with. Others might be *difficult* to deal with. Still others might be *impossible* to deal with. For each scenario I describe, all four judges are to display their answer by holding up one of the cards signifying if they think the decision is easy, difficult, or impossible."
4. Before starting to read statements to the panel, reinforce that there are no "right" or "wrong" answers. Students will be asked to share why they voted as they did. Because students bring a variety of backgrounds, cultural and religious beliefs, and values, they may make different decisions. Reinforce the following rules related to the class discussion:
   - You can disagree, but please be respectful of other people's right to their own opinion.
   - No put-downs are allowed.
   - At any time, if you feel you must pass on a question or response, you have the right to do so.
   - Agreeing to disagree is an effective relationship management skill.
5. Start the activity by reading one of the statements. Once students on the panel have voted and explained their thinking, open up the discussion to the class. After some discussion, move on to the next statement.
6. After reading and discussing a few statements, thank the panel and request four new volunteers. Continue the same process with the new panel.

7. After all of the statements you selected have been discussed, allow enough time to conclude the day's lesson by reviewing the processing questions.
8. Before the lesson ends, assign a journal entry for homework. For this entry, students each are to choose one of the scenarios that they rated as being either difficult or impossible and write a journal entry of at least three paragraphs. Within these paragraphs, students should state reasons why their chosen scenario would be difficult or impossible for them to deal with. Volunteers may be solicited to share their journal entry during the next lesson if they are comfortable doing so.

Processing

1. Out of all the statements discussed during the activity, which ones were the easiest to decide on? Why?
2. Out of all the statements discussed during the activity, which ones were the most difficult to decide on? Why?
3. Was your being a male or a female a factor in some of the decisions? Explain.
4. What role did internal influences, such as personal values, self-image, or your sense of right and wrong, play in your decision making?
5. What role did external influences, such as the media, family, peers, or laws, play in your decision making?

Assessment

- Students actively participate in the panel discussion.
- Students complete a journal entry of at least three paragraphs for homework.

Easy, Difficult, or Impossible: Values Voting

How difficult would it be to . . .

1. Remain abstinent until marriage?
2. Ask someone out whom you are attracted to?
3. Kiss and touch a partner in a sexual way, and then stop before actually going further?
4. Tell someone you have been dating that you want to have sex with him or her?
5. Have a one-night stand?
6. Break up with a boyfriend or girlfriend you still like, yet whom you see as more of a "friend" than a boyfriend or girlfriend?
7. Date your best friend's ex?
8. Tell your mom you had sex with someone?
9. Become a parent at this stage of your life?
10. Tell your dad you had sex with someone?
11. Discuss birth control with your partner before having sex?
12. Tell your partner you may have infected him or her with an STI?
13. Go to a clinic because you suspect you might have contracted an STI?
14. Buy and carry condoms with you in the event that you might have sex?
15. Tell your mom you are pregnant or got someone pregnant?
16. Tell your dad you are pregnant or got someone pregnant?
17. Do something that is against your religious beliefs?
18. Have a baby and give it up for adoption?
19. Break up with someone you have dated for six months by sending him or her a text message?
20. Break up with someone you have dated for six months by telling him or her in person?

LESSON 13: WHAT AM I? THE 411 ON CONTRACEPTION

Level: High school

Time: 45 minutes

National Health Education Standards

1. Core Concepts
3. Accessing Information

National Sexuality Education Standards: Performance Indicators

- Compare and contrast the advantages and disadvantages of abstinence and other contraceptive methods, including condoms.
- Define emergency contraception and describe its mechanism of action.
- Access medically-accurate information about contraceptive methods, including emergency contraception and condoms.

Rationale

Most men and women, at various times in their lives, need to make decisions about birth control. Having a baby can be one of life's greatest gifts and pleasures; but for teens, dealing with an unplanned pregnancy can be confusing and stressful. This lesson will provide students with information related to various methods of preventing pregnancy, including abstinence. Students will discuss the advantages and disadvantages of various forms of contraception. Most important, they will come to understand that the most effective forms of birth control are those that are used correctly and consistently every time. They will also learn that the only 100 percent effective form of birth control is abstinence.

Materials and Preparation

Small slips of paper, one for each student

Bag or box to hold slips of paper

Copies of "Fact Sheet: The 411 on Birth Control and Contraception" handout

Teacher copy of "What Birth Control Method Am I?" to be read as part of the review game

Anatomical models or slides of the male and female reproductive systems

Procedure

ACTIVITY 1: LECTURE AND DISCUSSION ABOUT BIRTH CONTROL METHODS

1. Ask the class, "How many of you think you might want to be a parent someday?" After a show of hands, ask, "How many of you would like to be a parent now?"
2. Facilitate a general discussion about why most teens do not want to be parents at this time in their lives. State: "For many adults, finding out they are going to have a baby is a happy occasion. For many teenagers, getting pregnant (or getting someone pregnant) is not such a joyous experience."
3. Explain that many high school students wait to have sex. Abstaining from sex is a healthy choice for teens. Teens who do choose to begin a sexual relationship, however, need to be aware of the various methods of birth control to avoid an unplanned pregnancy and sexually transmitted infections.
4. Hand out a small slip of paper to each student. Ask students to anonymously write down two things they know about birth control on their paper. Collect all papers when students have finished and place them in a bag (or box).
5. Reach into the bag and read one slip of paper. Initiate a class discussion on the accuracy of the statements, clarifying any misinformation. Continue reading the other slips of paper until all have been read and discussed. Often, a number of students will have the same or very similar statements. When you come to a statement that has already been discussed, note that this is the case and move on to the next.
6. Distribute the "Fact Sheet: The 411 on Birth Control and Contraception" handout. Ask a volunteer to read the information aloud while the other students follow along on their own copy. Answer any questions students have about any of the methods.
7. When all methods have been discussed, explain that the fact sheet does not go into detail about some of the side effects, rates of effectiveness, laws and regulations, and costs associated with many of these methods. Encourage students who would like more information to visit their doctor or local clinic for further information and counseling. There are also several websites with more detailed information about all of these methods. One of the most commonly used and reliable sites is www.plannedparenthood.org.

ACTIVITY 2: REVIEW GAME—WHAT BIRTH CONTROL METHOD AM I?

1. Break the class up randomly into two coed teams, and have them stand on either side of the room.
2. Explain that they are going to play a review game, What Birth Control Method Am I? In this game, you will describe a type of birth control. Each turn, one person on each team will be chosen to guess which form of birth control is being described. The contestant must answer the question himself, and may not receive assistance from anyone on his team. If he gives the correct type of birth control, his team will get one point. If his guess is incorrect, the team will not get a point, and you will give the correct answer.

3. After the first team has gone, follow the same procedure with one of the students on the other team. Continue with the game until all the methods of birth control have been explored. The team with more points at the end wins.
4. Ask the processing questions.
5. In a future class session, give the class a quiz or test based on the information brought out in the review game.

Processing

1. What forms of birth control is the class most familiar with? Why do you think this is?
2. What forms of birth control is the class least familiar with? Why do you think this is?
3. Where can people receive more information about birth control and their sexual health?

Assessment

- Students write anonymous comments on their knowledge of birth control.
- Students give answers in the review game.
- Students actively participate in a discussion of the processing questions.
- Students take a quiz or test based on the information provided in the lesson during a future class session.

Fact Sheet: The 411 on Birth Control and Contraception

The term "contraception" generally means preventing the male's sperm from meeting the female's egg, and usually refers to some type of chemical or device. "Birth control" is a broader term for controlling the birth of children and planning families. Teens who choose to be sexually active need to make decisions about what forms of birth control to use each time they have sexual contact. Following is information to help teens decide which forms of birth control might be most appropriate for them:

- Many contraceptive devices will not protect a person from sexually transmitted infections (STIs), so to prevent the transmission of STIs, the use of a condom is a positive choice. Many people will combine the use of a condom with another method of birth control, such as the birth control pill. Combining two different forms of contraception is referred to as "dual protection."
- To be effective, birth control must be used correctly and consistently. Some birth control methods are more reliable than others, and may offer protection against STIs.
- If pregnancy is not desired, it is important to choose a method you and your partner will use every time you have intercourse.
- Some teens are able to talk to a parent or guardian about birth control; others cannot. Talking to a trusted adult is recommended to ensure that you receive proper information. You can get information and counseling at most local health clinics or from your doctor.

Available Forms of Birth Control

There are many available forms of birth control and, as science and technology advance, new forms of birth control are introduced. There is no one "best" form of birth control; what forms people choose to use depend on their age, lifestyle, and future goals. Each individual and couple should discuss the forms of birth control that they are most comfortable with. Several of the methods listed here may not be appropriate for teens. As your life changes, you may need or want to use different birth control methods. Most types of birth control have some negative side effects. These should be discussed with your doctor or health care provider. Once counseled about birth control options, teens should choose whichever methods they feel are best for them. Consistent and correct use is the key to effective birth control. The following is a list and brief description of common forms of birth control:

Abstinence—can mean different things to different people. In regard to pregnancy prevention, it means choosing not to engage in sexual intercourse—or, more specifically, vaginal intercourse. Abstinence can be a healthy choice for many teens, and it has many advantages, including these: (1) it is free, (2) it does not require a prescription, and (3) it is 100 percent effective.

Birth control patch—a thin, square patch that is placed on the female's skin. It works by slowly releasing hormones that prevent eggs from leaving the ovaries. It also thickens cervical mucous, which helps block sperm from reaching the egg. A patch is placed on the female's arm, leg, or other body part for a week. The patch is replaced every week for three weeks,

Fact Sheet: The 411 on Birth Control and Contraception (*continued*)

then the female goes "patchless" for the fourth week. The patch requires a checkup and a prescription from a doctor. The patch is 91 to 95 percent effective.

Birth control pill—also referred to as "oral contraceptives"; one of the most common methods used by teens. The pill works by releasing hormones that prevent ovulation and by making cervical mucous thicker. The pill is taken every day, with twenty-one "active" pills and seven "reminder" pills. Each month, a new prescription is needed. The pill is about 91 percent effective with typical use, accounting for human error like forgetting to take the pill every day. If used correctly, the pill can be up to 99 percent effective in preventing pregnancy. It does not prevent STIs. The pill requires a checkup and a prescription from a doctor.

Birth control sponge—a small, round piece of foam inserted into the vagina up to twenty-four hours prior to intercourse. It works by covering the cervix and blocking sperm from entering the uterus. It also releases a spermicide, keeping sperm from moving. It must be left in place for at least six hours after intercourse. It is available without a prescription.

Depo-Provera—an injection or shot that a female gets every three months. The shot contains a hormone that prevents the ovaries from releasing eggs. It also thickens cervical mucous, reducing the chance of a sperm reaching an egg. The injection requires a checkup from a doctor. Every three months, the female must return to the doctor to get another shot. Depo-Provera is about 94 percent effective.

Diaphragm—a shallow silicone cup inserted into the vagina before having intercourse. It is used with a spermicide. The diaphragm works by blocking sperm from entering the uterus; also, the spermicide kills sperm. The diaphragm requires a checkup and proper fitting from a doctor.

Emergency contraception (EC)—referred to as the morning-after pill; used as a "backup" method for preventing unintended pregnancy. A female might use EC after having sex if a condom breaks or slips off, when no birth control was used at all, or if she was raped. To be most effective, EC should be taken within 120 hours after intercourse. EC is presently available over the counter. The most commonly used brand is called Plan B.

Female condom—a polyurethane pouch with a flexible ring at each end. It is inserted into the vagina prior to intercourse. It can sometimes be difficult to use properly. It can be purchased without a prescription. An advantage of the female condom is that it helps reduce the risk of sexually transmitted infections.

Implant—a thin rod about the size of a cardboard matchstick. It is made from a flexible plastic and is surgically inserted just under the skin on the

(*continued*)

Fact Sheet: The 411 on Birth Control and Contraception (*continued*)

inner side of the female's upper arm. It works by releasing hormones that keep the ovaries from releasing eggs and also thickens cervical mucous. Once implanted, it is up to 99 percent effective in preventing pregnancy for up to three years. Because it needs to be inserted, it requires a visit to a doctor or health clinic.

Intrauterine device (IUD)—a small, "T-shaped" plastic device inserted into the uterus for an extended period, usually several years. IUDs work mainly by affecting how sperm move so they cannot join with an egg. A female needs to go to a doctor for the insertion.

Male condom—a "barrier method" of birth control; provides a barrier by covering the penis. Male condoms are a common method of birth control for teens. Condoms are generally made from latex, lambskin, polyurethane, or nonlatex natural rubber. Lambskin condoms are generally not recommended because they do not offer as much protection in preventing STIs. Having the penis covered helps prevent the male's sperm from reaching the female's egg. Condoms need to be used properly to be effective (directions are often in the box they are bought in). In general use, male condoms are about 82 percent effective. If used correctly and consistently, effectiveness rates can be above 90 percent. They are inexpensive and do not require a prescription. Beside abstinence, condoms are the most effective protection against STIs, but hormonal methods are more effective in preventing pregnancy.

Spermicide—a foam, cream, or gel containing chemicals that kill sperm or keep sperm from moving. Spermicides are not very effective by themselves. They are most effective when used in combination with another method, such as a condom or other barrier method. They are available without a prescription.

Vaginal ring—a small, flexible ring inserted into the vagina for three weeks. On the first day of the fourth week, the female removes the ring to have her menstrual period. The vaginal ring works by releasing hormones that prevent ovulation. The vaginal ring requires a checkup and a prescription from a doctor.

Vasectomy and tubal ligation—surgical procedures blocking sperm (vasectomy) or eggs (tubal ligation) from being released. They are usually permanent and 100 percent effective.

Withdrawal—when a male withdraws or pulls his penis out of the female's vagina before ejaculation. Withdrawal is one of the least effective methods of birth control because even if a male pulls out before he ejaculates, pregnancy can still occur. Often a tiny amount of pre-ejaculate will be released from the urethra before ejaculation. This pre-ejaculate often has enough sperm in it to cause a pregnancy

What Birth Control Method Am I?

1. I am the only natural method of preventing pregnancy that is 100 percent effective. I am free and do not require a visit to a doctor. What method am I? **(Abstinence)**
2. I slowly release hormones from the skin into the bloodstream. I am effective for one week, and then I must be replaced. After three weeks of this, I take a week off and a female gets her period. I am 91 to 95 percent effective. What method am I? **(Birth control patch)**
3. I must be fitted by a doctor. I am most effective if used along with a sperm-killing cream or jelly. I look like a small rubber dome. What am I? **(Diaphragm)**
4. I am a lubricated polyurethane pouch inserted into the vagina before intercourse. I provide some protection against STIs. What am I? **(Female condom)**
5. I am an injectable form of birth control administered by a doctor every three months. One of the side effects while taking me is that some females stop having periods. What am I? **(Depo-Provera)**
6. I am the most common form of birth control for males and usually made of latex. I prevent sperm from entering the vagina. I am available without a prescription and can help protect against sexually transmitted infections. I am most effective when used correctly and consistently every time. What am I? **(Male condom)**
7. An applicator is used to insert me into the vagina right before sex. I contain chemicals that kill sperm. I am most effective when used with a condom or other barrier method. I can be purchased over the counter. What am I? **(Contraceptive foam or jelly)**
8. I consist of high concentrations of hormones that keep the ovary from releasing an egg. I can be used up to 120 hours after unprotected sex, but am most effective if used as soon as possible after unprotected sex. Although there are several forms, the most common brand is Plan B and can be bought at a pharmacy. What am I? **(Emergency contraception or morning-after pill)**
9. I am one of the most popular methods of birth control for females. I should be taken at the same time every day for twenty-eight days, with twenty-one "active" pills that release hormones and seven "reminder" pills. The female gets her period every month. What am I?
(Birth control pill or oral contraceptives)
10. I am a thin rod about the size of a cardboard matchstick. I am surgically inserted just under the skin on the inner side of the female's upper arm. I am up to 99 percent effective in preventing pregnancy for up to three years. What am I? **(Implant)**
11. I am not very effective. I rely on perfect timing and self-control. Sperm can be present without the male feeling anything. What am I? **(Withdrawal)**
12. I am a surgical procedure that makes a man sterile. I am generally considered a permanent form of sterilization. I am rarely used by teens. What am I? **(Vasectomy)**

LESSON 14: UP CLOSE AND PERSONAL

Level: Middle school, High school

Time: 40 minutes

National Health Education Standards

1. Core Concepts
4. Interpersonal Communication

National Sexuality Education Standards: Performance Indicators

- Demonstrate ways to communicate decisions about whether or when to engage in sexual behaviors.
- Explain the health benefits, risks and effectiveness rates of various methods of contraception, including abstinence and condoms.
- Demonstrate the use of effective communication and negotiation skills about contraception including abstinence and condoms.

Rationale

This Up Close and Personal (UCP) lesson encourages students to engage in open, honest discussion by completing sentence stems. It allows for the integration of the affective (emotional) and cognitive (informational) domains. In addition, students will practice positive communication skills, including active listening, interpreting verbal as well as nonverbal messages, asking for clarification, and using "I" messages to assertively state their feelings and opinions on topics related to pregnancy and reproduction.

Although the format for this activity is relatively simple, the rules must be followed for the activity to be effective, and you, as the facilitator, must ensure that they are strictly enforced.

Materials and Preparation

Small lamp (optional)

Up Close and Personal sheet with several UCP sentence stems. (*Note:* Prior to teaching this activity, you should familiarize yourself with "Facilitating a UCP Session," which can be found at the end of the lesson.)

Procedure*

1. Ask students to form a circle with their chairs. Turning off the overhead lights and using a lamp may make the environment more conducive to an informal discussion.
2. Introduce the activity in the following manner:

   Today we are going to do an activity called Up Close and Personal. It is simple to do, but for it to go smoothly, there are some rules to follow.

---

*Unfinished sentences have been a useful learning tool for many years. The specific format used in this lesson has been adapted from the book *Up Close and Personal: Effective Learning for Students and Teachers* (Raleigh, NC: Lulu Press, 2007), by teacher, colleague, and friend Robert Winchester. Robert can be contacted at trustinbob@aol.com.

First, understand this is not group therapy. Instead it is an opportunity for you to talk about how you feel about yourself, relationships, likes, dislikes, things that have come up in class, memories, and life in general. Although I will be facilitating the activity, I will also be sitting in the circle and participating along with everyone else.

The activity is in the following format: I will read an unfinished sentence. Each of you will think about how you would finish this same unfinished sentence. Someone in the circle will then raise his or her hand and state his or her completed sentence. He or she will point to his or her right or left to determine which way around the circle we will proceed.

When going around the circle, there should be no talking by anyone else. If something is said that you want to respond to or comment on, you must wait until we have gone all the way around the circle. If you cannot think of anything to say, or choose not to respond when it is your turn, you may simply say, "Pass" or "Come back to me." Everyone, including the teacher, is allowed to pass.

When we have gone around the entire circle, I will ask anyone who passed if he or she would like to respond at this time. I will also ask for any questions or comments about anything that was said when going around the circle. At this point, there can be open discussion.

Please note that during this activity, no names should be mentioned at any time. Instead, say something like, "I know someone who . . ."

In addition, as with other lessons, what is said in class stays in class. However, please do not share anything that is too personal, that makes you feel uncomfortable, or that you wish to keep to yourself.

3. Once the rules have been explained and agreed on, read the first sentence stem aloud. After allowing a few moments for reflection, ask a student volunteer to start by stating his completed sentence. That student will then point to his left or right to note in which direction the remaining students will be given a chance to complete the sentence. Students then give their responses until everyone around the circle has spoken or passed.
4. At times, a student may simply not be ready to respond to a particular question. When this happens, remind her to pass, noting that she can answer after everyone else has spoken. It is also not unusual for many students to have the same response to a question or statement. "Repeats" reinforce the important concept that although all people are unique, they often share many of the same thoughts, feelings, and values.
5. After all students have responded, open up the discussion by asking if anyone has any questions or comments about anything that was said. Encourage students to talk in more detail about why they completed the sentence the way they did. Students may also ask others in the circle, including the teacher, to expand on their answer. Students may do so, or they may choose to pass.
6. Continue the circle discussion for as long as it is viable, constantly monitoring and enforcing the rules. When the discussion on a given sentence has run its course, move on to the next unfinished sentence.

7. Share the processing statements.
8. All UCP sessions should end with some brief closure in the form of another unfinished sentence. Examples include the following: "Today I learned . . ." "I learned that I . . ." "Right now I feel . . ." and "Something I want to say to one of my classmates is . . ."
9. Conclude the day's activity by summarizing what occurred in the session, making appropriate connections to the subject matter and curriculum. Then thank the class and say, "This ends our Up Close and Personal class for today."

Processing

1. If anyone has any concerns or questions about what was discussed during our UCP session today, he or she can speak to me privately after class or can bring it up for discussion during our next class session.
2. There are many people, including teachers, coaches, counselors, or school psychologists, who can assist you with any personal issues that you may want to share with them. Keep in mind that these individuals, as mandated reporters, *must* report any verbalization or indication that you may want to hurt yourself or hurt others, or revelations of abuse of any kind, to the appropriate authorities for follow-up and counseling services.

Assessment

- Students actively participate in the UCP activity. Even though some students may decide to pass on one or more questions, as long as they are actively listening and following the ground rules, they are "actively participating."

Facilitating a UCP Session

- Facilitation is a skill that you can improve with practice.
- Silence is not a negative phenomenon. Silence often indicates that higher-level thinking is taking place.
- Going over ground rules at the beginning of each session is a needed and helpful technique to prevent inappropriate behavior.
- Unacceptable behavior should be stopped the moment it is recognized. To do this, pause the activity and point out the offense to the individual. For example, say, "What was just said is a put-down (or personal name), and it is not allowed in the circle discussion. Please do not do it again," or "Please do not talk to your neighbor when you should be listening to the one person who is supposed to be talking."
- If a student persists in breaking the activity's rules, talk to him one-on-one after class. Let the student know that if his behavior continues, he may not be able to participate in the future. This almost always stops the offensive behavior.
- Remind students of the information teachers *must* report if shared:
  1. If they are going to hurt themselves
  2. If they are going to hurt others
  3. If they are being abused

Possible UCP Sentence Stems: Pregnancy, Reproduction, and Parenting

1. At this instant, I feel . . .
2. Messages found in the media tell us that sex is . . .
3. You are ready to start a sexual relationship when . . .
4. You are ready to become a parent when . . .
5. At this point in my life, if I got pregnant or got someone pregnant, I would . . .
6. For teens who are sexually active, the best type of birth control is . . .
7. In my opinion, abortion . . .
8. Emergency contraception, or the morning-after pill, . . .
9. If I have kids someday, I will try to . . .
10. If I have kids someday, I will never . . .
11. The best thing parents or guardians can teach their kids is . . .
12. One thing I learned today is . . .

LESSON 15: HOME-SCHOOL CONNECTION

TALKING ABOUT PREGNANCY AND REPRODUCTION

Level: Middle school, High school

Time: Varies

National Health Education Standards

2. Analyzing Influences
5. Decision-Making

National Sexuality Education Standards: Performance Indicators

- Analyze factors that influence decisions about whether and when to become a parent.
- Assess the skills and resources needed to become a parent.

Rationale

Being a parent is one of life's most important jobs. All children deserve parents or guardians who are loving, caring, and nurturing. Communication with parents or guardians can help teens postpone becoming parents until they are more mature, responsible, and ready to handle the demanding roles of parenthood.

The main purpose of this Home-School Connection activity is to give teens and their parents or guardians the opportunity to privately discuss issues related to parenting.

After completing the assignment, parents or guardians are requested to sign on the bottom. All responses from teens and parents or guardians on the Home-School Connection activity will be kept confidential. It will not be turned in to the teacher or graded. On the due date, students will be asked to *voluntarily* share any interesting comments or insights they learned or observed by participating in the assignment. Students *and* parents or guardians can choose to pass on any discussion they wish to keep private.

With family input and support, the overall goal is to encourage teens to become well-informed, caring, respectful, and responsible adults.

Materials and Preparation

Copies of "Parent or Guardian Interview: Talking about Pregnancy and Reproduction" worksheet

Procedure

1. Explain to the class they are going to have an assignment to complete with one or more parents or guardians.
2. Hand out the Home-School Connection worksheet to each student and assign a due date.
3. On the day the assignment is due, check to see if students have completed the assignment by noting whether or not it was signed on the bottom. Do not collect or grade it. Explain that all students are required to complete the assignment, but are not required to share the information on the due date unless they voluntarily choose to do so.
4. Ask for student volunteers to share results of the discussions they had with the adult or adults they interviewed. This discussion should include asking the processing questions. Remind students that answers are voluntary and that no personal information needs to be shared.
5. Complete the discussion by having students participate in a class whip, using a specific sentence stem pertaining to the topic. Each student will quickly make one brief statement related to the activity, such as "I learned . . ." "I feel (or felt) . . ." or "I was surprised . . ."

Processing

1. Which family members did you choose to speak with?
2. How did you feel talking to family members about this topic? Were you comfortable with this discussion? Were the family members comfortable with this discussion?
3. What are some of the biggest changes the family members you talked to mentioned when they discussed becoming parents or guardians?
4. What did the family members you interviewed describe as the most rewarding part of being parents or guardians?
5. What did they say are some of the biggest challenges?
6. How did the parents or guardians you interviewed feel about the statement "Most teens are unprepared for the responsibility of becoming a parent"?
7. Did anything surprising come up during the conversation?
8. What did you learn from doing this assignment?
9. What did you learn from our follow-up class discussion?

Assessment

- Students bring completed and signed assignments to class.
- Students voluntarily participate in the follow-up discussion related to the assignment.
- Students participate in the class whip.

Parent or Guardian Interview: Talking about Pregnancy and Reproduction

Directions: Interview one or both parents or guardians and ask the questions that follow (they may pass on answering any question). Write brief answers.

1. When you first became a parent or guardian, what were the biggest changes in your life?

____

____

2. What do you think is the most rewarding part of being a parent or guardian?

____

____

3. What do you think is the most difficult part of being a parent or guardian?

____

____

4. What do you think are the most important personality traits a parent or guardian should display?

____

____

5. "Most teens are unprepared for the responsibility of becoming a parent." Explain whether you agree or disagree with this statement.

____

____

6. Parent-teen communication is sometimes difficult, especially when it comes to talking about sexual issues. What message would you like to give about what it means to be a responsible parent?

____

____

____

____

____

____

Parent or guardian signature(s): ______________________________

Student signature: ______________________________

5 Sexually Transmitted Infections and HIV

Sexually transmitted infections, or STIs, are transmitted from an infected person to an uninfected person through an exchange of bodily fluids, most often through sexual contact. Many STIs can also be transmitted from blood-to-blood contact and through the sharing of contaminated drug equipment.

In recent years, experts in the area of public health have suggested replacing the term "STD" with "STI." To many people this change in terminology is not an issue, and the terms tend to be used interchangeably. In the National Sexuality Education Standards, the term "sexually transmitted diseases" is used as one of the seven major topics areas. We, however, have chosen to use the term "sexuality transmitted infections." What terminology is used, though, does not matter. What *does* matter is students' being educated on STIs. This involves giving students accurate information about STIs, discussing attitudes and feelings about that information, and empowering students with the functional knowledge and skills they need to maintain their sexual health.

A number of activities in Chapter Five focus on the "need to know" functional knowledge that is developmentally appropriate for middle and high school students. Other activities stress the importance of the affective or "feeling" domain, and use stories, simulations, and values-clarification strategies. Life skills, such as accessing information, interpersonal communication, decision making, and self-management, are integrated and practiced throughout the lessons in this chapter.

Because information related to STIs and HIV is constantly changing, teachers are encouraged to stay up to date on the latest scientific research and effective teaching strategies. In addition, as with all sexuality education materials, educators need to check with state mandates and local guidelines on what is deemed appropriate to teach at different grade levels. Although concern about HIV/AIDS has led to more open discussions about safer sex, there may be resistance in some school districts to teaching about certain preventative measures, including condom use. A truly comprehensive human sexuality education curriculum includes activities that focus on reducing the risk of contracting STIs and HIV as well as abstinence.

Before implementing sexuality education lessons, especially when dealing with the topic of HIV/AIDS, please ensure that you have the support of school and district administrators, parents or guardians, and community members.

LESSON 1: TRANSMITTING STIs

Level: Middle school

Time: 40 minutes

National Health Education Standard

1. Core Concepts

National Sexuality Education Standards: Performance Indicators

- Define STIs, including HIV, and how they are and are not transmitted.
- Compare and contrast behaviors, including abstinence, to determine the potential risk of STI/HIV transmission from each.

Rationale

The risk for HIV among youth typically begins when they become sexually active or start using drugs. This lesson attempts to illustrate the rapid progression possible in transmitting HIV. Variations of this lesson have been used by health and sexuality educators for years to demonstrate this point. In the lesson, students will be moving around the room exchanging index cards with three different people, which will simulate exchanging bodily fluids that may transmit HIV.

Materials and Preparation

Front board with "HIV" and "AIDS" written on it

Index cards, one for each student. The cards should have lines on one side and be blank on the other, and should be set up in the following manner:

1. On the blank side of three index cards, in the bottom left-hand corner, print a small letter *H*.
2. On the blank side of two index cards, in the bottom left-hand corner, print a small letter *A*.
3. On the blank side of two index cards, in the bottom left-hand corner, print a small letter *C*.
4. As the class enters the room, make a mental note of the total number of students in the day's session. Subtract from that total the number seven, then count out the remaining number in blank index cards. These blank cards should then be mixed with the seven marked cards to complete the "deck" to be used for the lesson. (For example, if there are thirty students, the seven marked cards will be mixed in with twenty-three blank cards.)

Procedure

1. Begin the class by asking students to define what HIV and AIDS are (the human immunodeficiency virus [HIV] and acquired immune deficiency syndrome [AIDS]).
2. Next, place one index card with the lined side up on the desk of each student.
3. Instruct students to write their name in the top right-hand corner of the lined side of their card. Then instruct them to write "1" on the first line, "2" on the second line, and "3" on the third line.

4. Tell the students that when they hear the word "go," they should get up, walk around the room, and find someone to pair up with. (*Note:* If there is an uneven number of students, you can pair off with one of the students.)
5. Once students are paired off, say, "You will have one minute to discuss the differences between the human immunodeficiency virus (HIV) and acquired immune deficiency syndrome (AIDS) with your partner." After the time is up, instruct the students to sign each other's cards on the first line.
6. Next, instruct the students to take their original card and find a new partner. Explain that this time they will have one minute to discuss the different ways HIV is spread. When the time is up, they should sign each other's cards on the second line.
7. Finally, tell students to find a third partner. This time, explain that they will have one minute to discuss ways to prevent or reduce the spread of HIV. As they did with their first two partners, students should sign each other's cards on the third line. When this has been done, ask students to take their card and return to their seat.
8. Engage students in a discussion of the three topics they addressed with their partners, making sure to clarify any misinformation or answer any questions students may have.
9. Then tell students to turn over their index card. Ask them to look for a small letter *H* in the bottom left-hand corner. Ask the students who have an *H* on their card (there should be three of them) to stand up. Ask the students what they think the *H* stands for. (It stands for HIV positive.)
10. Explain to the class that they should imagine that the three students who had an *H* on their card were infected with HIV. Tell the students to pretend that instead of signing other students' cards, they engaged in sexual contact with them. Ask that any students who had their card signed by a person who is standing (has an *H* on his card) also to stand up, because they may now be HIV positive.
11. Say to the class, "If anyone still sitting had his or her card signed by anyone who is *now* standing, please stand at this time." Explain that they need to stand because they, too, *may* have become HIV positive.
12. Continue with this process. Generally, most students in the class will be standing in the end. Stress that only three people were infected at the start of the exercise, yet virtually the entire class may have become infected by the end of the activity.
13. At this point, ask the students to once again look at the back of their card, and tell the two students who have the letter *C* on their card to raise their hand. Ask students to guess what the *C* stands for. (It stands for having used a condom properly.) The two students with a *C* on their card may sit down because in this simulated exercise, they used a condom correctly when they had contact with their partners.

    Note: Because the people who used condoms properly may not have been infected, the people they came in contact with may also have avoided becoming infected. It may also be possible that some people standing may not have become infected, depending on the *order* in which the names are listed on their card. Explain this concept to the class. Also, state that the use of condoms is often referred to as "safer sex," because using condoms can reduce, but not eliminate, the risk of getting HIV.

14. Now ask the students to once again look at the back of their card. There should be two students with the letter *A* on their card. Ask students to guess what the *A* stands for. (It stands for abstinence.) The two students with an *A* on their card may sit down because they abstained from sexual contact and prevented the spread of HIV. In this exercise, if a person had her card signed by one of these two students, she was not at risk of contracting HIV from either of them. However, if this person had exchanged cards with someone else who was infected, she might have become infected.
15. Involve the class in a discussion of the activity by asking the processing questions.
16. Give the homework assignment, based on the activity done in class. For homework, students are to write an essay of at least fifty words discussing three or more ways to avoid or reduce the risk of getting HIV or other sexually transmitted infections. They are also to explain how each of these ways reduces the risk of contracting an STI.

    Possible answers for this homework assignment include

    - Practicing abstinence
    - Using condoms correctly and consistently
    - Being in a faithful, monogamous relationship
    - Not sharing drug equipment or having sexual contact with anyone who has shared drug equipment
    - Avoiding sexual contact with multiple partners
    - Not engaging in sexual contact while under the influence of alcohol or other drugs

Processing

1. Why were most students standing up by the end of the activity?
2. Was it possible to tell who had an *H* on their card? Is it possible in real life to tell if someone is HIV positive?
3. Discuss this statement: "When you have unprotected sex with someone, it's like having sex with anyone he or she has ever had sex with."
4. What does the word "monogamous" mean? (It means being faithful and committed to only one partner.) Why do people in a monogamous relationship have a decreased risk of contracting an STI?
5. Do condoms eliminate the risk of contracting HIV? Explain. (Condoms' efficiency lessens if they are expired, break, or are used incorrectly or inconsistently.)
6. Does abstinence eliminate the risk of contracting HIV? Explain.
7. How did it feel to imagine you might have contracted HIV?

Assessment

- Students participate in the class activity and follow-up discussion.
- Students complete the homework assignment.

LESSON 2: STI SCENARIOS—MAKING HEALTHY DECISIONS

Level: Middle school, High school

Time: 40 minutes

National Health Education Standards

1. Core Concepts
2. Analyzing Influences
3. Accessing Information
5. Decision-Making

National Sexuality Education Standards: Performance Indicators

- Describe the signs, symptoms and potential impacts of STIs, including HIV.
- Analyze the impact of alcohol and other drugs on safer sexual decision-making and sexual behaviors.
- Identify local STI and HIV testing and treatment resources.
- Apply a decision-making model to choices about safer sex practices, including abstinence and condoms.

Rationale

All people, regardless of sexual orientation or age, can become infected with an STI if they are involved in behaviors that put them at risk. In this lesson, students will examine scenarios involving sexually transmitted infections. This includes accessing accurate information related to each scenario, and then applying a decision-making model to each.

Materials and Preparation

Teacher copy of "STI scenarios," cut into nine separate sections

Copies of "Decision-Making Guide" worksheet (one per group)

Resource materials, such as health texts, brochures, or websites

Procedure

1. Divide the class into nine groups.
2. Provide each group with a different slip describing one of the STI scenarios.
3. Give each group a copy of the "Decision-Making Guide" worksheet.
4. Explain that as a group, students will read the scenario and brainstorm how to complete their worksheet. For each group, ask one student to be the recorder and two other students to be the spokespeople.
5. Remind the groups that although there may be many alternatives, they are to attempt to come up with the *most health-enhancing decision* in response to their scenario.

6. Allow students to use resources (texts, brochures, and websites) to assist them in making the best, most health-enhancing decision as they complete the "Decision-Making Guide" worksheet. Give groups fifteen minutes to complete the worksheet.
7. When the fifteen minutes are up, have the spokespeople from the first group (Scenario 1) read their scenario. They should then go through the steps in the decision-making process, discussing how group members came to their decision.
8. Ask if there was any disagreement among group members on any steps in the decision-making process. If there was a disagreement, afford any individuals in the group the opportunity to express differing points of view as well as their reasoning.
9. Open up the discussion to the class. Survey the class to determine if they felt the decision that the first group made was the most health enhancing. Ask, "Were there any other options or alternatives that could have also been considered healthy decisions?"
10. After the first group's scenario and decision have been discussed, move on to the other groups and follow the same steps.
11. After all groups have spoken, ask the processing questions. Conclude with the point that the need to practice safer sex applies to *all* people, regardless of gender identity or sexual orientation.

Processing

1. How common do you think the provided scenarios are in real life?
2. How often are these scenarios shown in the media? Explain.
3. Some of the scenarios did not involve exclusively heterosexual couples. *Some* involved lesbian couples, gay couples, or bisexual couples. Which messages or decisions were similar for both lesbian, gay, and bisexual couples and heterosexual couples? What messages or decisions were different? Explain.
4. What local resources exist for teenagers to obtain sexual health information?
5. When a teenager goes to a clinic or doctor about his or her sexual health, will his or her parents or guardians find out?

   Note: There are many federal and state laws and regulations related to teens and sexual health. These laws vary from state to state and occasionally from county to county within the same state. Information on access to confidential health services in your area may be found on either of the following websites:

   - Advocates for Youth, www.advocatesforyouth.org
   - Planned Parenthood, www.plannedparenthood.org

Assessment

- Students participate in the group decision-making scenarios and follow-up discussion, with each group providing correct information pertaining to the assigned scenario.

STI Scenarios

Scenario 1

Jessica went to a party at the house of her best friend, whose parents were away for the weekend. She met this guy, and they started talking. He asked if she wanted a beer, but Jessica said that she does not drink alcohol or do other drugs. He offered to get her a soda, and she said "yes." The next morning Jessica woke up undressed in one of the upstairs bedrooms. She felt confused and did not remember anything from the night before. What should Jessica do?

Scenario 2

Sasha and Tiffany are juniors in college. They have been in a monogamous relationship for six months. One weekend when Sasha was away, Tiffany met a former friend, Blake, at a party. They wound up having oral sex. A few weeks later, Tiffany got a call from Blake saying he found some small growths on his genitals. After seeing a doctor, Blake was diagnosed with genital warts (HPV). Blake suggested that Tiffany go to a doctor to get tested. Tiffany has not noticed any symptoms, and has not said anything to Sasha. What should Tiffany do?

Scenario 3

Rick has had unprotected sex with three different girls in the last year. Three months ago, he noticed blisters on his penis. He was diagnosed as having genital herpes. Since his diagnosis, he has been abstinent. He recently started dating a girl that he really likes. What should Rick do?

Scenario 4

Alex and Pat have not had intercourse, but have engaged in oral sex. Alex had had several sexual partners before meeting Pat. Pat had been abstinent from all types of sexual contact prior to meeting Alex. Pat is worried about getting an STI from oral sex and wants them both to get tested. Alex says you cannot get an STI just from oral sex. What should Pat do?

Scenario 5

Maria is fifteen and has been going out with a guy who is nineteen. She thinks she might have an STI. She talked to Angela, her eighteen-year-old sister, about her concerns. Maria does not know where to go to get tested. She also does not want her parents to find out she got tested. What should Maria do?

STI Scenarios (*continued*)

Scenario 6

Last month, Han went to a fraternity party, got drunk, and had unprotected sex with a girl he'd just met named Heather. There is a rumor going around campus that Heather uses drugs and is HIV positive. What should Han do?

Scenario 7

In his high school health class, Tom was only taught about "abstinence until marriage," and never discussed condoms or safer sex. He signed a pledge to stay abstinent until he got married. When he got to college, however, he fell in love with Kristen, and decided it would be okay to have sex because they were in love. Kristen said that he should use a condom because she was not on the pill. Tom never learned the proper way to use a condom, but is embarrassed to admit it. What should Tom do?

Scenario 8

At the age of seventeen, Bob confided in his parents that he is gay. He has a boyfriend, but they are not "exclusive." Bob's parents know that gay men are at a higher risk for contracting HIV than any other group. They want to discuss safer sex with him, but do not know how to start this conversation. They love him very much and want him to be happy—and safe. What should they do?

Scenario 9

Cindy's boyfriend told her he has chlamydia, but she does not know what this means. He told her it is one of the most common STIs around. When he noticed a discharge from his penis and burning when he urinated, he thought he might have gonorrhea. But when he got tested, it came back positive for chlamydia. The doctor told him he was fortunate, because most men and very few women actually show symptoms. His doctor also said that if chlamydia is untreated it can be serious. Cindy and her boyfriend have had unprotected sex. What should they do?

Names: ____

____

Decision-Making Guide

1. Clearly state the decision to be made.

____

____

____

____

2. List the possible choices or alternatives involved in your decision.

____

____

____

____

3. Consider the short- and long-term consequences (advantages and disadvantages) of each choice.

____

____

____

____

4. Make a decision, and list your reasons for your choice.

____

____

____

____

5. Evaluate your decision.

____

____

____

____

LESSON 3: DEAR DR. SPLENDID SIMULATED STI INFORMATION WEBSITE

Level: Middle school

Time: Two 40-minute sessions

National Health Education Standards

1. Core Concepts
3. Accessing Information
4. Interpersonal Communication

National Sexuality Education Standards: Performance Indicators

- Describe the signs, symptoms and potential impacts of STIs, including HIV.
- Compare and contrast behaviors, including abstinence, to determine the potential risk of STI/HIV transmission from each.
- Identify medically-accurate information about STIs, including HIV.
- Demonstrate the use of effective communication skills to reduce or eliminate risk for STIs, including HIV.

Rationale

This lesson allows students to become "health experts" by responding to questions about STIs. Using age-appropriate classroom or Internet resources, students will share correct information and advocate for healthy decision making. In addition, students will be asked to perform a brief skit reinforcing the correct information and skill development from their original response.

Materials and Preparation

Copies of "Guidelines for Accessing Reliable Health Information and Services" handout

Brochures, pamphlets, or websites containing information about local, state, and national resources on STIs

Copies of "Dear Dr. Splendid Group Worksheet" (one per group)

Teacher copy of "Sample E-mail Questions," cut into six pieces

Procedure

ACTIVITY 1: DAY 1—ACCESSING RELIABLE HEALTH INFORMATION AND SERVICES

1. Begin the lesson by distributing the "Guidelines for Accessing Reliable Health Information and Services" handout to each student. Depending on prior student knowledge and discussion, it should take approximately ten minutes to review the information on the handout.

2. Divide the class into six small groups.
3. Explain to the students that they will be involved in a small group activity in which they are "health experts" working for a website, responding to e-mails sent to Dr.Splendid@STIs.org. Explain that Dr. Splendid is an imaginary, internationally known expert on STIs with several medical degrees. He started his nonprofit website to address the many questions teens have about STIs. As hired health experts, students will write a meaningful response to a realistic problem submitted to Dr. Splendid.
4. Each group's goal is to properly answer one of the six e-mails received at Dr. Splendid's website, finding their answer in the pamphlets, brochures, and websites (if available) provided for the class.
5. Hand out the "Dear Dr. Splendid Group Worksheet" and a slip of paper with a different e-mail question to each group. Group members should place their names and the number of the e-mail they will be researching at the top of the page. Read the directions on the worksheet along with the class. Ask the groups if they have any questions and clarify as necessary.
6. Give groups twenty minutes to research the correct information and advice to give, and to compose a written response. Each group should designate one person to write the response and another person to read it. All group members should participate in researching and formulating the group's answer.
7. Once the response to the e-mail has been written, each group should use the remainder of the period to create a very brief skit related to their scenario, which they will present during the next class. The skit should be one to two minutes in length, provide accurate information, have a positive or healthy message or theme, and demonstrate at least one of the following skills: healthy decision making or accessing reliable information.

ACTIVITY 2: DAY 2—DEAR DR. SPLENDID GROUP ANSWERS AND SKITS

1. Give students the first five to ten minutes of class to reconvene their group, finalize their answer, assign roles, and practice their brief skit.
2. When ready, have each group read their assigned e-mail to Dr. Splendid, along with their reply. Your role is to clarify and correct all information during presentations.
3. Groups will then take turns acting out their skits. The class will offer a critique of the information and skill development illustrated as part of an overall discussion following each skit. For each skit, the class discussion and evaluation should focus on the following:
   a. Did the skit illustrate the skill of accessing accurate information related to the group question and scenario?
   b. Did the skit have a positive or healthy message?
   c. Did the skit illustrate healthy decision making?
4. Conclude the lesson by asking the processing questions.

   Note: If none of the groups' responses or skits included an HIV testing site in their region, refer students to http://HIVtest.cdc.gov. It is also possible to use a cell phone to find a local testing site simply by texting their local five-digit zip code to KNOWIT (566948).

Processing

1. What did you know about the STI that your group was assigned *before* researching the correct information in your group?
2. What did you learn about your assigned STI *after* researching in your group and performing in your skit?
3. Based on the information you learned from the other groups, which of the STIs are most common for teens and young adults? (Chlamydia, HPV, and herpes)
4. Which of the STIs do you feel are the most serious? Explain your answer.
5. What did you learn about accessing reliable information? How can you tell if a website is reliable? What are some things to look for that might indicate that a website is *not* reliable?
6. How would you complete the following sentence? "If I thought I might have contracted an STI, I would . . . because . . ."

Assessment

- Students participate in group research and the formulation of their group's response.
- Groups meet all requirements on their worksheet for composing their response, and the response is accurate.
- Groups present their skit, with feedback provided from peers and the teacher.

Guidelines for Accessing Reliable Health Information and Services

Knowing how to find correct health information and how to choose a health-related product or service is an important health skill. Knowing how to access health information can better prepare you to make healthy choices. When trying to determine whether health information is reliable or not, it is important to check the validity of the source. For example, Joe Shmo might have a website called justlikesteroidsbutsafe.com. This is probably a business that sells nutritional supplements that may be of questionable value.

Reliable sources of information generally include

- Parents or guardians, counselors, and other trusted adults
- Newspaper or magazine articles by health professionals or experts
- Library sources, such as science books, encyclopedias, or consumer or medical newsletters

The following guidelines should help you determine whether your sources of information from the **Internet** are credible:

- URLs ending in .com are usually from commercial businesses that provide a service or are selling something. They **may** or **may not** be accurate and credible.
- URLs that end in .org are usually from community organizations, such as the American Cancer Society.
- URLs that end in .gov are from government agencies.
- URLs that end in .edu are from colleges or other educational institutions.

These designations can sometimes provide you with clues as to the validity of the site. Because .com sites are generally trying to sell something, they may not always be reliable. **Websites that end in .org, .gov, and .edu tend to be more reliable.**

The date the website was created or revised can tell you how up to date it is. Information about the author of the site can also give you clues about the validity of the information. By typing in the author's name in a search engine (sometimes referred to as "googling someone"), you can often find out more background information about this individual. Finding out who is providing the information is probably the most important part of evaluating a site's validity.

It is also good practice to use at least **two** sources when accessing health information. If the information from both sources is in agreement, it is an indication that the sources are reliable.

Names: ____

____

Question number: ____________________

Dear Dr. Splendid Group Worksheet

Directions: Your group's task is to properly answer one of the many e-mails received at Dr. Splendid's website. Answers can be found in the pamphlets, brochures, and websites provided for the class.

Your group should read and respond to the e-mail sent to Dr. Splendid. Your reply should

- Be a minimum of one hundred words
- Include accurate, up-to-date information that directly answers the question or addresses the problem
- Stress that most young adolescents do not engage in risky sexual behaviors
- Include how the STI involved can be prevented, treated, or cured
- Use communication skills to persuade the individual who wrote the question to act in ways that will promote his or her health and the health of others
- Include at least one local, state, or national resource that this person can contact for additional information

Your group will have twenty minutes to research the correct information and advice and compose a written response. Each group should designate one person to write the response and another person who will read the response to the class during the next class session. All group members should participate in researching and formulating the reply. You may continue on the next sheet to reply to the person who sent the e-mail to Dr. Splendid.

Dear ______________________,

____

____

____

____

____

____

____

(*continued*)

Names: ____

____

Question number: ____________________

Dear Dr. Splendid Group Worksheet (*continued*)

Sample E-mail Questions

Question 1

To: DrSplendid@STIs.org

I am in eighth grade and a virgin. My friend has been going out with a tenth grader, and he has been trying to get her to have sex. I heard a rumor that he has used needles to shoot heroin. My friend says she thinks she will probably have sex, because most teenagers are having sex anyway.

I am afraid that she might be putting herself at risk for AIDS. She is a good friend, but she has been hanging out with a different crowd.

My question is . . . Can she get AIDS from him? If I cannot talk her out of having sex, is there anything she can do to reduce her risk? What can I say or do to help her?

Signed,

ScaredSuzie@aol.com

Question 2

To: DrSplendid@STIs.org

I read something in the newspaper about herpes. The article claimed it was a sexually transmitted infection, but I thought it was a cold sore that people got around their mouth. I presently have a cold sore on my lip. Does this mean I have herpes? Could you clear this up for me? How did I get it? How long will it last? Can it be cured? Should I see a doctor? By the way, I am fifteen and have never had any type of sex. Help!!

Signed,

ConfusedKyle@optonline.net

Question 3

To: DrSplendid@STIs.org

My friend says he has "crabs." He claims he got it from a toilet seat or from towels that he shared at his gym. My other friend said this is not true; that you can only get crabs from having sex. Who is right? I do not even know what crabs are. I kind of heard that you get them from sex, but I do not really know. My friend has tried using soap and water in the shower, but he still itches like crazy. What should he do?

Signed,

CrablessChris@aol.com

(continued)

Sample E-mail Questions (*continued*)

Question 4

To: DrSplendid@STIs.org

I had sex with a guy about a month ago. I went to a party and got a little drunk, and . . . well . . . you know . . . it just happened. Today I got a call from him telling me that he has something called chlamydia. I do not know anything about it. I never even heard of it before. I feel fine and do not have any symptoms, but he says I should still get a checkup. He was the first guy that I ever had sex with, so I am pretty sure I am okay. But I thought I would check with you just to be sure. What is this "chlamydia" stuff anyway, and what should I do?

Signed,

NervousNellie@comcast.net

Question 5

To: DrSplendid@STIs.org

My partner and I have been going out for about a month. The other day we were arguing about what abstinence means. I think it means not having sexual intercourse. She thinks it also means not having oral sex. I told her there is no way she can get any diseases just from oral sex, and she says that is not true.

We make out and do other stuff, but to this point it has always been with our clothes on! I respect her and would never force her to do something that she is not comfortable with, but I am ready to take it to the next level. So I guess my question is, Is oral sex safe? And if that's all you're doing, is it still considered abstinence?

Signed,

TestingTaylor@aol.com

Question 6

To: DrSplendid@STIs.org

On spring break last month, my older sister went to Florida and had a really good time, if you know what I mean! One night she got stoned on pot and had sex with some guy she did not even know. She said he looked clean so they did not use a condom. Anyway, she said she has these small bumpy things around her vagina—they look like warts! She is grossed out because they are really nasty looking and are starting to itch. I had a wart on my foot last year and used some stuff from the drugstore that made it fall off. She asked me if she could treat these the same way. What do you think?

Signed,

Worriedaboutwarts@comcast.net

LESSON 4: BODILY FLUIDS—HOW YOU CAN AND CANNOT SPREAD HIV

Level: Middle school, High school

Time: 40 minutes

National Health Education Standards

1. Core Concepts
2. Analyzing Influences

National Sexuality Education Standards: Performance Indicators

- Define STIs, including HIV, and how they are and are not transmitted.
- Evaluate the effectiveness of abstinence, condoms and other safer sex methods in preventing the spread of STIs, including HIV.
- Analyze factors that may influence condom use and other safer sex decisions.

Rationale

Although HIV/AIDS has been around since the 1980s (and possibly earlier), myths about the human immunodeficiency virus and how it is passed still exist. The objective of this lesson is to distinguish myths from facts in regard to the transmission of HIV.

One activity will demonstrate which bodily fluids can and cannot spread the virus. A second activity will allow students to simulate an exchange of bodily fluids to observe how the sharing of saliva can lead to colds and flu, but not HIV.

Materials and Preparation

Ten index cards. On each card, write one of the bodily fluids listed here in large letters with a marker:

Blood	Semen	Breast milk	Saliva	Cough droplets
Tears	Sweat	Vaginal fluids	Sneeze droplets	Urine

Three small, clear plastic cups

Bottled water, enough to half-fill the three plastic cups

Procedure

ACTIVITY 1: HIV TRANSMISSION AND BODILY FLUIDS

1. State to students: "There are many myths about how HIV can and cannot be transmitted from one person to another. The reality is that HIV is a virus that cannot live outside the body and dies quickly when exposed to the air. The virus is found in certain bodily fluids. Some bodily fluids can transmit the virus, and others cannot."

2. Ask for ten volunteers. Each volunteer will be given one of the cards with a bodily fluid written on it and should stand in the front of the room, facing the class.
3. Have one of the students step forward. Ask the class if the bodily fluid written on the student's index card can transmit HIV. Allow students to explain why (or how). If there is any disagreement, or if students are unsure, you should explain the correct answer.
4. If it is determined that a bodily fluid *can* transmit HIV, the student with that card should remain at the front of the room. If the fluid *cannot* transmit HIV, that student should hand her card to you and take a seat. Continue this process with each of the ten students.
5. At the conclusion of the activity, there should be only four students left in front of the room. Their cards will read: "Blood," "Semen," "Vaginal fluids," and "Breast milk." Explain that although things like coughing and sneezing may cause the spread of other infections, like colds and flu, they cannot spread HIV.
6. Explain the following concept:

   HIV cannot be spread if an infected person sneezes or coughs near someone else. Although HIV can be an extremely dangerous virus, it is also a very fragile virus. It takes very specific types of behaviors to transmit the virus from one person to another. Those behaviors involve direct sexual contact (vaginal, anal, or oral), whereby the infected fluid is spread from one person to another. Sharing needles is also a risky practice because a small amount of blood stays in the hollow core of the needle and is not exposed to air. If a person with HIV uses a needle to shoot heroin, steroids, or other drugs, the small amount of blood that remains in the needle may contain HIV. The virus can then be passed on to anyone else who shares that needle or potentially other types of drug equipment with the already infected user.

   The transmission of HIV from an HIV-positive mother to her child during pregnancy, labor, delivery, or breastfeeding is called mother-to-child transmission. With early detection, an HIV-positive mother may be given medications that greatly reduce the risk of transmission. Because of this early intervention, risk of giving birth to an HIV-positive baby is less than 5 percent in the United States. In Africa and other areas of the world where access to early diagnosis and treatment is not readily available, many thousands of babies are born HIV positive each year.

7. Allow the remaining students to return to their seat.

ACTIVITY 2: "SWAPPING SPIT"

1. Fill three clear plastic cups halfway with bottled water. (Students can watch you do this.)
2. Ask for three volunteers. Give each of them one of the plastic glasses.
3. Now say: "As you see, this cup is filled with plain water from the original water bottle. Would you all be willing to take a sip of the water and swallow it?" If volunteers agree, have them take a sip. If a volunteer does not agree, he does not have to take a sip.

4. Then ask: "Now, would you be willing to take another sip, swish it around in your mouth, and then spit it back into your glass?" Again, if they agree, they should do so. If they do not agree, they can abstain.
5. Continue with, "Now, are you willing to take another sip of water from your glass and swallow it? If yes, please do so. If not, you can abstain." If they agree, they can do so.
6. At this point, take the glasses and exchange water from one glass into another, mix up the glasses, and hand them back.
7. Say: "Now, **I do not want you to do this!** However, would any of you be willing to drink out of the glass you have now?"

   Note: Almost all students will decline. If a student is actually willing to drink from the glass, **do not allow this.**
8. Ask students why they would not drink out of the glass. ("It's got germs!" "It's gross!")
9. So that students will come to understand how people who think they are being safe might not actually be safe, ask the processing questions.
10. Explain further for those who *do* choose to engage in sexual behaviors that when there may be an exchange of bodily fluids, they can reduce their risk by using condoms. Condoms provide a barrier to help prevent bodily fluids from spreading from one person to another. They are not 100 percent effective, but using them consistently and correctly greatly reduces the risk. Regarding drug use, remind students that sharing drug equipment is a very dangerous practice and poses a high risk of contracting many infections, including HIV.
11. Bring closure to the lesson by summarizing both activities: "We have demonstrated how certain behaviors (for example: coughing, sneezing) can spread illnesses like colds and flu. However, HIV can only be spread by direct contact with infected blood, semen, vaginal fluids, and breast milk. Condoms may reduce the risk, and using them is referred to as practicing 'safer sex.' The only 'safe sex' is no sex, or sexual abstinence. For most teens, waiting to have sex until they are older, more mature, and more responsible is the safest, healthiest choice."
12. Give the following homework assignment to the class (students must answer all parts of the question to get credit for the assignment): "Many teens feel pressure to have sex before they are ready. Describe one internal (attitudes, values, religious beliefs) and one external (peers, TV, movies, music, the Internet) factor that may influence or pressure a young person to become sexually active before he or she is ready. Explain how each factor could cause a teenager to make a decision about sex that may put him or her at risk for a sexually transmitted infection."

    Possible answers include

    - Seeing celebrities on TV or in movies who are sexually active. The answer should include a specific example of a particular person, TV show, or movie.
    - Being pressured by a boyfriend or girlfriend to be sexually active.
    - Knowing peers who are sexually active or who encourage sexual activity.
    - Being teased by peers about not being sexually active.
    - Having curiosity about being—or the desire to be—sexually active.

Processing

1. How do the different forms of sex (oral, anal, and vaginal) allow HIV to be passed? (HIV transmission involves the exchange of certain bodily fluids—blood, semen, vaginal fluids, and breast milk. Although saliva does not transmit HIV, if these other fluids get into the mouth [during oral sex, for example], it may be possible to transmit HIV in this way. Any open sores or cuts in the mouth increase the risk.)
2. When you were first told to take a sip of water, you assumed it was safe to drink it. How do you know that I did not use the leftover fluids from the last class that did this activity?
3. Do you think people are always honest when talking about past sexual partners? Explain.
4. Why are teens advised *not* to engage in sexual activity? (The decision to engage in sexual activity is a big one and should not be taken lightly. Abstaining from sex, especially for young teens, is the safest decision. If a person does not share drug equipment or chooses not to have vaginal, anal, or oral sex, that individual does not have to worry about getting a sexually transmitted infection.)

Assessment

- As part of the class discussion, students note medically accurate information about HIV and forms of transmission.
- Students complete the additional homework assignment.

LESSON 5: STIs AND HIV— WHAT I KNOW, WHAT I WANT TO KNOW, WHAT I LEARNED

Level: Middle school

Time: 20–30 minutes

National Health Education Standards

1. Core Concepts
4. Interpersonal Communication

National Sexuality Education Standards: Performance Indicators

- Define STIs, including HIV, and how they are and are not transmitted.
- Demonstrate the use of effective communication skills to reduce or eliminate risk for STIs, including HIV.

Rationale

The objective of this lesson is to determine what students already know, or think they know, about sexually transmitted infections, including HIV. This lesson can be used at the beginning of a unit to separate myths from facts.

Materials and Preparation

Soft "sponge-type" ball or beanbag

Copies of "HIV/AIDS and Other STIs" worksheet

Procedure

1. Explain to the class that the objective of the day's activity is to find out what they already *know* (or think they know) or *want to know* about sexually transmitted infections, or STIs. Students may have also heard STIs being referred to as sexually transmitted diseases, or STDs.
2. On the front board, write "STIs, Including HIV" as a heading. Below that, write three headings, with vertical lines to form columns: "What I Know," "What I Want to Know," and "What I Learned."
3. Ask students each to move their desk so all students can form a large circle in the center of the room while standing. Join the circle to demonstrate how the activity will work, holding the soft ball (or beanbag).

4. Give the following directions:

   We are about to begin to explore the topic of sexually transmitted infections, including HIV and AIDS, by finding out what people in this class have heard about them. We will also find out what you would *like* to know, and hear any questions you may have about HIV or other STIs.

   As you can see, I have a soft ball in my hand. What I am going to do is say my name, then gently toss the ball underhand to someone else in the circle. After I toss the ball, I will fold my arms across my chest, indicating that I have already gone. No one should toss the ball to someone whose arms are crossed.

   The second person will catch the ball (ideally) and then say her name. Please remember to whom you tossed the ball and that person's name. This is very important. The second person will then toss the ball to anyone on the circle, remember to whom she tossed it and that person's name, and fold her arms across her chest.

   The game will continue until everyone has gone. When the last person has caught the ball and said his name, he will toss the ball back to me.

5. After everyone has gone, give the following instructions for the second time around: "The second time around, the same order should be followed—you will toss the ball to the same person and receive it from the same person. This time, however, instead of saying *your* name when you have the ball, you will call out the name of the person you tossed the ball to the first time around, tossing the ball to that person. Because you should know to whom you are supposed to toss the ball, you do not have to fold your arms after you toss the ball."
6. Continue around the circle until everyone has gone and the ball gets back to you. (At this point, step outside the circle and go to the front of the room to act as recorder.)
7. Explain that the third time around, again following the same order and starting with the first student, students will continue to toss the ball. This time, students should take turns stating one thing they *know* or *want to know* about STIs. It could be something they have heard from others, seen on TV, read about, learned in school, and so on. If a student is not sure about something, that is okay. The point of this activity is to separate myths from facts in regard to infections that can be spread by sexual contact. If students are having difficulty coming up with something to say, they can repeat a statement or question that has already been mentioned. For example, if a student says, "I want to know if the sores you get on your mouth are herpes," and another student has the same question, the second student can then say, "I also want to know if the sores on your mouth are herpes."
8. While students are verbalizing their comments or questions, you should record all statements under the first column ("What I Know") or the second column ("What I Want to Know"). Once the ball has gone all the way around the circle, students will have a chance to make additional statements or ask additional questions by raising their hand and having the ball tossed to them. You should continue to record facts and questions under the appropriate column.
9. When all statements and questions have been verbalized, have students return to their seat. Distribute the "HIV/AIDS and Other STIs" worksheet to each student.

10. Refer to the front board, starting with the first column, "What I Know." Read the first statement and allow students to discuss whether or not they believe the statement is accurate. If you confirm that it is accurate, ask them to write it down in that column on their worksheet. If it is a myth or an incorrect statement, students will not write it down, and it will be erased from the board. Continue this process with all statements from the first column.
11. Move on to the second column, "What I Want to Know." Start off by asking if anyone in the class thinks she knows the answer to the first question. Discuss possible answers. You can clarify any information, and then have students write in the correct answer in the appropriate column on their worksheet. Continue this process for all the questions in the second column.
12. Move on to the third column, "What I Learned." For this column, go around the room in a "class whip," having students state one thing they learned about STIs, including HIV/AIDS. After verifying that these statements are correct, record them on the board, and ask students to copy them down on their worksheet.
13. Conclude the activity by asking the processing questions.

Processing

1. Why is knowing the correct information about STIs important for teens and adults?
2. There is a lot of misinformation about HIV, AIDS, and other STIs. Why do you think this is so?
3. Were you surprised about anything that you learned today? If so, what was it?

Assessment

- Students actively participate in the ball toss.
- Students are involved in the discussion of the worksheet, including the class whip.

Name: ______________________________

HIV/AIDS and Other STIs

What I Know	What I Want to Know	What I Learned

LESSON 6: TEN WISHES FOR YOUR FUTURE
HOW HIV CAN CHANGE YOUR LIFE

Level: Middle school

Time: 30 minutes

National Health Education Standards

1. Core Concepts
3. Accessing Information
4. Interpersonal Communication
6. Goal Setting

National Sexuality Education Standards: Performance Indicators

- Describe the signs, symptoms and potential impacts of STIs, including HIV.
- Identify medically-accurate information about STIs, including HIV.
- Demonstrate the use of effective communication skills to reduce or eliminate risk for STIs, including HIV.
- Develop a plan to eliminate or reduce risk for STIs, including HIV.

Rationale

The objective of this lesson is to have students describe what they *wish* their future would be like, and compare that with what their future might be like if they contracted HIV.

Note: Students should have had some introductory lessons on HIV, including instruction on how it is transmitted; how to reduce the risk of contracting the virus; the short- and long-term effects of HIV on one's immune system and overall health; and treatment options. It is also important to stress in this lesson the physical, mental, emotional, social, and spiritual impact that being HIV positive might have on their lives.

Materials and Preparation

Copies of "Ten Wishes for Your Future" worksheet

Scrap paper for students' replies to the concluding question

Guest speaker from a local organization who will discuss how being HIV positive has an impact on one's personal life (optional)

Procedure

ACTIVITY 1: TEN WISHES

1. Distribute the "Ten Wishes for Your Future" worksheet to all students. Allow approximately five to seven minutes for students to complete the first section.
2. When students are done, have students volunteer to share some of the items on their list. Make note of some of the items most students have in common.
3. After a brief discussion, explain that students are going to imagine one change to their lives: that they are HIV positive. Ask students to refer back to their original list and make necessary adjustments based on the impact that HIV could have on them physically, mentally, emotionally, and socially. Again, allow approximately five to seven minutes for the completion of this part of the activity.
4. Ask for volunteers to share what items on their first list are *still* on their HIV-positive list. Then ask which items from their first list are *not* on their HIV-positive list.
5. Interject factual information to clarify how HIV might have an impact on their lives, especially in regard to their physical, mental, emotional, social, and spiritual health; dating; having children; and any future goals.
6. Ask students to complete the remainder of the worksheet. They should list some ways that their parents or guardians and peers would react to the news of their being HIV positive.
7. Continue the discussion by asking the processing questions.

ACTIVITY 2: ROLE-PLAY ABOUT BEING HIV POSITIVE

1. Ask for two students to volunteer to be in a brief role-play: Student A is HIV positive, and Student B is the potential new boyfriend or girlfriend.
2. Read the following scenario:

   You are HIV positive, are currently on medication, and show no outward signs of being infected. You meet someone and decide to go on a date. The first date goes well, but there is no physical contact. You agree to go out again, have a good time, and realize that you really like this person.

   Here is your dilemma: your new friend calls and asks you to come over for dinner. Your friend mentions that no one else will be around, and it will give you both some time to "be alone."

   You decide to go, but are determined to reveal your HIV status to this person before the relationship goes any further.

   The night of the dinner invitation arrives. After a nice dinner and friendly conversation, you both sit on the couch. Your new friend leans over and kisses you.

   What do you do?

3. Ask the volunteers to act out the conversation the person who is HIV positive (Student A) might have with the potential new boyfriend or girlfriend (Student B).
4. Then have a class discussion on the outcome of the role-play. Was it realistic? What were the options for the person who is HIV positive? Would other students in the class have enacted this scenario differently?

5. End the lesson by having students anonymously answer the following question on scrap paper, which will be collected as they leave the classroom: "Why is it important for someone to reveal his or her HIV status before starting a sexual relationship?"
6. As an optional additional activity, invite someone who is HIV positive to speak to the class. Planned Parenthood or another local HIV support service agency may know of volunteers who are willing to share their personal story with students. Such speakers often have a very powerful and long-lasting effect on their audience.

   Note: Each school district has its own approval process for bringing in guest speakers. Check with your administration before having any guest speakers come to your school and classroom.

Processing

1. What emotions would the people in your life possibly feel if you were HIV positive? Who would be supportive?
2. Do you believe your friends would feel the same way about you? Why or why not?
3. How would it affect your present relationships? Would it affect your plans for getting married or being in a long-term relationship? Having children? Finances?
4. If you met a potential long-term partner, when would you tell him or her about your HIV status? On the first date? Once you got "serious"? Before you had sex for the first time?
5. Contracting HIV can have an impact on your short- and long-term goals in life. What are three ways that you can eliminate or reduce your risk of contracting STIs, including HIV?

Assessment

- Students complete the "Ten Wishes for Your Future" worksheet and actively participate in the follow-up discussion.
- Students observe the role-play and participate in the class discussion.
- Students provide anonymous answers to the final question.

Name: ___________________________

Ten Wishes for Your Future

Directions: If you could see into your future, what would be there? Please take a moment to look into your future, and list ten things you would like to accomplish in your life. You can go anywhere or do anything.

1.	6.
2.	7.
3.	8.
4.	9.
5.	10.

Your Future with HIV

You have just been told that you have HIV and are very sick. How will this diagnosis change your ten wishes from the previous list? Please rewrite your future wishes in the list that follows, and be sure to include a short paragraph about how you feel your parents and friends would react to the news that you are HIV positive.

1.	6.
2.	7.
3.	8.
4.	9.
5.	10.

Name: ______________________________

Ten Wishes for Your Future (*continued*)

Parents

____

____

____

____

____

____

____

____

____

Friends

____

____

____

____

____

____

____

____

____

LESSON 7: AGREE—DISAGREE—NOT SURE ATTITUDES ABOUT HIV AND AIDS

Level: Middle school, High school

Time: 30–40 minutes

National Health Education Standards

1. Core Concepts
3. Accessing Information

National Sexuality Education Standards: Performance Indicators

- Compare and contrast behaviors, including abstinence, to determine the potential risk of STI/HIV transmission from each.
- Describe the signs, symptoms and potential impacts of STIs, including HIV.
- Access medically-accurate prevention information about STIs, including HIV.
- Explain how to access local STI and HIV testing and treatment services.

Rationale

Individuals with HIV/AIDS are often stigmatized and discriminated against. In this lesson, students will have an opportunity to express their personal opinions and values related to HIV and AIDS. Throughout this discussion, any misinformation will be corrected to ensure that students have a proper understanding of the virus. Students must be aware that people living with HIV/AIDS need help, love, and support. They should also be aware of the laws protecting people with HIV/AIDS from discrimination.

Students will be given a homework assignment that involves writing a letter from one friend to another who may be engaging in sexual behaviors that put him at potential risk for HIV infection.

Materials and Preparation

Three extra chairs placed at the front of the room for volunteers to sit in

Nine large index cards or pieces of construction paper. Each volunteer should have a set of three cards that have "Agree," "Disagree," or "Not Sure" written on them in marker.

List of eleven values statements (samples provided at the end of this lesson)

Procedure

1. Ask three volunteers to sit at the front of the room. You will read these volunteers some statements related to HIV/AIDS, in response to which they will have to express their personal opinion by holding up the "Agree," "Disagree," or "Not Sure" card.

2. Review the rules for discussion:
   - You have the right to pass on any statement.
   - Listen to each other, and do not interrupt.
   - *No put-downs.* If you disagree with someone, simply state why you disagree. Everyone has the right to his or her own opinion.
3. Explain the activity: "Today I would like to learn your opinions and attitudes about HIV/AIDS. I am going to read a statement, and when I am finished, I would like you to hold up one of your cards, informing me as to whether you *agree, disagree,* or are *not sure.* I will then give each of you a chance to explain why you feel the way you do. After your explanation, we will ask if anyone in the class has additional comments. After the statement is fully discussed, we will move on to another statement." Begin reading the statements.
4. After two statements have been read and discussed, thank the volunteers, and ask for three different volunteers. Continue using different students until all statements have been discussed.
5. Within the discussion, allow students to express their opinions, making sure to correct any inaccurate *information* that may come up in the class discussion. For example, in regard to the fourth values statement included at the end of this lesson, it is true that very few teens die from AIDS-related diseases, but this is because the time between infection and the onset of symptoms may be five years or more. Many people who have full-blown AIDS in their twenties could have become infected with HIV as teenagers. Also, although students are entitled to their own opinions, you should attempt to focus on health-enhancing behaviors (you cannot get HIV from sharing a can of soda, but you can spread other germs), and to encourage compassion for anyone with this disease (no one *deserves* to die from AIDS, regardless of how it was contracted).
6. Conclude the activity by asking students the processing questions.
7. Assign students an extended response question for homework, sharing the following scenario and directions:

   > Rick and Jason have both played on the high school football team since freshman year and are good friends. They both served as volunteers for today's "agree—disagree—not sure" activity in health class. Rick thinks Jason has some misconceptions about HIV/AIDS, and is worried because Jason has had unprotected sex with at least two different girls at their school.
   >
   > Write a letter from Rick to Jason. In the letter, Rick should tell Jason three ways that HIV can be transmitted and three ways that HIV cannot be transmitted. Rick should also tell Jason two ways that he can reduce his risk of getting HIV.
   >
   > Also include in your letter one reliable *resource person* or *place* that Jason can go to for more information and advice on HIV prevention, including where he can be tested in his community.

   In assessing student homework, look for accurate information about transmission:

Ways that HIV can be transmitted:

- Through any sexual contact whereby bodily fluids are exchanged, including vaginal, oral, or anal sex
- By sharing needles or other drug equipment with an infected person
- From an HIV-infected mother to her baby during pregnancy, birth, or breast-feeding
- Through any type of direct blood-to-blood contact

Ways that HIV cannot be transmitted:

- By sneezing or coughing or breathing the same air as someone who is infected
- By shaking hands
- By hugging or kissing
- By using the same toilet seat as an infected person
- By sharing a towel or washcloth

Ways that Jason can reduce his risk of infection:

- He can abstain from all forms of sexual contact in which bodily fluids are exchanged.
- If sexually active, Jason can always use a latex condom—and use it correctly.
- Jason can have a mutually faithful, monogamous, long-term relationship in which both partners are uninfected.
- Jason can avoid engaging in sexual activity while under the influence of alcohol or other drugs, because this increases the risk of unprotected sex or incorrect condom use.
- Jason can never share drug equipment.

When identifying resource people and places for accurate HIV information, the student should:

- Identify specific people or places and evaluate the validity of those sources. Examples include a health teacher, school nurse, guidance counselor, local clinic, hospital, or private physician.
- Identify the type of assistance available from each source.

Note: If students have difficulty in determining how to find a local HIV testing site, make sure they have the following information at their disposal: students can log onto www.cdc.gov/hiv/topics/testing/index.htm and find a testing site by entering their zip code.

Processing

1. Why do you think myths about HIV exist?
2. How often do you hear about HIV and AIDS? More or less often than in the past?
3. What person in your family would you feel comfortable asking additional questions about HIV? What about an adult in your school? In the community?

Assessment

- Students participate in the "agree—disagree—not sure" activity and discussion.
- Students complete the homework assignment.

Values Statements about HIV and AIDS

1. Some people who contract HIV/AIDS deserve to get it.
2. It should be a law that all newborn babies be tested for HIV.
3. High school students who are HIV positive should not be allowed to attend school or play sports.
4. Very few teenagers die from AIDS, so they do not really have to worry about safer sex.
5. People who know they are HIV positive and spread the virus to someone else by having unprotected sex should be sent to prison.
6. Teaching high school students about abstinence from sex is a waste of time.
7. Classroom demonstrations on the correct way to use a condom encourage students to have sex.
8. I would not share a can of soda with someone I knew was HIV positive.
9. A teacher who is HIV positive should tell his or her students.
10. If a cafeteria worker who serves food in the lunchroom is HIV positive, this person should reveal his or her status to a supervisor or the principal.
11. An employer has the right to ask about the HIV status of a potential job applicant.

LESSON 8: CHRIS'S STORY—WHAT IT'S LIKE TO HAVE HIV

Level: Middle school, High school

Time: 30–40 minutes

National Health Education Standards

1. Core Concepts
8. Advocacy

National Sexuality Education Standards: Performance Indicators

- Describe the signs, symptoms and potential impacts of STIs, including HIV.
- Describe common symptoms of and treatments for STIs, including HIV.
- Advocate for sexually active youth to get STI/HIV testing and treatment.

Rationale

Although HIV/AIDS has been around for many years, there currently is no cure or vaccine. The good news is that with early detection and medical support, many people with HIV/AIDS are living longer, healthier lives. Also, people experience HIV differently. Some people develop AIDS within a few months as the virus quickly weakens their immune system. Others live with HIV for decades and have a normal life expectancy. The same is true in regard to symptoms of HIV—some people become ill shortly after infection, whereas others may not show signs of HIV for years after infection.

By reading a fictional story of a person infected with HIV and then responding to questions, students will gain a better understanding of what it might be like to be a person living with HIV.

Materials and Preparation

Front board or newsprint and markers

Copies of "Chris's Story: What It's Like to Have HIV" handout

Procedure

1. Write "HIV Positive" on the front board (or newsprint).
2. Have students brainstorm a list of words or phrases they associate with this term. Students should copy the list into their notebook.
3. Begin a discussion by asking the following questions:
   a. What is your perception of the daily life of someone living with HIV?
   b. Where do these ideas come from?
   c. Can you think of examples from the media that portray the life of someone living with HIV?

4. Explain to the students that they will now read a story about a person named Chris. Although the story is fictional, it is based on a compilation of true stories of people currently living with HIV.
5. Distribute the "Chris's Story: What It's Like to Have HIV" handout. Allow students seven to eight minutes to read the story.
6. When students have finished reading the story, ask the processing questions.
7. Conclude the class by assigning one of the following advocacy projects:
   a. Students may choose to volunteer and write an awareness paper about their experience. Many towns and counties across the country have support centers for people living with HIV/AIDS. They are often looking for volunteers to assist with their services (for example, the provision of food, transportation, and child care).
   b. Students can arrange an HIV/AIDS Awareness Day by asking for support from the school's administration. Preparing for this day can include inviting someone living with HIV to speak at the school; having a voluntary agency set up a booth in a common area to distribute pamphlets or other information about HIV, including where to get tested locally; or both.
   c. Students can participate in an AIDS Walk, and then write an awareness paper about their experience. Many areas of the country, especially larger cities, have an annual AIDS Walk. These fundraisers promote awareness of the problem while raising money to help agencies that provide support services for people with AIDS.
   d. Students can write an article for the school newspaper on HIV and AIDS. This article should incorporate important facts and statistics, including (1) how HIV is and is not transmitted; (2) medically-accurate information about HIV; (3) an explanation of how to access local HIV testing and treatment services; (4) advocacy for sexually active teens to get HIV testing and treatment; and (5) a description of the laws pertaining to sexual health care services, including patient confidentiality in regard to HIV testing and treatment
   e. Students can create a video project or an audio announcement developed for the school PA system by using "new media" tools or interactive forms of communication via the Internet. These might include a school-approved Facebook posting, blog, podcast, mass text message, and more.

   Any of these activities can be planned anytime during the school year, but may be especially effective in conjunction with World AIDS Day, which is held annually on December 1.

Processing

1. How old was the person in the story when he or she contracted HIV?
2. How did the person contract HIV? What might have reduced this person's risk of contracting HIV? (Abstinence, condoms)
3. How did the person find out he or she had HIV? How did he or she feel at first? Have those feelings changed over time? If so, how?
4. How did friends and family members react?

5. How has this person's day-to-day life changed? Physically? Mentally? Socially? Emotionally? Spiritually?
6. How is the reality of Chris's life similar to the terms listed on our brainstormed list from the beginning of the lesson? How is it different?
7. What types of treatment does this person receive? What is it like to receive this treatment?
8. Compared to the early days of the AIDS epidemic in the 1980s and 1990s, what have been the biggest advances in the diagnosis and treatment of HIV and AIDS? What has been one of the biggest disappointments in regard to HIV and AIDS?
9. What is the difference between being HIV positive and having AIDS?
10. When you read the story, did you picture Chris as a male or a female? What difference, if any, would it make?
11. What is the best thing you can do to protect yourself from getting HIV/AIDS?
12. What is one thing you can do to help someone living with HIV or AIDS?

Assessment

- Students participate in the brainstorm activity and follow-up discussion, and make a list of the brainstorm items in their notebook.
- Students read "Chris's Story" and participate in a follow-up discussion.
- Students complete an assigned advocacy project.

Chris's Story: What It's Like to Have HIV

My name is Chris. I am twenty-one years old, and I found out about a year ago that I am HIV positive.

Last year I got "the worst flu ever" and decided to go to a doctor. When I first was tested, my CD4 cell (T-cell) count was around 300 cells per cubic millimeter of blood. Three hundred is low, which means that the virus was attacking my immune system. Normal T-cell counts can range from around 500 to 1,000. The good news was that my count was not below 200, and I had no signs of an opportunistic infection, like pneumonia. So, technically I am HIV positive but do not have AIDS. I started on treatment right away, and my T-cell count is up to 650. That means that the drugs are helping my body fight the virus and strengthening my immune system.

Another test I have to take is a viral load test. This test measures the level of HIV in your blood. My latest test showed that my viral load is "undetectable." That does not mean that I do not have HIV—just that it is so low that they cannot measure it. I still can pass HIV to someone else.

At first I was scared and angry. I thought it was a death sentence. I had had unprotected sex because I just did not like using condoms. I did not think it could happen to me. To this day, I do not really know whom I got it from. I guess I learned my lesson about safer sex.

Anyway, I'm sure you're wondering what it's like being HIV positive. Well, at first I freaked out. I didn't know whom I could talk to or what I should do. Then I learned that with positive medical support, I can live a long time. I have joined a support group, and some of the people in the group have lived with this for over twenty years. Unfortunately, some people do not respond well to the meds, develop full-blown AIDS, and die within a few years of being diagnosed.

One thing that is difficult is being tested every few months, because I don't know if my T-cell count will go up (that's good!) or down. I also don't know if my viral load will go up (that's bad) or down. I also have had to change my meds a couple of times. I got really, really sick with bad side effects from one of the drug combinations prescribed to me, so I had to go on some other meds. They seem to be helping and don't make me sick.

I get tired sometimes, and if I'm not careful about taking my medications and eating healthy, I start to lose weight. The mental and social part of this is probably the worst. I get depressed a lot. My parents have been supportive, but I lost some of my so-called friends when they found out I was HIV positive. I had goals of getting married and even being a parent, but I'm not sure if that will happen. I don't date because, well, how do you tell someone you like that you are HIV positive? I can just see the first date: "Hi, I'm Chris, and I have HIV." I don't think so! That's one of the hardest parts of living with HIV—disclosing my status.

To help other people not become infected with HIV, I decided to obtain a bachelor's degree in health education at a local university. I figured one positive thing to come out of my experience will be to advocate to others about knowing correct facts plus ways of preventing HIV transmission.

LESSON 9: GETTING HOOKED ON THE STEPS OF PROPER CONDOM USE

Level: Middle school, High school

Time: 40 minutes

National Health Education Standards

1. Core Concepts
3. Accessing Information
4. Interpersonal Communication
5. Decision-Making
6. Goal Setting
7. Self-Management

National Sexuality Education Standards: Performance Indicators

- Describe the steps to using a condom correctly.
- Develop a plan to eliminate or reduce risk for STIs, including HIV.
- Demonstrate skills to communicate with a partner about STI and HIV prevention and testing.
- Access medically-accurate prevention information about STIs, including HIV.
- Apply a decision-making model to choices about safer sex practices, including abstinence and condoms.
- Describe a range of ways people express affection within various types of relationships.

Rationale

If used consistently and correctly, condoms can be a very effective method of preventing pregnancy and sexually transmitted infections. Most condoms fail because of human error. By talking openly about condoms, students who decide to become sexually active will have a better understanding of their proper use. In this experiential group activity and discussion, students will explore the steps to using a condom correctly. After students "fish" for the individual steps for proper condom use, they will work cooperatively as a class to place all steps in the proper order.

Materials and Preparation

Small fabric, foam, or cardboard "fish," big enough for one statement to be written on one side. Sample statements are included at the end of this lesson, but they should not be numbered on the fish. (*Note:* If you do not have the materials or time for the fishing activity, simply create a set of cards from card stock or construction paper, with each one containing a step for proper condom use. These can be randomly handed out to students.)

Fishing rod or stick with fishing line

"Dot" magnets glued to fish to represent eyes (available in many craft stores). Also needed are additional magnets, attached to the fishing line.

Front board. Before class, ensure the board is able to hold magnets. If it is not, provide masking tape to affix fish to the board.

Condoms for demonstration (optional)

Procedure

1. Introduce the activity by providing brief facts about teen pregnancy and STIs, including HIV. One point to stress is that *abstinence* is the only 100 percent effective method of preventing pregnancy and STI transmission. However, for those people who choose to be sexually active, condoms may provide protection against pregnancy and HIV and some other STIs (although they are not 100 percent effective).
2. Ask the class to form a circle with their desks. Students each can sit on top of their desk, facing the center of the circle.
3. In the center, place the "fish" on the floor, making sure to have the statements facing the floor so students cannot see what is written on them.
4. Explain that the objective of the lesson is for students to understand the proper steps for using a condom. One by one, volunteers will attempt to catch a fish using the fishing rod (or stick). To catch a fish, students must allow the magnets on the fishing line to line up with the fish's eye.

   Note: Request that students not fling the line behind or in front of them. Although this activity simulates fishing, these fish need the participants to be gentle, just like a person needs to be careful with condoms.
5. Have students begin fishing. As fish are caught, they should be placed on the front board.
6. After all of the fish have been caught, allow the class to work cooperatively to put the fish in order. This might entail your choosing a leader to call on others for suggestions.
7. Once the fish have been organized into a chosen order, have students comment on the sequence and add suggestions. Then ask the processing questions.
8. After the proper sequence has been discussed, teachers have the option of demonstrating proper condom use, based on the correct sequence of cards. (A condom may be rolled onto fingers for this activity, simulating how it would be rolled onto the penis.)

   Note: Depending on the developmental level of the students, state mandates or regulations, and local district policy, the condom demonstration activity may or may not be appropriate or permitted. Teachers should check with their administration or district health advisory committee to determine whether a condom demonstration is acceptable to use in their classroom. It is strongly recommended that each school district have an AIDS Committee, a Wellness Advisory Committee, or both, through which such decisions can be made, with input from parents or guardians and the community in determining what is most developmentally appropriate for students.
9. Review steps for proper condom use, clarifying any questions students may have.

Processing

1. Do you agree or disagree with the order of the steps? Which cards are out of order? Why?
2. Is it possible to have more than one "correct" answer? Why?
3. If a person does not remember the proper steps for using condoms, where might he or she find the information? (Inside the box of condoms, from a reliable website, from a health teacher)
4. Were there any steps that surprised you? Explain.
5. Why are the steps for proper condom use important for sexually active people to know?

Assessment

- Students participate in making decisions to put the steps in the correct order.
- Students actively participate in the class discussion.
- If the optional condom demonstration is given, students actively participate by observing the demonstration and asking any questions they may have about proper condom use.

Sample List of Steps for Proper Condom Use

1. Meet someone you are attracted to.
2. Decide to have sexual intercourse.
3. Talk to your partner about using condoms.
4. Purchase latex condoms (check the expiration date on the outside of the box).
5. Store condoms in a cool, dry, place.
6. Kiss, hug, and touch (arousal).
7. Get an erection.
8. Check the expiration date on the condom wrapper.
9. Carefully open the package (teeth or fingernails can tear the condom).
10. Check the condom for leaks and tears.
11. Place a drop of water-based lubricant on the inside tip of the condom.
12. Pinch the condom at the tip to leave space at the end.
13. Unroll the condom on the erect penis, all the way to the base.
14. Have intercourse.
15. Ejaculate.
16. After ejaculation, hold the rim of the condom while the penis is still erect, and withdraw.
17. Wrap the condom in a tissue and throw it away in the garbage (not in a toilet bowl).

LESSON 10: UP CLOSE AND PERSONAL

Level: High school

Time: 40 minutes

National Health Education Standard

4. Interpersonal Communication

National Sexuality Education Standards: Performance Indicator

- Demonstrate the use of effective communication skills to reduce or eliminate risk for STIs, including HIV.

Rationale

STIs, including HIV, have reached epidemic proportions in the United States and around the world. Teachers need to be sensitive to the possibility that some children and teens may have parents or guardians, other family members, or friends who have HIV or AIDS. Although there is still no cure or vaccine, people who have HIV or AIDS can enjoy happy and productive lives due to advances in medical treatment.

Although the format for this activity is relatively simple, the rules must be followed for the activity to be effective, and you, as the facilitator, must ensure that they are strictly enforced.

The Up Close and Personal (UCP) activity is designed to create an atmosphere of trust and mutual support within the group. Confidentiality is inherent in the activity, and it is possible that students will disclose personal information about themselves or about someone close to them. You should be prepared for this possibility by checking the school policy and state education law on disclosure of HIV status. Every employee has a duty to treat as highly confidential any knowledge concerning the HIV status of a student.

Note: It is unlikely that you will get through all sentence stems in one class session. You can decide which statements would be most appropriate for your students. Choices may be based on background information discussed in previous lessons, students' developmental level, restrictions you may have concerning what topics *can* and *cannot* be discussed, and your own comfort level in facilitating discussion.

Materials and Preparation

Small lamp (optional)

Up Close and Personal sheet with several UCP sentence stems. (*Note:* Prior to teaching this activity, you should familiarize yourself with "Facilitating a UCP Session," which can be found at the end of the lesson.)

Procedure*

1. Ask students to form a circle with their chairs. Turning off the overhead lights and using a lamp may make the environment more conducive to an informal discussion.
2. Introduce the activity in the following manner:

   Today we are going to do an activity called Up Close and Personal. It is simple to do, but for it to go smoothly, there are some rules to follow.

   First, understand this is not group therapy. Instead it is an opportunity for you to talk about how you feel about yourself, relationships, likes, dislikes, things that have come up in class, memories, and life in general. Although I will be facilitating the activity, I will also be sitting in the circle and participating along with everyone else.

   The activity is in the following format: I will read an unfinished sentence. Each of you will think about how you would finish this same unfinished sentence. Someone in the circle will then raise his or her hand and state his or her completed sentence. He or she will point to his or her right or left to determine which way around the circle we will proceed.

   When going around the circle, there should be no talking by anyone else. If something is said that you want to respond to or comment on, you must wait until we have gone all the way around the circle. If you cannot think of anything to say, or choose not to respond when it is your turn, you may simply say, "Pass" or "Come back to me." Everyone, including the teacher, is allowed to pass.

   When we have gone around the entire circle, I will ask anyone who passed if he or she would like to respond at this time. I will also ask for any questions or comments about anything that was said when going around the circle. At this point, there can be open discussion.

   Please note that during this activity, no names should be mentioned at any time. Instead, say something like, "I know someone who . . ."

   In addition, as with other lessons, what is said in class stays in class. However, please do not share anything that is too personal, that makes you feel uncomfortable, or that you wish to keep to yourself.

3. Once the rules have been explained and agreed on, read the first sentence stem aloud. After allowing a few moments for reflection, ask a student volunteer to start by stating his completed sentence. That student will then point to his left or right to note in which direction the remaining students will be given a chance to complete the sentence. Students then give their responses until everyone around the circle has spoken or passed.

---

*Unfinished sentences have been a useful learning tool for many years. The specific format used in this lesson has been adapted from the book *Up Close and Personal: Effective Learning for Students and Teachers* (Raleigh, NC: Lulu Press, 2007), by teacher, colleague, and friend Robert Winchester. Robert can be contacted at trustinbob@aol.com.

4. At times, a student may simply not be ready to respond to a particular question. When this happens, remind her to pass, noting that she can answer after everyone else has spoken. It is also not unusual for many students to have the same response to a question or statement. "Repeats" reinforce the important concept that although all people are unique, they often share many of the same thoughts, feelings, and values.
5. After all students have responded, open up the discussion by asking if anyone has any questions or comments about anything that was said. Encourage students to talk in more detail about why they completed the sentence the way they did. Students may also ask others in the circle, including the teacher, to expand on their answer. Students may do so, or they may choose to pass.
6. Continue the circle discussion for as long as it is viable, constantly monitoring and enforcing the rules. When the discussion on a given sentence has run its course, move on to the next unfinished sentence.
7. Share the processing statements.
8. All UCP sessions should end with some brief closure in the form of another unfinished sentence. Examples include the following: "Today I learned . . ." "I learned that I . . ." "Right now I feel . . ." and "Something I want to say to one of my classmates is . . ."
9. Conclude the day's activity by summarizing what occurred in the session, making appropriate connections to the subject matter and curriculum. Then thank the class and say, "This ends our Up Close and Personal class for today."

Processing

1. If anyone has any concerns or questions about what was discussed during our UCP session today, he or she can speak to me privately after class or can bring it up for discussion during our next class session.
2. There are many people, including teachers, coaches, counselors, or school psychologists, who can assist you with any personal issues that you may want to share with them. Keep in mind that these individuals, as mandated reporters, *must* report any verbalization or indication that you may want to hurt yourself or hurt others, or revelations of abuse of any kind, to the appropriate authorities for follow-up and counseling services.

Assessment

- Students actively participate in the UCP activity. Even though some students may decide to pass on one or more questions, as long as they are actively listening and following the ground rules, they are "actively participating."

Facilitating a UCP Session

- Facilitation is a skill that you can improve with practice.

- Silence is not a negative phenomenon. Silence often indicates that higher-level thinking is taking place.

- Going over ground rules at the beginning of each session is a needed and helpful technique to prevent inappropriate behavior.

- Unacceptable behavior should be stopped the moment it is recognized. To do this, pause the activity and point out the offense to the individual. For example, say, "What was just said is a put-down (or personal name), and it is not allowed in the circle discussion. Please do not do it again," or "Please do not talk to your neighbor when you should be listening to the one person who is supposed to be talking."

- If a student persists in breaking the activity's rules, talk to him one-on-one after class. Let the student know that if his behavior continues, he may not be able to participate in the future. This almost always stops the offensive behavior.

- Remind students of the information teachers *must* report if shared:

    1. If they are going to hurt themselves
    2. If they are going to hurt others
    3. If they are being abused

Possible UCP Sentence Stems: STIs and HIV/AIDS

1. If I had to use one word to describe how I am feeling right now, it would be . . .
2. When I hear the words "sexually transmitted infections" or "STIs," the first thing I think of is . . .
3. People with STIs or HIV need . . .
4. If someone in this school were HIV positive, most kids would . . .
5. In regard to talking about HIV/AIDS, my parents or guardians . . .
6. When it comes to condoms, most teenagers . . .
7. A drug addict who gets HIV from sharing drug equipment . . .
8. One of the reasons why teenagers might not use protection is . . .
9. If a close friend confided in me that he or she was HIV positive, I would . . .
10. If I had to be diagnosed and treated for an STI in this town or county, I would . . .
11. One thing that I can personally do to reduce my risk of contracting an STI is . . .
12. Talking with your partner about sex is . . .
13. If my partner were pressuring me to become sexually involved and I wasn't ready, I would . . .
14. Something I learned today . . .

LESSON 11: HOME-SCHOOL CONNECTION

TALKING ABOUT SEXUALLY TRANSMITTED INFECTIONS—WHAT DO YOU KNOW?

Level: Middle school, High school

Time: Varies

National Health Education Standards

1. Core Concepts
4. Interpersonal Communication

National Sexuality Education Standards: Performance Indicators

- Define STIs, including HIV, and how they are and are not transmitted.
- Evaluate the effectiveness of abstinence, condoms and other safer sex methods in preventing the spread of STIs, including HIV.
- Demonstrate the use of effective communication skills to reduce or eliminate risk for STIs, including HIV.

Rationale

Parents or guardians and schools are vital partners in helping young people take responsibility for their health. The primary role of the school is to provide students with accurate information as well as engage them in developing and practicing interpersonal skills. It is the responsibility of parents or guardians to communicate family values and beliefs. The main purpose of this Home-School Connection activity is to give teens and their parents or guardians an opportunity to privately discuss their current level of knowledge about HIV/AIDS and other STIs.

After completing the pretest questions with their child, parents or guardians are requested to compose a brief message they would like to send their son or daughter about keeping healthy and avoiding or reducing the risk of contracting an STI. Parents or guardians are also requested to sign the bottom of the page to verify that the student has completed the assignment at home. All responses from teens and parents or guardians on the Home-School Connection activity will be kept confidential. It will not be turned in to the teacher or graded. On the due date, students will be asked to *voluntarily* share any interesting comments or insights they learned or observed by participating in the assignment. Students *and* parents or guardians can choose to pass on any discussion they wish to keep private.

By working together, schools and parents or guardians can assist young people in adopting attitudes and behaviors that reduce their risk of contracting STIs or HIV.

Materials and Preparation

Copies of "Talking about Sexually Transmitted Infections" worksheet

Teacher copy of "Answers to 'Talking about Sexually Transmitted Infections'" for use during the follow-up discussion

Procedure

1. Explain to the class that they are going to be given an assignment to complete with one or more parents or guardians.
2. Distribute the Home-School Connection worksheet and assign a due date.
3. On the day the assignment is due, check if students have completed it by noting if the sheet was signed on the bottom. Do not collect or grade the assignment.
4. Go over each statement from the Home-School Connection worksheet to ensure students and their respective families have the correct answers (provided at the end of this lesson). Discuss any points students are unsure about. Students should share the correct answers from the pretest with the adults who assisted them with the assignment.
5. After all statements have been discussed, ask for student volunteers to share any interesting points from the discussion they had with the adult or adults they interviewed. Within this discussion, ask the processing questions.
6. Conclude the discussion with a "class whip." Each student will make one brief statement related to the activity. Examples may be "I learned . . ." "I feel (or felt) . . ." or "I was surprised . . ."

Processing

1. Which family members did you choose to speak with?
2. How did you feel talking to your parents or guardians after they and you took this quiz about sexually transmitted infections? Were you comfortable with this discussion? Were your parents or guardians comfortable with this discussion?
3. Did you and your parents or guardians agree on all the answers? If not, what were some questions that you disagreed on?
4. What were some of the messages you received about abstinence and growing up to be a sexually responsible adult?
5. How did you feel about the messages or advice that your parents or guardians shared with you?
6. Did anything surprising come up during the conversation?
7. What did you learn from doing this assignment?
8. What did you learn from our follow-up class discussion of the correct answers?

Assessment

- Students complete the Home-School Connection assignment.
- Students participate in the follow-up discussion related to the assignment, including the sharing of correct answers.
- Students participate in the class whip.

Talking about Sexually Transmitted Infections

School health programs help youth adopt attitudes and behaviors that can reduce their risk of HIV and other sexually transmitted infections (STIs). These programs should be developed with the active involvement of parents or guardians to ensure that they are consistent with the local community's values.

Directions: Parents or guardians and their child should complete and discuss the following questions together. Under the heading "Student Answer," the student should write whether he or she believes the statement is true or false. In the "Adult Answer" column, the adult should write whether he or she believes the statement is true or false. If more than one adult completes the sheet, additional answers can fit on the "Adult Answer" line, and adults should initial their respective responses. Alternately, the second adult may write his or her answers on the back of the worksheet. After all statements are completed, please discuss your answers. This Home-School Connection activity is designed to give parents or guardians a chance to share not only their knowledge about sexuality but also their opinions and values. When the pretest is completed, it should be signed by all parties. One parent or guardian is then asked to write on the other side of the paper a brief response to the question that follows the pretest.

During a future class, the correct answers will be given to your child. Students will then be encouraged to continue discussing the statements at home, sharing any needed corrections.

Thank you in advance for your cooperation.

	Student Answer	Adult Answer	
1.	________________	________________	The symptoms of STIs can very often be absent or hidden, especially in women.
2.	________________	________________	The risk of becoming infected with HIV can virtually be eliminated by not engaging in sexual activities in which bodily fluids are exchanged and by not using intravenous drugs.
3.	________________	________________	Many STIs simply go away by themselves.
4.	________________	________________	Being under the influence of alcohol or other drugs can increase a teen's risk of having unprotected sex.
5.	________________	________________	In most states, teens must obtain the permission or consent of a parent or guardian to get tested and treated for STIs.
6.	________________	________________	Genital herpes and genital warts (HPV) are caused by bacteria. They can usually be cured easily.
7.	________________	________________	Although there are now more effective treatments, there is still no cure or vaccine for HIV/AIDS.
8.	________________	________________	HIV can be contracted by donating blood.
9.	________________	________________	Latex condoms, when used correctly and consistently, can reduce the risk of contracting an STI.
10.	________________	________________	The birth control pill and other hormonal types of contraception are also effective in preventing STIs.

Parent or Guardian Question

What **message** do you want your child to get from **you** about sexually transmitted infections, including HIV? (Please write your answer on the back of this page.)

Parent or guardian signature(s): ____

Student signature: ____

Answers to "Talking about Sexually Transmitted Infections"

1. **True.** Many STIs do not show any early symptoms in both males and females. Females, because of their internal reproductive system, are less likely to notice such symptoms as sores, blisters, or urinary problems.

2. **True.** These are the most common ways that HIV is transmitted.

3. **False.** The germs that cause STIs stay in the body once infected. Untreated STIs can lead to serious health problems, including infertility.

4. **True.** Being under the influence of alcohol or other drugs may affect judgment as well as safer sexual decision making.

5. **False.** In most states, teenagers can get tested and treated for STIs without the permission or consent of a parent or guardian.

6. **False.** These infections are caused by a virus and have treatments to relieve symptoms, but no cure.

7. **True.** Medications can reduce symptoms and extend lives, but are not a cure. There is presently no vaccine to prevent contracting HIV.

8. **False.** All needles used when donating blood are prepackaged, sterile, and disposed of after one use. You cannot get HIV, hepatitis, or any other infectious disease from donating blood.

9. **True.** Although not 100 percent effective, latex condoms, when used consistently and correctly, reduce the risk of STI transmission.

10. **False.** Birth control pills, when used correctly, are effective in preventing pregnancy, but offer no protection against STIs.

Healthy Relationships

6

Relationships play a major role in our lives, especially during the teen years. Although there are many types of relationships (with family, friends, peers, and others), most of the lessons in Chapter Six focus on comparing and contrasting the characteristics of healthy and unhealthy romantic relationships. In a classroom environment that promotes mutual respect and trust, students will be able to practice communication skills that foster healthy relationships.

Romantic relationships exist on a continuum from healthy to unhealthy to abusive, and everywhere in between. Dating is an important process for young people because it is a way for them to learn about other people and their feelings toward them. Because of their inexperience in dating, however, it can be difficult for teens to determine whether their relationships are healthy or not.

Readiness for dating varies among individuals. Before getting involved in a romantic relationship, many teens start off as friends, spending time together to get to know each other, often in group activities. Dating is also a way to learn about romantic and sexual feelings, setting boundaries in regard to sexual activity, and what it is like to be in an intimate relationship.

Teens live in a society that sends them mixed and often negative messages about sexuality. In this fast-paced world of information technology, teens are bombarded with distorted messages about relationships in advertising, on social networking sites, on television, in movies, and in music. To counter these images and messages, it is important to give students a positive view of human sexuality, arming them with interpersonal communication and self-management skills to enhance their own health and avoid risky behaviors. Several lessons in Chapter Six give students opportunities to practice interpersonal communication and self-management skills related to

- Creating healthy relationships
- Ensuring that personal boundaries are respected in intimate relationships
- Ending a relationship
- Using social media in respectful and appropriate ways

Note: In planning lessons and activities related to relationships and dating, you should be aware that gay, lesbian, and bisexual youth, like heterosexual youth, may or may not date. Gay, lesbian, or questioning teens are not yet likely to have come out to their peers. Because of their desire to "fit in," often their first experiences are with partners of the other sex. When setting up scenarios or role-plays, you should endeavor not to disenfranchise students who may be gay or questioning their sexuality. This can be done by using gender-neutral names in scenarios, and by using the term "partner" rather than "boyfriend" or "girlfriend."

LESSON 1: WHOSE RELATIONSHIP IS THE HEALTHIEST?

Level: High school

Time: 40–50 minutes

National Health Education Standards

1. Core Concepts
7. Self-Management

National Sexuality Education Standards: Performance Indicators

- Describe characteristics of healthy and unhealthy romantic and/or sexual relationships.
- Explain the criteria for evaluating the health of a relationship.

Rationale

It is important for teens and adults to understand that both partners share responsibility for the quality of a relationship. In this lesson, students will brainstorm a list of qualities and characteristics that distinguish healthy relationships from unhealthy ones. Students will be involved in a group activity in which they must rank six fictional relationships in order of which is the healthiest, first individually and then in groups. This lesson can be followed by Lesson 3, "Components of a Healthy Relationship," to review what was discussed in class.

Materials and Preparation

Copies of "Whose Relationship Is Healthiest?" worksheet

Front board

Procedure

1. Explain that today's topic for discussion will be distinguishing healthy from unhealthy romantic or dating relationships.
2. Ask students to start a new page in their notebook and copy down the chart that you will draw on the front board.
3. Write and underline the word "Relationships." Under that word, draw a vertical line down the center of the board. Under the left side of the word Relationships, write the word "Healthy." On the right side under the word Relationships, write the word "Unhealthy."
4. Explain that over the next five minutes, you would like students to brainstorm words or actions that they associate with either side. Students can volunteer a word or action on either side, allowing free thought and word association. At this point in the brainstorm, there will be no discussion or disagreement among students. You should write all terms on the appropriate side (as suggested by the student) on the front board. Students will copy down this list in their notebook.

5. After the five minutes is up, end the brainstorm. Ask students to look at both lists and allow open discussion on why items were placed on one side or the other. Allow students to explain and expand on reasons why they feel certain qualities or behaviors are placed on one side or the other. Although there may be some disagreement, most often the students will accept that there are certain characteristics of healthy and unhealthy relationships that they can all pretty much agree on. The following are common items that may be found on each side of the list:
   - *Healthy relationships:* Respecting each other, trusting each other, having fun and enjoying being with each other, mutual attraction, communication, compromise, setting boundaries and respecting privacy, spending time together and time alone or with family and friends, respecting sexual limits, feeling comfortable and safe
   - *Unhealthy relationships:* Jealousy or possessiveness, lack of respect, lack of privacy, texts or calls to check up on you, putting you down or calling you names, accusations of flirting or cheating, trying to control what you do or whom you see, being angry one minute and apologetic the next, emotional or physical abuse
6. After completing the discussion of the characteristics of healthy and unhealthy relationships, distribute copies of the "Whose Relationship Is Healthiest?" worksheet, Explain to students that they will be reading about six different relationships. When they have finished reading, they should individually rank the relationships described based on how healthy they feel each relationship is.
7. Students should begin by ranking the six fictional relationships from 1 (the healthiest) to 6 (the unhealthiest), writing brief explanations for their answers on their worksheet.
8. Groups of four to five students will then be formed, in which students will create an overall group ranking. Ask students to attempt to agree within their group on how to order the relationships from the healthiest to the unhealthiest. Give groups ten minutes for this discussion.
9. On completing their rankings, groups should write their answers on the front board and then explain them to the rest of the class. Ask the processing questions to ensure that the concept of relationship health is expanded on and discussed.
10. After asking the processing questions, ask students to complete sentence stems and share them in a "class whip." They may also complete the sentence stems for homework and bring them to the next class for a follow-up discussion. Possible sentence stems may include "I learned . . ." "I learned that I . . ." "I feel . . ." "In my opinion . . ." and "I was surprised that . . ."
11. To conclude the activity, ask students to describe in their journal or notebook the components of a healthy dating relationship.
12. As an additional activity, students can ask a peer, family member, or other adult to complete the worksheet to gain another person's perspective. Students can then either share this insight during a future class or write about it in their journal.

Processing

1. What rankings did group members agree on?
2. Which did you not agree on? Explain your group's decision making.
3. How do you determine if a relationship is healthy?
4. How much time is needed for people to know they are in a healthy relationship? Is there a time requirement?
5. Does having an illness, like HIV, stop people from having dating relationships? Explain.
6. What characteristics from the descriptions do you not like? Why?
7. In scenarios C and E, the genders of the partners were not clearly defined. All four names can be gender neutral (male or female). Who assumed that both people in scenarios C and E were two males? Who assumed they were two females? A male and a female? Did anything in either story lead you to believe certain people were male or certain people were female? If so, what characteristics or "stereotypes" led you to make these assumptions?
8. Would your ranking of all six couples change, based on whether the couples in scenarios C and E were both female? Both male? If so, explain your rationale for your new ranking. (Virtually all of the characteristics of a healthy relationship are the same for gay, lesbian, or bisexual youth as they are for heterosexual youth.)
9. How did you feel completing this activity?

Assessment

- Students assess fictional descriptions to describe characteristics of healthy and unhealthy relationships.
- Students write independently in their journal about the components of a healthy dating relationship.
- Students complete sentence stems, either in a class whip or for homework.
- Students complete the additional activity.

Name: ___________________________________

Whose Relationship Is Healthiest?

Directions: Rank the following situations from one to six, with one being the healthiest and six being the unhealthiest. *Write an explanation on the back of this sheet justifying your ranking.*

A. Brian is eighteen years old and has been dating Cindy for two years. They have an occasional disagreement but seem to get along well, especially because they have many common interests, including bowling and photography. Recently, Cindy has been pressuring Brian to have sex, something they have never done with one another before. Brian reminded her that he wants to wait until marriage, but Cindy wants to rent a hotel room the night of their senior prom for a "special night." When Brian did not agree to this, Cindy cheated on him with another guy because she got tired of waiting. She has not told Brian about her having had sex with another guy. ____

B. Rob and Barbara, both high school seniors, have been dating for a little over six months. Rob is on the football, wrestling, and baseball teams, and loves watching any sporting event on TV. Barbara is the editor of the yearbook, is on the speech and debate team, and babysits for her neighbors' three children every Friday night. Because their time is filled with other obligations, Rob and Barbara see each other Saturday evening for a weekly date and have lunch every other day in the cafeteria. Last month they went to "third base" and are considering going "all the way" if Barbara goes on the pill. ____

C. Dakota is an eleventh grader and just started seeing Riley two weeks ago. Neither of them has ever had any form of sex, yet they are considering it with each other on their three-month anniversary. Both are really into each other, calling and texting throughout the school day. They rarely have disagreements and can see spending the rest of their lives with each other. Both Dakota and Riley feel they are in love. ____

D. Maria is a twenty-year-old junior at a community college who is very popular. She has many good friends and has been dating Pat for eight months. She was diagnosed with HIV last year and always takes her medication, follows a healthy diet, and exercises three times during the week. She also attends a local religious meeting at her temple. On their third date, Maria told Pat about her HIV-positive status; Pat responded that she still wanted to pursue a relationship with her and, when both were ready, would speak to a local health educator about how to lower her risk of contracting the virus when they were to have sexual contact. ____

E. Harley and Ali are both college freshmen who have been "hanging out" almost every day for two months. Harley sends Ali flirty text messages throughout the day. Last week, Harley checked Ali's phone for text messages when Ali was using the restroom. While doing this, Harley deleted some of the phone numbers of Ali's friends. Harley has fallen in love and this weekend is taking Ali to a romantic restaurant. Harley is hoping that Ali feels the same way and that they can become an "exclusive" couple. ____

F. Steven and Kathy have been dating for close to three years. Because they have known each other since middle school, they feel they are best friends and can trust one another completely. Both have friends of the opposite sex and can hang out with each other's friends comfortably. Recently Steven started texting some of his female friends jokes about sexual acts and asked Kathy to send a photo of her breasts through a photo text. ____

LESSON 2: MY PERFECT ROMANTIC PARTNER

Level: Middle school, High school

Time: 40 minutes

National Health Education Standards

1. Core Concepts
2. Analyzing Influences
4. Interpersonal Communication
5. Decision-Making

National Sexuality Education Standards: Performance Indicators

- Compare and contrast the characteristics of healthy and unhealthy relationships.
- Explain the criteria for evaluating the health of a relationship.
- Analyze the ways in which family, friends, peers, media, society and culture can influence relationships.
- Demonstrate communication skills that foster healthy relationships.

Rationale

People define and describe their "perfect" partner differently. Because people have different values, belief systems, personalities, and histories, characteristics found in significant others will also be different. To demonstrate this, students will visually represent their perception of a "perfect" potential romantic partner, and then will compare and contrast their perceptions with those of their peers. Although no person is "perfect," students can believe that a person is "perfect" for them. This lesson allows students to note how other people, including those of their own and the opposite gender, define a "perfect" dating partner. This activity also encourages students to reflect on the qualities they feel are important in personal relationships.

Materials and Preparation

Scrap paper, one eight- by ten-inch piece per student

Markers or colored pens and pencils (optional)

Tape

Procedure

1. Begin the lesson by asking students to define the word "perfect." After they have decided on a brief definition, ask them to discuss whether a romantic partner is able to be "perfect." This discussion will usually lead to the conclusion that no person is perfect, but that a person with specific qualities or characteristics can be "perfect" for someone.

2. Explain that students are going to be sharing with their peers their vision of the "perfect" romantic partner. To do this, they will each draw their ideal romantic partner as best they can, with the option of using descriptive words on their drawing. For example, if a student believes her perfect romantic partner is generous, she may draw a gift being given to another person with the word "generous" written by it. Request that *no names* be written on students' drawings. Students should take no more than ten minutes to complete their drawing.
3. After students have finished drawing, ask them to display their work somewhere on a classroom wall with a piece of tape.
4. After all drawings are posted (unless some students have requested not to share theirs), allow the students to walk around the room to look at their peers' work. Remind students to be respectful when giving any feedback. Five minutes should be enough time for students to compare and contrast their peers' drawings.
5. Have students return to their desk. Ask the processing questions, giving students time to come up with their responses.
6. For the next class, ask students to process what their peers drew and discussed in class in a journal writing assignment. Students should explain their reactions to what other people noted as important characteristics of a potential romantic partner, as well as reactions from their peers to their own drawing.

Processing

1. What were some common qualities your classmates looked for in a romantic partner?
2. What is something that surprised you from this activity?
3. How are you and your peers similar in regard to what you hope for in a dating relationship? How are you different?
4. In general, were qualities males preferred different from the qualities females preferred? If so, in what ways?
5. What influences what you perceive to be a "perfect" romantic partner? (Examples may include friends or the media.)
6. After thinking further about what you initially drew, what, if anything, would you change in your diagram? Why?
7. What did you learn from this activity?

Assessment

- Students draw their "perfect" romantic partner and participate in the class discussion of the drawings.
- Students compare and contrast people's ideas of ideal romantic partners.
- Students write in their journal about what their peers drew and stated in class.
- Students communicate effectively during the class discussion. (The rubric from Chapter Three may be referred to.)

LESSON 3: COMPONENTS OF A HEALTHY RELATIONSHIP

Level: Middle school, High school

Time: 30–40 minutes

National Health Education Standards

1. Core Concepts
7. Self-Management

National Sexuality Education Standards: Performance Indicators

- Compare and contrast the characteristics of healthy and unhealthy relationships.
- Analyze the similarities and differences between friendships and romantic relationships.
- Explain the criteria for evaluating the health of a relationship.
- Describe characteristics of healthy and unhealthy romantic and/or sexual relationships.
- Explain how media can influence one's beliefs about what constitutes a healthy sexual relationship.

Rationale

Many lessons on human sexuality focus on the prevention of pregnancy and sexually transmitted diseases. Yet students often want to discuss and learn what it takes to have healthy relationships, including dating relationships. This lesson allows students to create web diagrams, noting the essential components of healthy relationships. In this lesson, students will visually see the characteristics of healthy relationships, practice effective communication, and demonstrate mutual respect.

Materials and Preparation

Large poster paper, one piece for each group

Two markers of different colors for each group

Tape

Procedure

1. On the front board, draw a basic web diagram (a sample is included in this lesson) with "Healthy Relationships" written in its center. Explain to the class that web diagrams will be created during the class session to note components of healthy relationships.
2. Separate the class into three groups by having students count off around the room by three. After students form their groups, distribute the large pieces of poster paper, one per group, and give each group a colored marker. Tell students that they will be taking turns writing on their poster.
3. Ask each group to write the same term from the board, "Healthy Relationships," in the middle of their poster. Each group should then create their own web diagram, writing components they perceive to be part of a healthy relationship. Ask the groups to think

of all different types of relationships, not just romantic relationships. These include relationships with parents or guardians, siblings, peers, friends, teachers, and coaches.

To help groups create their original web diagram, ask the following questions:

a. What qualities do you want in your friends?
b. What qualities do you expect your teachers and coaches to have?
c. What skills do you want people you have relationships with to have?
d. Think of a strong friendship. How would you describe it?
e. What has stopped you from having a relationship with someone?
f. How does the media define healthy relationships?
g. What characteristics do you admire in a friend's family?

4. After the groups have written some components on their web diagram, distribute a second marker of a different color to each group. Explain that groups are now to *add* further components, if there are any, needed for healthy *dating* relationships. (*Note:* Students may write the word "sex" on their web diagram. If they do this, ask the group to process and write what is needed to ensure the relationship remains healthy.)

   To help students create the next section on their web diagram, ask the following questions:

   a. Think of a romantic couple that has been together for a long period. How would you describe their relationship?
   b. What has stopped you from having a dating relationship with someone?
   c. Are there additional skills you would expect from a dating partner?
   d. How does the media define healthy dating relationships?
   e. What characteristics do you admire in the relationship between a friend's parents or guardians?
   f. Think of some grandparents who have been together for a long period. What characteristics do they have?

5. After all groups complete both parts of the web diagram, have them display their poster for the other groups to view. (A sample web diagram is shown in Figure 6.3.1.) Follow with a group discussion using the processing questions.
6. Allow the posters to remain displayed until the end of the unit or semester, for reference when completing other lessons dealing with relationships.
7. Ask students to continue to process the concept of healthy relationships by writing in their journal. The reflection can include how they know if their own relationships are healthy.

Processing

1. What are the common components of healthy relationships listed across the groups?
2. What did your group not list that you want to add to your own poster after seeing another group's poster? (Groups can add these qualities to their poster.)
3. What do you think was the purpose of this activity?

4. Are there any listed characteristics on the web diagrams that you think are unhealthy? Explain.
5. Would having arguments or conflicts be a common or normal part of a healthy relationship? Explain.
6. Does the media correctly portray healthy relationships?
7. Looking over the components of healthy relationships, can any of you share a real-life example of a healthy relationship you have seen in your own life? Explain how you know the relationship is healthy.

Assessment

- Groups complete their web diagram, noting characteristics of healthy relationships (including dating or romantic relationships).
- Students reflect in their journal about the concept of healthy relationships, including how they know if their own relationships are healthy.

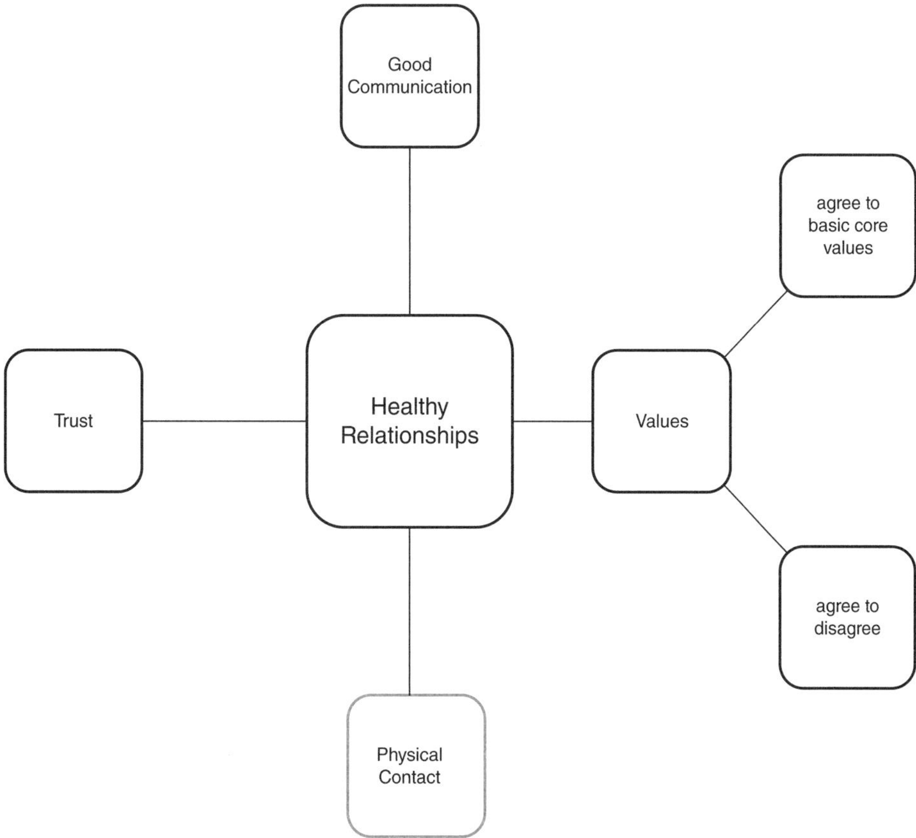

Figure 6.3.1 Sample Healthy Relationships Web Diagram

LESSON 4: WHAT IS LOVE? PART 1

Level: Middle school, High school

Time: 30–40 minutes

National Health Education Standards

1. Core Concepts
2. Analyzing Influences
7. Self-Management

National Sexuality Education Standards: Performance Indicators

- Describe characteristics of healthy and unhealthy romantic and/or sexual relationships.
- Analyze the ways in which family, friends, peers, media, society and culture can influence relationships.
- Describe the potential impacts of power differences such as age, status or position within relationships.
- Describe a range of ways people express affection within various types of relationships.
- Explain the criteria for evaluating the health of a relationship.
- Explain how media can influence one's beliefs about what constitutes a healthy sexual relationship.

Rationale

The term "love" is often used in greeting cards, on TV, in music, and in other forms of media. This lesson allows students to begin to process what they believe love is and is not. Although the statements may seem simple, each requires reflective thinking during as well as after the lesson.

Note: There is no "correct" answer for what love is, although there are many definitions written in dictionaries. Therefore, it needs to be pointed out that the definition of the word "love" differs depending on who is defining it.

Materials and Preparation

Copies of "What Is Love?" worksheet

Signs reading "Agree," "In the Middle," and "Disagree" that students can see from any seat in the classroom

Tape

Front board

Procedure

1. On the board in front of the room, write "Love" in large letters. Explain to the class that the day's lesson is going to help clarify how each person defines love.
2. Distribute the "What Is Love?" worksheet to each student and ask students to complete the ten statements by circling to indicate if they *agree, disagree,* or are *in the middle.* They should do this without any peer input.
3. As students are filling in their answers, tape the three signs up in the room. It is best to spread them out such that students can stand close to—but not actually by—a sign to show some indecision. If necessary, move chairs and desks to make a larger space so that students will be able to move about freely.
4. Explain that the statements about love from the worksheet will be read aloud. Students then need to indicate whether they agree, disagree, or are in the middle about each statement. To show their answer, they should stand under the sign indicating how they feel about the statement. Explain that there are no "correct" answers. These are their opinions, and the purpose is to generate a class discussion. Yet their goal is to be able to explain their position well enough for other students to understand their point of view.
5. Read the first statement and allow the students to move to the area of the room displaying their chosen answer. After all students are standing in place, ask them to explain why or how they made their decision to stand there. Students who are swayed by an argument can move to a new position. Having students explain what convinced them to change their mind often leads to insight. When the statement has been adequately addressed, move on to the next.
6. After all ten statements have been read aloud and answered through the walking activity, ask students to go back to their seat for the final class discussion. Within the discussion, ask the processing questions, giving students time to think of their answers.
7. Before the class ends, note the homework assignment also listed on the worksheet.

Processing

1. What is something surprising or shocking that you heard today?
2. What is something you heard that made you rethink one of your decisions?
3. Where do you think you learned what love is?
4. How often do you hear the term "love" referred to in the media? How do you feel about this?
5. Some people say teenagers cannot be in love. What do you think about that?

Assessment

- Students complete the "What Is Love?" worksheet.
- Students participate in the class discussion and walking activity, noting and understanding the range of opinions pertaining to relationships.
- Students complete the homework assignment, which allows them to individually define love.

Name: ______________________________

What Is Love?

Directions: Circle the answer that best describes your beliefs about love.

1. Everyone experiences love.
   Agree **In the middle** **Disagree**
2. People can fall in love at first sight.
   Agree **In the middle** **Disagree**
3. All people need is love.
   Agree **In the middle** **Disagree**
4. Love and infatuation are the same thing.
   Agree **In the middle** **Disagree**
5. Love is needed to get married.
   Agree **In the middle** **Disagree**
6. If you are in love, you should get married.
   Agree **In the middle** **Disagree**
7. Love can be bought.
   Agree **In the middle** **Disagree**
8. You should only have sex if you are in love with the person.
   Agree **In the middle** **Disagree**
9. People of different races can fall in love with each other.
   Agree **In the middle** **Disagree**
10. People of different ages (generations) can fall in love with each other.
    Agree **In the middle** **Disagree**

Homework

For next class, write your own definition of love. In addition, ask two other people to give you their definition of love.

LESSON 5: WHAT IS LOVE? PART 2

Level: Middle school, High school

Time: 40–50 minutes

National Health Education Standards

1. Core Concepts
2. Analyzing Influences

National Sexuality Education Standards: Performance Indicators

- Describe characteristics of healthy and unhealthy romantic and/or sexual relationships.
- Analyze the ways in which family, friends, peers, media, society and culture can influence relationships.
- Describe the potential impacts of power differences such as age, status or position within relationships.
- Describe a range of ways people express affection within various types of relationships.
- Explain the criteria for evaluating the health of a relationship.
- Explain how media can influence one's beliefs about what constitutes a healthy sexual relationship.

Rationale

Continuing on from Lesson 4, "What Is Love? Part 1," this lesson allows students to process what the term "love" means to them. For this, students will analyze verses pertaining to love.

Employing the Socratic method for the discussion enables students to question one another, allowing for higher-level, critical thinking. This lesson follows a Socratic seminar format, in which students are asked questions and then given a few moments to think about their answers. People often answer questions quickly without thought—but the Socratic method requires students to think. As a question is posed, silence may occur for a brief period; this is natural. Eventually a student will say something that initiates another student's comment. Arriving at a final answer is not the goal; the process of how things are discussed is what is important, as well as students' coming to understand that they may have to "agree to disagree." Because the provided examples are opinions formed by people's own experiences, disagreements may occur during a discussion.

Materials and Preparation

Ice in a glass, a container of water, and a teakettle arranged on a table in the center of the room. These items should be displayed in an artistic fashion to add to the discussion. (*Note:* Please follow building regulations in regard to what is and is not allowed in the classroom.)

Desks and chairs, organized in a circle around the table so that students are able to see everyone in the room

Teacher copy of "Verses about Love." This should be printed on large paper for the class to see or displayed on the front board. Copies can also be made for students.

Scrap paper for exit card responses (optional)

Copies of "Love in the Media" homework

Procedure

1. Begin the lesson by reviewing what students learned from the previous lesson. (Comments may range from "People define love differently" to "I never realized how this term can make people talk and think so much.")
2. Ask students to take out their definitions of love from the previous lesson's homework assignment, and ask volunteers to read aloud their own or another person's definition of love.
3. After a few examples are shared, refer to the middle table with the ice in a glass, the water in a container, and the teakettle. Tell the class the display is one person's answer for her definition of love. Allow the students to then state what this person's message might be. Answers may include the following:
   - Love can change, just as water can change its form.
   - For some people, love can be cold.
   - For some people, love can be steamy.
   - Some people may not see any difference—water is water.

   As in many discussions employing the Socratic method, students may ask each other questions and disagree.
4. Display one of the examples from "Verses about Love" (or another example of your choosing). Individual copies could also be handed out, but addressing only one reading at a time allows for higher-level thinking and understanding. Ask the processing questions one at a time, allowing students time to respond. Socratic learning requires patience, including having students think for a longer period of time. If the chosen verse does not illicit discussion, choose another verse.
5. Toward the end of the class, ask students to reflect on the discussion, either in their journal or on an exit card.
6. For an additional assignment, hand out the "Love in the Media" homework and have students find a media source dealing with love. These can be played for the class and discussed. A grading rubric is provided for students' benefit.

Processing

1. What does this verse say about love?
2. What was the author feeling when writing this?
3. Is "love" a verb? A noun? An adjective? Explain.
4. After our discussions, how has your viewpoint on love changed, if at all?

Assessment

- Students participate in the class discussion, noting the variety of ways that love is defined and expressed.
- Students reflect on the lesson in their journal or on an exit card.
- Students complete the "Love in the Media" homework.

Verses about Love

A passage from *The Velveteen Rabbit*, written by Margery Williams, often used in wedding ceremonies:

"What is REAL?" asked the Rabbit one day, when they were lying side by side near the nursery fender, before Nana came to tidy the room. "Does it mean having things that buzz inside you and a stick-out handle?"

"Real isn't how you are made," said the Skin Horse. "It's a thing that happens to you. When a child loves you for a long, long time, not just to play with, but REALLY loves you, then you become Real."

"Does it hurt?" asked the Rabbit.

"Sometimes," said the Skin Horse, for he was always truthful. "When you are Real you don't mind being hurt."

"Does it happen all at once, like being wound up," he asked, "or bit by bit?"

"It doesn't happen all at once," said the Skin Horse. "You become. It takes a long time. That's why it doesn't happen often to people who break easily, or have sharp edges, or who have to be carefully kept. Generally, by the time you are Real, most of your hair has been loved off, and your eyes drop out and you get all loose in the joints and very shabby. But these things don't matter at all, because once you are Real you can't be ugly, except to people who don't understand."

A verse from 1 Corinthians 13:4–7, also commonly used in wedding ceremonies (found at www.biblestudytools.com):

Love is patient and kind; love is not jealous or conceited or proud; love is not ill-mannered or selfish or irritable; love does not keep a record of wrongs; love is not happy with evil, but is happy with the truth. Love never gives up; its faith, hope, and patience never fail.

A quote from comedian Rita Rudner (found at www.searchquotes.com):

I love being married. It's so great to find that one special person you want to annoy for the rest of your life.

A quote from Plato (found at www.searchquotes.com):

Love is a grave mental disease.

(continued)

Hindu Marriage Poem (found at www.spiritualcelebrations.com):

You have become mine forever.
Yes, we have become partners.
I have become yours.
Hereafter, I cannot live without you.
Do not live without me.
Let us share the joys.
We are word and meaning, unite.
You are thought and I am sound.

May the nights be honey-sweet for us.
May the mornings be honey-sweet for us.
May the plants be honey-sweet for us.
May the earth be honey-sweet for us.

Name: ______________________________

Love in the Media

Directions: Messages of "love" are found in different forms in the media. Choose one media source to analyze and answer the following questions.

1. What media source did you find? Supply a URL if the source was found online. If a URL is not available, explain how you found the source.

____

____

____

____

2. According to this media source, what is love?

____

____

____

____

3. Do you agree or disagree with the message? Explain.

____

____

____

____

4. How do you think this message influences others' beliefs about relationships?

____

____

____

____

In addition, you may be asked to present your media source to the class for additional credit. If you choose to do this, be prepared to explain your answers to the preceding questions.

(continued)

Name: ______________________________

Love in the Media (*continued*)

The assignment will be graded according to the following rubric:

Love in the Media Rubric (4 Points Total; 6 Points Total with Bonus)

	2 POINTS	1 POINT	0 POINTS
Media source	The student fully explained how love is depicted in the source. The location of the source was also provided.	The student stated how love is depicted in the source. The location of the source was also provided.	The student didn't provide any statement or explanation. No source was provided, or the source did not pertain to the topic.
Personal opinions	The student explained how he or she felt about the message, expanding on his or her own viewpoint. Thoughts were also provided on how the message can influence others.	The student stated how he or she felt about the message, yet should have explained further. Also, the student briefly stated how the message could influence others.	No personal opinions were provided, or opinions provided did not pertain to the topic.
Presentation to class (BONUS CREDIT)	The media source was shown to or played for the class (for a maximum of thirty seconds to prove points). The student verbally explained his or her answers to the homework questions.	The media source was shown to or played for the class (for a maximum of thirty seconds to prove points). The student only briefly stated his or her viewpoint.	The student chose not to present.

LESSON 6: MINE, YOURS, AND OURS WHOSE DECISION IS IT?

Level: Middle school, High school

Time: 30–40 minutes

National Health Education Standards

5. Decision-Making
7. Self-Management

National Sexuality Education Standards: Performance Indicators

- Describe the potential impacts of power differences such as age, status or position within relationships.
- Apply a decision-making model to various sexual health decisions.
- Demonstrate respect for the boundaries of others as they relate to intimacy and sexual behavior.

Rationale

In the excitement of romantic relationships, people sometimes compromise on their own wishes, which can include individuals' feeling that they have less power than their partner or not speaking up when they disagree. This lesson attempts to explain how people in healthy relationships allow their partner to make their own decisions and set boundaries. Students first brainstorm common decisions made within a dating relationship, and then discuss who in the relationship should make each decision. Overall, students will discover possible factors having to do with control within relationships, as well as come to understand that both partners have rights.

Materials and Preparation

Front board or large poster paper for the brainstorm activity

Set of three signs for each student, reading "Mine," "Yours," and "Ours"

Copies of "Letter to a Friend" homework

Procedure

1. Have students arrange themselves in a circle formation, with a section of the circle open so students can view the front board (or poster paper).
2. Begin by asking students to list in their notebook all the possible decisions that may be made within a dating relationship. After some minutes have passed, ask students

to write one of their listed decisions on the front board without repeating one already listed. Decisions might include

- Who should pay for a date
- Who decides where to go for the first date
- Who should ask whom out
- Who should kiss whom
- Whose decision is it to have a form of sex
- Whose decision is it to choose a form of birth control
- How a person should dress
- With whom a person can hang out
- How a person should act in front of others
- When to call or text each other
- How much time to spend together

3. Distribute the sets of signs to students. Explain that the signs will be used for students to note who is responsible for each specific decision in a dating relationship they are in or may eventually be. Specifically, the "Mine" sign will be raised by students who feel particular decisions are to be theirs within a dating relationship. The "Yours" sign will be raised by students who feel particular decisions are to be made by their partner. And the "Ours" sign should be raised by students who feel that particular decisions are to be made by either partner or both partners.
4. Begin by going over the decisions listed in the brainstorm, one at a time, in whatever order you think is most appropriate. For each decision, ask students to note who in the relationship should make the stated decision by raising one of the three signs ("Mine," "Yours," or "Ours"). Once all students have raised their chosen sign in response to a given decision, ask volunteers to discuss why they chose the particular person in the relationship to make that decision.

   Note: Students may at times be hesitant to display their decisions. It may therefore be helpful to have them respond to initial, "warm-up decisions" before moving on to those pertaining to more intimate decisions. Examples include

   - Who should pay when going to a movie
   - Who should call the other person first

   Then refer to the decisions noted on the board, perhaps beginning with ones for which students may find it easier to provide an answer.
5. If students disagree on who is responsible for the stated decision, allow them to express their viewpoint. For example, if the decision of whether or not to take the contraceptive pill arises in a heterosexual relationship, allow students to process if this decision is the male's responsibility, the female's responsibility, or the responsibility of both partners. Another example is the question of who should pay for a date in a same-sex

relationship. Allow students to process whether a specific person should pay for a date or whether either person in the relationship can pay.

Note: Students may disagree; however, they need to understand that not allowing a partner to make independent decisions creates an unbalanced and unhealthy relationship.

6. After many decisions have been discussed, ask the processing questions. Ensure that the following points are raised:
   - Allowing one person to make the majority of decisions in a relationship can alter the power balance within it.
   - Both people in the relationship have the right to make their own decisions about sexual behaviors. Each partner needs to respect the other's decision.
   - A decision pertaining directly to a person's physical, mental, or emotional health should not be taken lightly. Nobody has the right to demand that a person do anything he or she does not want to do.
7. Hand out the "Letter to a Friend" homework and ask students to complete it for the next class, during which letters may be shared.

Processing

1. How do you determine who is to decide certain things in a dating relationship?
2. Who taught you about decision making in dating or romantic relationships? Do you agree with what you were taught?
3. What decisions does the class agree on?
4. What decisions does the class *not* agree on? Why do you think that is?
5. If one person is given the responsibility of making particular decisions in a relationship, does that alter who has more power in the relationship? What is power in a relationship?
6. How does a power imbalance affect the health of a relationship?

Assessment

- Students participate in the class discussion and hold up their chosen signs.
- Students complete the "Letter to a Friend" homework assignment.

Name: ___________________________

Letter to a Friend

Directions: Your friend Pat just started dating Lee over three months ago. Because Pat does not want to cause any friction, Lee makes almost every decision in their relationship, including where to eat, what movies to see, and with whom to hang out. As more time passes, you notice Pat acting like a passive person, which is not like Pat at all. For the next class, write a letter to Pat that includes the following points:

1. Explain to Pat the lesson just completed in class, including the lesson's purpose.
2. Express your concern for Pat because Lee seems to have the "power" in their relationship.
3. Offer some suggestions for how Pat can talk to Lee about making more decisions.
4. Suggest one or more available resources for Pat to talk about the situation to gain additional input. Resources can include those discussed in earlier lessons.

The assignment will be graded according to the following rubric:

Letter to a Friend Rubric (16 Points Total)

	3–4 POINTS	1–2 POINTS	0 POINTS
Explanation of the day's lesson	The student explained the day's lesson and its purpose in his or her own words.	The student briefly stated what the day's lesson was about, but seemed confused about its purpose.	The student's explanation of the lesson was poor or not provided.
Description of power	The student correctly explained how a power imbalance can occur in a relationship and how one seems to be present in Pat's relationship.	The student raised the concern of a power imbalance, but did not explain his or her thoughts in sufficient detail.	The power imbalance was described incorrectly or was not referred to at all.
Advice	The student provided positive advice concerning what Pat can do about the situation, including noting a viable resource.	The student provided some advice to Pat, but information was brief. A resource was provided.	Advice was not provided or did not pertain to the situation. No resource was provided.
Overall presentation	The letter was written in a positive manner. The student included his or her own thoughts and feelings.	The letter was written in a fair manner. More could have been included in reference to thoughts and feelings.	The letter was poorly written, and no personal thoughts and feelings were included.

LESSON 7: BEING "IN THE MOMENT"—A STORYTELLING ACTIVITY*

Level: Middle school, High school

Time: 40–50 minutes

National Health Education Standards

1. Core Concepts
4. Interpersonal Communication
5. Decision-Making
7. Self-Management

National Sexuality Education Standards: Performance Indicators

- Explain the criteria for evaluating the health of a relationship.
- Describe characteristics of healthy and unhealthy romantic and/or sexual relationships.
- Demonstrate ways to communicate decisions about whether or when to engage in sexual behaviors.
- Demonstrate effective ways to communicate personal boundaries and show respect for the boundaries of others.
- Demonstrate effective ways to communicate personal boundaries as they relate to intimacy and sexual behavior.
- Demonstrate respect for the boundaries of others as they relate to intimacy and sexual behavior.

Rationale

The phrase "in the moment" is often used when a person attempts to explain a decision that was not thought out thoroughly. This lesson seeks to demonstrate this occurrence. In this lesson, students hear of a teenage couple that may eventually become sexually active. Students will then explore and describe what the couple needs to consider before doing anything physical with each other, including writing a skit (for homework) that incorporates refusal skills and performing a role-play during a future class.

Materials and Preparation

Dice (one for each student)

Name tags or sticky notes with one name from the included story written on each

Teacher copy of "In the Moment . . ."

Music

---

*This lesson uses ideas found in "How Crowded Is Your Bed?," a lesson from the following source: Montana Office of Public Instruction, HIV/AIDS/STD Program, *HIV/AIDS Prevention Education: K–12 Teaching Strategies for the Prevention of Unintended Pregnancy and HIV/AIDS/STD* (Helena, MT: Author, n.d.), 75–78, http://opi.mt.gov/pdf/hived/K–12OPIActivities.pdf.

Blanket

Pieces of clothing in a bag

Front board or newsprint and markers

Copies of "Refusal Skills: Ways to Say 'NO'" handout

Copies of "We Need to Talk" homework

Procedure

1. After students have entered the room and are settled, give each student one die. Ask students to roll their die six times and record their results in their notebook.
2. Next inform the class that you will tell them a story about two high school students who are in a heterosexual dating relationship. For this story, volunteers are needed for the main characters as well as others. After assigning two students as the main characters, Barbara and Tom, have those students hand out the name tags to others in the class. Depending on the class size, some students may not be given a name tag.
3. Ask "Barbara" and "Tom" to stand in the front of the class. Begin to explain the situation they are in, as mentioned in Part 1 of the included story, "In the Moment . . ." For added affect, ask the characters particular questions; for example, you can ask what meal Tom is going to prepare for Barbara (the most common answer tends to be macaroni and cheese).
4. Continue reading the story as both main characters act out their role.
5. At the end of the first part of the story, stop Barbara and Tom from continuing the role-play. Each should remain at the front of the room.
6. Ask the class, "What should Tom and Barbara consider before continuing?" Have the class brainstorm all considerations Barbara and Tom should think about before continuing with their evening. Write this list on the front board (or newsprint). The list may include
   - Whom Tom or Barbara may tell later or the next day.
   - Their reputations.
   - Whether their feelings toward one another may change, for the better or for the worse.
   - Whether they should use a condom or other type of birth control.
   - Possible pregnancy occurrence. (At this point, ask those students who rolled a six with their die to stand up. This number represents who got pregnant or got someone pregnant.)
   - Possible STIs. (Ask anyone who rolled a five to stand. This number represents who got an STI.)
   - If they are being videotaped (unfortunately, people have done this without their partner's knowledge).
   - Their sexual histories.

   During this brainstorm, continue to ask whether the audience heard Tom or Barbara communicate with each other about any of the mentioned concerns while being "in the moment." For example, did Barbara ask about Tom's past, and vice versa?

7. After the brainstorm, explain that Tom and Barbara posted personal blogs online. They chose to note their respective sexual histories, which will now be revealed to the entire class.
8. Place the blanket on the floor in front of Tom and Barbara. Begin to read Part 2 of the story. As a new name is mentioned, the person with that name on her name tag should go toward the front of the room. If any form of sexual contact was mentioned with that character, ask the person to stand on the blanket. If there was no sexual contact, the person should stand near but not on the blanket.
9. Continue reading the rest of the story. Pause when students approach the blanket so they can determine whether they should be on or off the blanket. At the end of the story, this visual history of Tom and Barbara shows students how a person's past can have an impact on future relationships.
10. At the end of the story, ask the class to assess what they saw. Within this discussion, ask the processing questions. Also discuss whether or not people from either person's past who have an STI should be on the blanket.
11. Distribute the "Refusal Skills: Ways to Say 'NO'" handout to students. Discuss how each refusal technique helps avoid unhealthy or risky situations. Then ask students to reenact the lesson's story using effective communication skills to ensure healthier decisions (see the rubric that follows).
12. Assign students the "We Need to Talk" homework, which will be checked and discussed during the next class meeting.

For your reference, here is a rubric for both the role-play and the homework:

Role-Play and "We Need to Talk" Homework Rubric (4 Points Total)

	2 POINTS	1 POINT	0 POINTS
Consequences of engaging in sexual behavior	The scenario was realistic and contained two or more consequences of engaging in sexual behavior. Information was correct.	The scenario was somewhat realistic and contained one consequence of engaging in sexual behavior. Information was correct.	The answer was too brief, it was inappropriate, no consequences were given, or a combination of these issues.
Use of effective communication	The scenario contained the use of effective communication skills. Two specific refusal skills were noted.	The scenario contained the use of effective communication skills. One specific refusal skill was noted.	Inappropriate communication occurred, no refusal skills were shown, or both.

Processing

1. How realistic is this situation? Explain.
2. What could potentially happen in this situation?
3. Who rolled a six with the die? What does this mean? How do you feel about this?
4. Who rolled a five with the die? What does this mean? How do you feel about this?
5. Have you heard of this scenario happening in real life? Without mentioning names, what was the outcome?
6. Did Barbara and Tom communicate effectively about what they were doing? Explain.
7. What should Barbara and Tom have talked about before getting "in the moment"?
8. What are the risks involved in this moment? What do you think will happen next?

Assessment

- Students practice active listening during the scenario involving Barbara and Tom.
- In the follow-up discussion, students note the lack of communication skills within the role-play. Students offer suggestions for what should have been communicated.
- Students reenact the story using effective communication skills to ensure healthier decisions.
- Students complete the "We Need to Talk" homework. Within students' dialogue, effective communication skills are shown.

In the Moment . . .

Part 1

Barbara and **Tom** are both high school seniors and have been dating for a few months. In May, Tom's father needed to attend a work conference, which would last from Wednesday night until Saturday afternoon. Being a sweet boyfriend, Tom invited Barbara over to make her dinner on Friday night. His brother **Bob,** who is a junior in college, was supposed to watch over Tom for the weekend. Bob, however, felt Tom did not need a "babysitter" and made plans to hang out with his own friends elsewhere.

So, on Friday night, Tom made Barbara dinner. (Ask the person pretending to be Tom what he would make.) To set the mood, Tom lit some candles and put on some nice music. (Play the music.)

After dinner, they sat on the couch in the living room. They began to kiss, and then . . . (Explain to the class that to respect Tom and Barbara's privacy, you will hold a blanket in front of them, with the help of another person, so they cannot be seen by the rest of the class. After the blanket is blocking where both students are sitting or standing, quietly ask them to go through the bag of clothing and throw the pieces over the blanket toward the audience. This will generally elicit both shock and laughter from the class. After the last piece of clothing is thrown, announce to the class that suddenly Tom, Barbara, or both realized what was about to occur and said, "Stop.")

Part 2

The following is an overview of Tom's and Barbara's sexual history:

Tom: As a freshman, Tom dated **Emily** for half of the year. All they did was kiss. Tom wanted more, so he broke up with her and started dating **Joanne.** After a few months, they went all the way and had sex. Over the summer, Joanne told Tom she thought she was pregnant. After much stress and worry, Joanne finally got her period. Tom and Joanne broke up shortly thereafter because things seemed too intense.

Barbara: As a freshman, Barbara dated **Cody.** They engaged in open-mouth kissing.

Tom: As a sophomore, Tom did not officially date anyone. He occasionally made out with some girls, and had oral sex performed on him by **Sue, Peggy, and Casey.** Casey has oral herpes.

Barbara: As a sophomore, Barbara visited her sister in college, where she attended a college party. At this party, she drank *a lot.* Since she was so drunk, she does not remember much; but she *does* remember having sex with some college guy she'd just met. She is "pretty sure" his name is **Wayne.** Wayne is kind of a "player" and has had sex with several females. We will just call them **"A," "B," "C," "D," "E,"** and so on.

Tom: As a junior, Tom started to rekindle a relationship with Joanne. They dated for a few months, and then broke up before the summer.

Barbara: As a junior, Barbara hooked up with **Dominic, Jack, and Jill.** She had some form of sex with each of these three people.

Name: ______________________________

Refusal Skills: Ways to Say "NO"

1. Be like a broken record—say "no" over and over.

   "No. I said 'no.'"

2. Be assertive with your words and body language.

   "I'm not interested in doing that" (using a firm tone and assertive body language).

3. Give a reason.

   "That's illegal," or "That's not safe," or simply "I don't want to do that!"

4. Ask questions.

   "What are you asking me to do?" or "Why do you want me to do that?"

5. Suggest a healthier and safer alternative.

   "Why don't we just stop what we are doing and go see a movie?"

6. Change the subject—talk about something else.

   "Have you finished your chemistry project yet?"

7. Use humor or sarcasm.

   "Oh sure, that's a *great* idea! If we get caught I'll be grounded for life."

8. Leave the situation, but keep the door open.

   "I'm leaving. I'm gonna listen to music. If you want to come, let me know."

Name: ______________________________

"We Need to Talk"

One stereotype about heterosexual romantic relationships is that the male is always the aggressor, pressuring the female to have sex. For this situation, assume Barbara was the aggressor and was pressuring Tom to have sex. Also assume that Tom did not think he was ready to have sex with Barbara.

Directions: Prepare a brief conversation between Tom and Barbara illustrating two types of refusal skills. Include in the conversation at least two risks associated with unplanned sexual activity. The first sentence has been written to help get you started.

Barbara: Come on, Tom, what's the matter? Don't you find me attractive?

Tom: ____

____

Barbara: ____

____

Tom: ____

____

Barbara: ____

____

Tom: ____

____

Barbara: ____

____

Tom: ____

____

LESSON 8: RANKING RISKS

SEXUALITY AND RELATIONSHIPS

Level: High school

Time: 40–45 minutes

National Health Education Standards

1. Core Concepts
4. Interpersonal Communication
7. Self-Management

National Sexuality Education Standards: Performance Indicators

- Compare and contrast behaviors, including abstinence, to determine the potential risk of STI/HIV transmission from each.
- Evaluate the effectiveness of abstinence, condoms and other safer sex methods in preventing the spread of STIs, including HIV.
- Analyze individual responsibility about testing for and informing partners about STIs and HIV status.
- Define sexual consent and explain its implications for sexual decision-making.
- Describe a range of ways to express affection within healthy relationships.
- Demonstrate effective ways to communicate personal boundaries as they relate to intimacy and sexual behavior.
- Demonstrate respect for the boundaries of others as they relate to intimacy and sexual behavior.

Rationale

Relationships involve taking risks. These risks create consequences, both positive and negative. Because of these risks, students need to understand the importance of personal decision making while in a romantic relationship. The objective of this lesson is to engage students in discussing behaviors that are potentially risky (to one's physical, social, mental, emotional, and/or spiritual health), then ranking them from higher risk to lower risk. Small groups will share their rankings with other groups to compare and discuss their rationales. By doing this, students will analyze the short- and long-term consequences of safe, risky, or harmful behaviors.

Materials and Preparation

Two index cards or strips of card stock per group, one reading "Higher Risk" and the other reading "Lower Risk"

Copies of "Chris and Pat: Extended Response Essay" handout

Masking tape, cut into small strips

For each group, ten index cards or strips of card stock with one risky behavior (written in bold Magic Marker) on each. (Suggestions for risk cards are included at the end of this lesson; alternately, you can create some in accordance with the needs of the class.)

Procedure

1. Ask students to explain what it means to take a *risk*. Explain that we all take risks every day, such as asking a person out, sitting next to someone we do not know, not doing homework, or volunteering during a class presentation. Some risks have minor consequences, whereas others have major consequences.
2. State the following: "From the time people are young, they take risks every day, and each time they take a risk, they learn something and grow as people. Although people do not know for sure what will happen when taking a risk, it is important for them to think about the possible consequences of a risky behavior before doing it. Consequences can be positive or negative. Consequences can affect a person's physical, social, mental, emotional, and/or spiritual health. They can also have legal implications. Because of this, we will be assessing the levels of risk for a list of behaviors."
3. Divide the class into four or five mixed-sex groups. Assign a group leader for each group, and give this student a set of two cards. The "Higher Risk" card should be taped near the top of the wall, and the "Lower Risk" card should be taped toward the bottom of the wall. Also, give each group a set of ten risk cards.
4. Explain to each group that they will have five minutes to rank the ten behaviors from highest risk to lowest risk. They should start with what they believe is the riskiest behavior, tape that card under the "Higher Risk" card, and then move on to what they believe is the next riskiest behavior, placing it below the first card. Although group members may not agree on all rankings, they must come to some consensus on the order.
5. After five minutes have passed, ask one of the groups to display their list for the large group and provide a brief rationale for their rankings. The other groups should then, in turn, follow suit.
6. After all groups have presented, allow for cross-group discussion. The focus should not be on what the "correct" order is (there is none), but on *why* different groups and individuals perceive things differently. Answers can include personal experiences, family and individual values, and the setting; all play an important part in influencing an individual's choices. Remind students of the importance of health-enhancing behaviors when making all decisions.

   Note: Students should also understand that some of the risks on the cards could have positive consequences. Allow the groups to process how positive consequences influenced their rankings.
7. When all groups have shared their list, have students return to their seat; take out their notebook; and brainstorm whether each risk listed can have an impact on a person's *physical, social, mental, emotional,* and/or *spiritual health*—or a combination of these. They can also address any legal ramifications of certain risky behaviors.
8. Continue the discussion by asking the processing questions.
9. Conclude the lesson by assigning the "Chris and Pat: Extended Response Essay" homework. Also, ask students to complete a follow-up activity in which they are to write a journal entry titled "A Time When I Took a Risk." For this, students should write about a personal experience in which they took a risk, including a description of the consequences. The composition should answer the following questions:

a. What was at risk? Did the risk have an impact on your physical, social, mental, emotional, and/or spiritual health? Were there legal consequences?
b. What or who influenced your decision to take the risk?
c. What were the consequences? Were they positive, negative, or mixed? Explain.
d. Would you take that risk again if it came up in the future?
e. What did you learn from the experience? Did it help you grow as a person?

Note: Some students may be uncomfortable writing about themselves. Allow students the option of writing about a fictional person instead. As with any classroom activity, students should know that if they reveal personal information related to hurting themselves, hurting others, or being abused, you, as a mandated reporter, are required to follow up with proper guidance personnel.

Processing

1. What rankings did your group agree on? Why do you think this is so?
2. Which items led to the most discussion or caused the most disagreement in the group?
3. How did personal experiences or personal values affect your rankings?
4. How does your sex affect how you perceive risk?
5. How did your group incorporate positive consequences into your rankings?
6. What risks are worth taking?
7. What risks do you think a person should take more than once?
8. What risks have you seen your peers experience?

Assessment

- Students discuss the topic of assessing risks, in groups and as a class. Student knowledge should include correct information about sexual risks pertaining to STIs and protection as well as personal safety.
- Students each write a journal entry titled "A Time When I Took a Risk."
- Students write an essay to complete the "Chris and Pat: Extended Response Essay" homework. This assignment can be read aloud in a future class.

Suggestions for Risk Cards

- Going to someone's apartment after meeting him or her at a college party
- Asking someone you do not know to dance with you while at a dance club or party
- Telling a longtime friend that you want to be "more than friends"
- Saying "I love you" for the first time to someone you have been dating
- Telling a boyfriend or girlfriend that you have genital herpes
- Telling a parent or guardian that you are pregnant or got someone pregnant
- Getting drunk and going out to someone's car to "be alone"
- Communicating with a college-age boyfriend or girlfriend that you want to remain abstinent until marriage
- Engaging in unprotected oral sex with a boyfriend or girlfriend
- Having unprotected sex
- Having sexual intercourse one time using a condom
- Engaging in oral sex with a person you just met and using protection
- Being a fifteen-year-old female and accepting a ride home from a party by a person you do not know
- Going to a clinic or doctor's office to get tested for HIV
- Communicating with your partner about using condoms before having sex

Chris and Pat: Extended Response Essay

Chris and Pat are both seniors in high school. They have been dating for several months. Up until now they have enjoyed a physical relationship that involves kissing and cuddling, but have not yet had any sexual contact. Pat feels ready to have sex and wants to bring up the topic on their date tonight. Chris has enjoyed the physical closeness so far, but does not think it is the right time to start having sex.

Directions: Write a brief skit in which Chris explains to Pat the consequences of having sexual contact. These consequences should be described in detail, including what area or areas of health may be affected (physical, social, mental, emotional, and/or spiritual). Chris should use appropriate interpersonal communication skills, including using an assertive but respectful tone and showing care and consideration for Pat's feelings. Chris should also use "I" messages, and at least two accurate facts related to possible consequences of sexual activity should be included.

Extended Response Essay Rubric (4 Points Total)

	2 POINTS	1 POINT	0 POINTS
Consequences of engaging in sexual behavior	The scenario was realistic and contained two or more consequences of engaging in sexual behavior. Information was correct.	The scenario was somewhat realistic and contained one consequence of engaging in sexual behavior. Information was correct.	The answer was too brief, it was inappropriate, no consequences were given, or a combination of these issues.
Use of effective communication	The scenario contained the use of effective communication skills. Two specific refusal skills were noted.	The scenario contained the use of effective communication skills. One specific refusal skill was noted.	Inappropriate communication occurred, no refusal skills were shown, or both.

LESSON 9: "WHAT'S YOUR NUMBER?"

Level: High school

Time: 40–50 minutes

National Health Education Standards

2. Analyzing Influences
4. Interpersonal Communication
7. Self-Management

National Sexuality Education Standards: Performance Indicators

- Analyze influences that may have an impact on deciding whether or when to engage in sexual behaviors.
- Analyze individual responsibility about testing for and informing partners about STIs and HIV status.
- Explain the criteria for evaluating the health of a relationship.
- Demonstrate respect for the boundaries of others as they relate to intimacy and sexual behavior.

Rationale

Movies and TV programs involving new romantic relationships rarely show a couple having a conversation about their respective sexual histories. This lesson allows students to consider discussing a potential partner's history and to think about how learning that information might affect their relationship. During this lesson, the concept of "double standards" may arise for heterosexual couples. Allow students to process whether or not double standards exist and what, if anything, can be done about them.

Materials and Preparation

Copies of "What's Your Number?" worksheet

Signs reading "No" and "Yes," taped up on opposite sides of the room. A third sign reading "Not Sure" should be taped in another area of the room.

Scrap paper for exit card responses

Procedure

1. Start the lesson by reminding students of effective communication skills, including how to phrase statements of disagreement. If students have not yet had practice in assertiveness techniques, including the use of "I" statements, spend some time going over these important skills.
2. Distribute the "What's Your Number?" worksheet. Students should quietly read the scenario to themselves and answer the questions.
3. After students' worksheets are completed, note the signs reading "No," "Yes," and "Not Sure" in the three different sections of the room. Explain that you are going to read aloud the questions from the worksheet, and that students are to indicate their answer

to each by standing by the appropriate sign. Ask students to take a stand, but allow those who are undecided to stand under the "Not Sure" sign.

4. Read the first question aloud, and have students answer it by standing by their chosen answer's sign. As soon as all students are standing by their answer's sign, ask for volunteers to share why they have chosen their particular answer.
5. After students have expressed their opinions and given brief explanations, read the next question aloud. Follow the same procedure until all remaining questions have been asked and answered.
6. To conclude the lesson, ask the processing questions. Give students time to consider question 5 in particular, noting that what is shown on TV or in movies *does not* usually include a discussion about sexual histories.
7. With five minutes left, ask students to respond anonymously to the following exit card question: "How does knowing a romantic partner's sexual history influence your decisions in the relationship? Explain in at least two paragraphs." Tell students to consider such factors as
   - The number of past sex partners
   - If sexual partners were of the same sex, the opposite sex, or both
   - If a past pregnancy occurred
   - If a curable STI, like chlamydia, had been diagnosed and cured
   - If an incurable STI, like herpes type 2, genital warts (HPV), or HIV, had been diagnosed.

   On leaving, students should hand in their response, which will be shared during the next class.
8. As an optional assignment, ask students to share the scenario from the lesson with another peer, friend, or family member, noting that person's opinions. Students then are to journal about what was said and whether or not they agree.

Processing

1. What was your initial reaction to what Sam was asking? How appropriate was the question?
2. What *rights* do people have in regard to knowing their partner's sexual history?
3. What *responsibilities* do people have when it comes to revealing their personal sexual history?
4. How can discussing a partner's sexual past be made comfortable for both people?
5. In real-life situations, how often do you think people discuss their sexual histories? Why is this?
6. How does discussing sexual histories affect current romantic relationships?

Assessment

- Students explain their answers from the "What's Your Number?" worksheet.
- Through the in-class discussion, students address people's responsibility to inform potential sexual partners of important health information within romantic relationships.
- Students respond anonymously to the exit card question.
- Students share the lesson's scenario with another peer, friend, or family member, and journal about the experience.

Name: ______________________________

"What's Your Number?"

Kim recognized Sam as soon as she entered her friend's house. Sam was in her first-semester college English course, and for four months they had exchanged flirtatious glances across the classroom. Now she was able to really meet her crush, and they spent the next two hours talking about trivial factoids in each other's lives.

Having an early soccer game the next morning, Kim told Sam she needed to leave. "Hold on . . . before you leave . . . what's your number?"

Kim looked down and blushed, feeling her heart skip a beat. She had never had a real romantic relationship in high school, just people she hung out with. But the idea of falling in love before graduating from high school excited her. She began to answer, "212-555 . . ."

"No," interrupted Sam, "I mean your number of sex partners."

Kim was stunned. She had never been asked a question like this before and did not know how to answer. Luckily, Sam's phone buzzed, noting that a new text message was received, and before they could continue talking, Kim quickly left the house.

Directions: Circle your answers to the following questions to the best of your ability:

1. Does Sam have the right to ask Kim this question?	Yes	No	Not sure
2. Does Kim have the right to ask Sam this question?	Yes	No	Not sure
3. If Kim has never had any form of sex, should she answer?	Yes	No	Not sure
4. If Sam has never had any form of sex, does it matter?	Yes	No	Not sure
5. Does the situation change if "Sam" is the nickname for "Samantha"?	Yes	No	Not sure
6. Does the number of past sexual partners matter?	Yes	No	Not sure
7. Do people always tell the truth about this number?	Yes	No	Not sure

Final question: What does this number represent to you? If someone were a virgin, would this be a positive thing or a negative thing? If someone has had several sexual partners, would it bother you? Explain your answers.

LESSON 10: LOVE IN THE DIGITAL AGE HOW TECHNOLOGY CAN HELP OR HURT

Level: Middle school, High school

Time: 40–50 minutes

National Health Education Standards

1. Core Concepts
2. Analyzing Influences
4. Interpersonal Communication
5. Decision-Making

National Sexuality Education Standards: Performance Indicators

- Describe the advantages and disadvantages of communicating using technology and social media.
- Evaluate the potentially positive and negative roles of technology and social media in relationships.
- Analyze the impact of technology and social media on friendships and relationships.
- Demonstrate effective ways to communicate personal boundaries and show respect for the boundaries of others.
- Describe strategies to use social media safely, legally and respectfully.
- Develop a plan to stay safe when using social media.

Rationale

In today's times, technology has advanced, allowing people to obtain information on numerous subjects and communicate with others in a variety of ways. Although Internet sites can provide information on a variety of topics as well as support for specific groups, people need to recognize that some sites may be biased, possibly containing inaccurate information. In addition, social networking sites allow people to share personal information that can be used to coerce or harm them. The objective of this lesson is to allow students to process how current technology can offer advantages and disadvantages to personal relationships. In addition, students may be provided with additional activities to plan how to remain safe when using technology and social media.

Materials and Preparation

Front board, with the following written on it: "How does the use of technology and social media help or hurt possible romantic relationships?"

Large poster paper and markers for each group (with tape to hang the completed poster) or copies of "Love Today: How Technology Can Help or Hurt" worksheet (one per group)

Scrap paper for exit card responses

Bulletin board (optional)

Procedure

1. Begin the lesson by asking students to list the current forms of technology they use to communicate with others. The list should include cell phones (for calls, texting, and so on) and the Internet (for e-mailing, blogging, using social networking sites, and so on). As students name examples, write them on the board. Point out that technology has brought us many advantages, yet at the same time has created concerns, including ones related to romantic relationships.
2. Refer to the question written on the board, explaining that the day's lesson will provide additional insight into possible answers.
3. Create groups of four to five students and distribute to each group either the "Love Today: How Technology Can Help or Hurt" worksheet or markers and a piece of poster paper on which a chart can be drawn and filled in. Explain that each group will complete their chart by listing "pros" for how technology can help romantic relationships. After each pro, the group should write a corresponding con or cons. (An example is provided on the worksheet.)
4. Give the groups ten to fifteen minutes to complete their chart.
5. After the groups have completed their chart to the best of their ability, ask one group to share one of their pro-con pairs with the class. After their point is discussed, ask the next group to give another example. As groups explain what they discussed, ask the students to add new pros and cons to their chart. An overall list can also be written on a front board for students to see the many pros and cons when it comes to using technology within romantic relationships.
6. After all groups have shared their examples, ask the processing questions.
7. To conclude the activity, ask students to note on an exit card one strategy people should employ when using technology and social media. These can be read to students during the next lesson to remind the class what was discussed, or they can be used to fill a bulletin board on the topic.

   Note: Additional classroom activities focusing on online safety can be found at www.safesocialnetworking.org, where you can sign up to receive additional information on online safety by creating an account. After inputting your name and school information, you will receive an e-mail with links to resources. Resources include information for teachers and students as well as student worksheets and extension activities.

Processing

1. In your opinion, does technology help or hurt potential romantic relationships? Explain.
2. How does your use of technology help or hurt your personal relationships?
3. Has using technology or social media caused a problem for someone you know? Without using names, explain the situation.
4. When using technology to communicate with others, what do you do to ensure effective communication?
5. Imagine that you have a younger brother or sister. What strategies would you teach him or her to be safe online?

Assessment

- Groups note the advantages and disadvantages of communicating via technology and social media.
- Students participate in the class discussion.
- Students complete their exit card.
- Students complete worksheets and extension activities from www.safesocialnetworking.org (optional).

Names: ____

____

Love Today: How Technology Can Help or Hurt

Directions: Fill in the following table by listing the pros (how technology can help a possible romantic relationship). After each pro is listed, make sure to include any cons (how the listed pro can hurt).

PROS	CONS
For example: • Dating websites might help you meet a possible boyfriend or girlfriend.	• People may not tell the truth in personal online descriptions. • Online services can be expensive.

LESSON 11: COME-ONS AND PRESSURE LINES

COMMUNICATING ABOUT SEX

Level: Middle school, High school

Time: 40 minutes

National Health Education Standard

4. Interpersonal Communication

National Sexuality Education Standards: Performance Indicators

- Demonstrate effective ways to communicate personal boundaries and show respect for the boundaries of others.
- Demonstrate effective ways to communicate personal boundaries as they relate to intimacy and sexual behavior.
- Demonstrate effective skills to negotiate agreements about the use of technology in relationships.

Rationale

Assertive communication enables people to maintain self-respect and clearly and honestly state their needs, wants, and feelings without dominating or abusing others. This includes resisting pressure to engage in sexual activity. Within this lesson, students will observe and practice negotiation and compromising skills to understand their importance in building and maintaining healthy relationships. Students will also practice assertive communication skills by resisting pressure to become sexually involved.

Materials and Preparation

Masking tape, long enough to make a line down the center of the classroom

Copies of "Communication Styles: How to Be Assertive" handout

Copies of "Come-Ons and Pressure Lines" homework. In addition, there should be small slips of paper, each with a pressure line from the homework written on it.

Procedure

ACTIVITY 1: COME OVER TO MY SIDE

1. Without any introductory statements, ask for ten volunteers. The volunteers should form two lines of five people each; one line is to stand on one side of the tape; the other line should stand on the opposite side of the tape. Volunteers should each be facing a peer from the other line.
2. Ask students to pair off with the person opposite them.
3. Tell students that they are going to play a little game, the objective of which is to try to get their partner to cross over to their side of the line. If they can get their partner to

come over to their side, they will *win*. Competition is only with their partner, not with other pairs. Students can use whatever communication strategies they can think of to entice their partner to come over to their side (for example: offering money, begging, playing up sex appeal, making promises), but they may not use any form of *physical force* to drag their partner across the line. Tell students that they will only have one minute to do this.

4. Ask if they have any questions. If not, begin the game by saying, "Go!"
5. The rest of the class should observe the different tactics used to entice partners over the line. At the end of one minute, say, "Stop!"
6. Ask processing questions 1 through 4.
7. If there was a stalemate, explain that this was a lose-lose situation. Neither person got what he or she wanted. If one partner stayed in place and the other crossed, this was a win-lose situation (or a lose-win situation for the person who crossed over the tape).
8. Occasionally, there will be a pair of students who figured out how to have a win-win solution. If not, reveal the "secret" of the game by asking all students to stand in their original spot. Then ask everyone to cross over so everyone is then standing on the opposite side. By doing this, *everybody* wins!
9. Explain that this exercise required negotiation and compromise. In a disagreement or in a relationship, there often must be a willingness on the part of both parties to try to work out a win-win solution. Often, people do not get everything they want, but they can both get *some* of what they want from the other person.
10. Extended discussion can lead into characteristics of healthy and unhealthy relationships. Remind students that one of the most important aspects of a healthy relationship is the partners' willingness to compromise and assertively communicate their needs and wants to the other person.

ACTIVITY 2: BEING ASSERTIVE

1. Distribute the "Communication Styles: How to Be Assertive" handout.
2. Discuss and model the three types of communication styles. A simple example you could give is as follows:

   You are in a restaurant. You order a hamburger well done. When it arrives at your table, you realize that it is too rare and not cooked enough. You can respond to this dilemma using one of three common communication styles.

   A *passive response* would be to think, but not speak, "I do not like my food this rare, but I feel funny saying something, so I will just try eating it." An *aggressive response* would be to say, "Hey waiter. This burger is so rare that I can hear it moo! I demand to see the manager!" An *assertive response* would be to say, "Excuse me. I ordered this burger well done and it is rare. Would you please take it back and ask for it to be cooked a little bit more?"

3. Explain that sometimes in a relationship, one partner is interested in starting a sexual relationship and the other partner is not. In such situations, there are often common "pressure lines" people use to get their partner to have sex.

4. Go around the room and quietly distribute the slips of paper with the pressure lines, one to each student. Inform them that their task is to formulate a "comeback line" to the pressure line. In their response, they should communicate in an assertive manner that they do not want to engage in sexual activity at this time. Allow a few minutes for students to think of their comeback line.
5. Then begin to read the pressure lines aloud. For each one, the student who was assigned that pressure line should respond with an assertive comeback line.
6. Continue around the room until all students have gone and all pressure lines have been given a response.
7. Allow students to discuss the comeback lines by asking processing questions 5 through 8.
8. At the conclusion of the lesson, distribute copies of the "Come-Ons and Pressure Lines" homework, and ask students to write responses to all of the pressure lines for next class.

Processing

1. Of the five pairs, did any person convince his or her partner to change sides? If so, how did he or she do it?
2. Why did people refuse to cross the line?
3. What would you call a situation in which one person gains and the other doesn't? (Win-lose)
4. What would you call a situation in which both people gain? (Win-win)
5. Which comeback lines were most effective? Why?
6. Which were not effective? Why?
7. Who here has a friend who has been pressured to be sexually active? Without saying the person's name, what happened? Would you have done things differently?
8. Why do you think there are so many lines designed to pressure someone to have sex? Where are these lines heard?

Assessment

- Students understand the principles of compromise and negotiation based on the first activity.
- Students participate in the pressure lines activity, and demonstrate assertive communication in their response.
- Students give written responses to the pressure lines for homework.

Communication Styles: How to Be Assertive

Assertive communication skills are important ones to have in a healthy relationship. These skills can be learned and practiced, and they enable you to be more comfortable and capable when it comes to having a healthy relationship.

Overall, there are three main communication styles:

Passive: When being passive, you accept a situation or statement without resistance. You are afraid to say how you feel in a situation and don't stand up for yourself. You let something happen without communicating what you feel is the right thing to do.

Assertive: When being assertive, you know what you want to do in a situation, and you confidently communicate what you want or feel. You do not let something "just happen"; instead, you state your viewpoint confidently, maintaining good posture and eye contact.

Aggressive: When being aggressive, you state your feelings or opinions in a forceful way. You know what you want to communicate and choose to do so in an angry manner. You may accomplish expressing your opinion, but you do so in a disrespectful and potentially harmful manner.

When it comes to communication, being **assertive** allows you to effectively

- STATE how you think and feel without hurting the other person's feelings
- STAND UP for your values and beliefs without putting the other person down
- STAND UP for your rights without abusing or taking advantage of the other person
- STATE what you want in a way that the other person should be able to respond positively to

"I" Messages

Understanding "I" messages" can be helpful in learning how to be assertive.

Steps to an "I" Message

1. Always start with "I," not "you." "I" puts the focus on your feelings, wants, and needs.
2. Clearly and simply state **how** you feel.
3. Say **what** is occurring that you do not agree with.
4. Tell the person what you **want** or **need.**

Example of an "I" Message

"I feel disappointed and taken for granted when you pressure me to do something I don't want to do. I need you to respect my feelings and decision."

Tips for Communicating Assertively in a Romantic Relationship

- Use "I" messages as much as possible.
- Listen to your partner and ask that your partner listen to you. Respect your partner's limits and boundaries. This is what a healthy relationship is all about.
- Say what you mean, and mean what you say. Be firm in the volume and tone of your voice, your facial expressions, and your body language.
- Make sure that one person does not dominate the other. Being equal partners usually means having a better and healthier relationship.
- Remember that **respect** and **responsibility** are two of the most important characteristics of a healthy relationship.

Name: ______________________________

Come-Ons and Pressure Lines

One of the most difficult parts of choosing to delay sex may be learning how to deal with situations in which sex is all your friends and peers are talking about. The person you are dating may also pressure you. Educating yourself on effective ways to let someone know "you are just not ready" is the best way to stick to your personal decision.

Some of the most popular come-ons have been around since your parents or guardians were teenagers. They are the pressure lines people typically use to convince others that having sex (of any form) is okay. By knowing what some of these pressure lines are, you can develop and practice your responses before you might actually encounter them. Doing so allows you to more confidently and firmly say "no."

Good luck!

Pressure Lines

Directions: For each of the pressure lines that follow, come up with a response to communicate you are not ready to have sex at this time in your life.

1. "It will strengthen our relationship."

____

____

2. "Show me you love me."

____

____

3. "But I love you."

____

____

4. "I'll stop whenever you tell me to."

____

____

5. "I've done it with everyone I've ever been in a relationship with. It's no big deal."

____

____

Name: ___________________________

Come-Ons and Pressure Lines (*continued*)

6. "I'll break up with you if you don't have sex with me."

7. "Nothing will happen. I promise."

8. "What are you waiting for? You're not planning on being a virgin your whole life, are you?"

9. "What are you afraid of?"

10. "If you don't have sex with me, I'll find someone who will."

11. "Sex is normal and natural. It will make you feel good."

12. "I've been tested, and I'm clean."

13. "Don't worry. I always use condoms."

14. "Don't worry. I'm on the pill."

(*continued*)

Name: ______________________________

Come-Ons and Pressure Lines (*continued*)

15. "Let me share this with you. If you really love me, you'll do it."

16. "Everybody's doing it."

17. "Nobody has to know. It will be our secret."

18. "I thought you found me attractive."

19. "What are you, a prude? What are you waiting for?"

20. "I'll use two condoms just to make it safer!"

21. "You got me all hot and bothered. I need a release!"

Can you think of any other come-ons and pressure lines? Write them here, along with possible responses.

LESSON 12: RICH'S DILEMMA

Level: Middle school, High school

Time: 40–50 minutes

National Health Education Standards

1. Core Concepts
4. Interpersonal Communication
8. Advocacy

National Sexuality Education Standards: Performance Indicators

- Describe the potential impacts of power differences such as age, status or position within relationships.
- Demonstrate effective strategies to avoid or end an unhealthy relationship.
- Demonstrate ways to treat others with dignity and respect.

Rationale

One difficult part of some romantic relationships is when they end. Ending a relationship is painful and requires coping skills. To better understand this concept, students will evaluate an ending of a high school relationship by reading a letter written by a high school boy. After hypothesizing why the breakup occurred, students will role-play one of two scenarios, demonstrating effective communication skills. Students will receive critical feedback on their role-play from their peers.

Materials and Preparation

Copies of "Rich's Dilemma" worksheet

Any needed props for role-plays

Procedure

1. Begin the lesson by explaining that students will be exploring a situation that happened to a teenage boy. The situation caused distress in his life, as has been the case with many other teenagers who have had the same experience. Explain to students that the objective of the lesson is to better understand why breakups happen and to practice effective communication skills to lessen the distress in similar situations in the future.
2. Allow students to form groups of four or five people (or you can create the groups). Distribute a copy of the "Rich's Dilemma" worksheet to each student. Ask groups to read about the situation, and then discuss the listed questions in Part 1 of the worksheet. As they are doing this, walk around the room to ensure the groups are on task (and not jumping to Part 2).
3. After all groups have discussed the situation and questions, have a brief discussion with the whole class to ensure that students correctly understand the situation and the level of discomfort Rich experienced.

4. Continue the discussion by asking the first five processing questions. Allow students to hypothesize about what the cause of the breakup was.
5. Next, explain that the class will be given the opportunity to role-play one of two scenarios dealing with Rich's breakup. It might be helpful to review effective communication practices with students beforehand, including assertive body positioning, using "I" statements, and interacting with no or limited distractions.
6. Ask groups to complete Part 2, undertaking one of two role-plays pertaining to the situation. Allow the groups ten minutes to prepare their script and skit.
7. Students will then present their skit, as the other groups note down feedback on their worksheets. This feedback can either be shared after each individual group presents or after all groups have performed. You, as the teacher, can also provide feedback.
8. Complete the lesson by asking the remaining two processing questions.
9. Before students leave the classroom, collect their worksheets to read the notes on the role-plays. These can be summarized for students during the next class.

Processing

1. Why do you think Rich's relationship ended?
2. What influences can affect a dating relationship?
3. Does the person who ends a relationship have more "power" over the other person? Explain.
4. What advice do you have for Rich?
5. How can a person cope in a healthy manner when another person breaks up with him or her?
6. Explain the positive communication skills shown in the role-plays.
7. What suggestions do you have to strengthen these role-plays, and to improve these types of conversations?

Assessment

- Students complete the "Rich's Dilemma" worksheet within their group.
- Groups' role-plays and scripts demonstrate effective strategies for coping with a breakup, modeling how to treat others with dignity and respect.
- Students evaluate role-plays on their worksheet.

Name: ____________________

Rich's Dilemma

Directions: Imagine that the following message has been put into a Question Box for your health teacher to read to the class. The student, who signed the message as "Rich," is an eleventh grader and has not had a lot of experience dating. Can you help him out?

> I recently got out of a relationship and to be completely honest, I do not even know why. From the start me and her were just friends. We talked every day for about a week or two. So it's about the second week we've been talking and I ask her to be my girlfriend and she said "yes," and was so happy. A couple of days later she told me she was rushing into a relationship and needed time to think. So supposedly she likes her ex at this point and you can tell I'm probably ticked off. The whole point of this is just how it's weird because she liked me so much and it just ended and I don't know why. I thought it over like a million times and I didn't do anything to make her mad or upset—nothing happened. As I am writing this it's hard to say what happened. . . I just don't get girls right now and I don't know what to say right now. This isn't much but this is how I feel and I just can't write anymore. This girl still has me confused to this day and I don't know what to do.
>
> —Rich

Part 1: Discussion Questions

1. Why do you think Rich's relationship ended?

____

____

2. What influences can affect a dating relationship?

____

____

____

3. What advice do you have for Rich?

____

____

____

4. How can a person cope in a healthy manner when another person breaks up with him or her?

____

____

____

(*continued*)

Name: ____________________________________

Rich's Dilemma (*continued*)

Part 2: Role-Play

Please choose one of the following two options:

Choice 1: Recreate the last time Rich and his girlfriend spoke in person. Write a script to be read to the class in which Rich's girlfriend breaks up with Rich in a fair and caring manner.

Choice 2: Imagine that instead of writing his message, Rich actually said the words to you, a good friend, face-to-face. Write a script of the conversation you would have with Rich.

Part 3: Audience Feedback and Support

Write down examples of positive communication skills you heard in the presented scripts. In addition, list recommendations to improve these two types of conversations. Specify in your notes which groups demonstrated which skills. Use the back of this sheet if you need more space.

Positive communication skills demonstrated:

____

____

____

____

____

____

____

Recommendations for improving these conversations:

____

____

____

____

____

____

____

____

LESSON 13: TRAPPED
ENDING UNHEALTHY RELATIONSHIPS

Level: High school

Time: 40 minutes

National Health Education Standards

1. Core Concepts
4. Interpersonal Communication

National Sexuality Education Standards: Performance Indicators

- Describe characteristics of healthy and unhealthy romantic and/or sexual relationships.
- Demonstrate effective strategies to avoid or end an unhealthy relationship.

Rationale

Ending a relationship is a skill that people often wish they did not have to use. This can be particularly difficult when a partner displays aggressive behavior. The purpose of this activity is to simulate being "trapped" in an unhealthy relationship. Students will observe a role-play demonstrating a breakup, and then discuss the strategies needed to handle the situation.

Materials and Preparation

Two-foot piece of string or twine for each person. At each end of the string, make a loop big enough for a person's hand to fit through, and tie a knot.

Four cards (made of card stock or laminated paper if possible). There should be two "Student A" cards and two "Student B" cards, made up according to the samples at the end of this lesson.

Procedure

ACTIVITY 1: STRING GAME—TRAPPED IN A RELATIONSHIP

1. Give each student a two-foot piece of string (or twine), with a loop on each end.
2. Pair students off. Have one person from each pair put his hands through both loops of the string so the string is looped around his wrists. Have the second person put *one* hand through a loop on her string. Before the second person puts her hand through the other loop, the string should be threaded through the first person's string to connect the two people. Once they are connected, the second person should put her other hand through the open loop at the end of her string. Explain that the objective of the activity is to get "unattached." Students are not allowed to break or cut the strings, or to slide the loops off their wrists. Allow four to five minutes for the pairs of students to attempt to solve the problem.

3. After students figure out the solution, or become frustrated, stop the activity and show the class how it is done. (If any of the pairs have done it successfully, have *them* show the class how it is done.) The directions are as follows:
   a. One person makes a loop in the middle of her string.
   b. Starting from one "elbow" side, on top of the other person's wrist, she then slides the loop *under* the other person's loop.
   c. Once it is on the other side of the loop, she continues to pull it through, past the other person's fingers, and lowers it beneath his hand.
   d. Once the loop is under the hand, if the first person can pull away, she is free.

   Note: Before attempting to have students solve this string problem, it may be helpful for you to practice with another person outside of class to ensure you have the correct solution.
4. Let students attempt to articulate the point of the activity. (The activity was designed to make students feel frustrated and trapped because they could not get away from the other person.) Explain that sometimes in a relationship, like in this activity, a person feels trapped because he or she does not know how to get out of it. Generate a discussion about how it felt to be trapped in this "relationship."
5. Before continuing, ask processing questions 1 through 4.

ACTIVITY 2: ROLE-PLAYS—ENDING RELATIONSHIPS

1. Ask for four volunteers (two males, two females) to play the partners in two heterosexual couples.
2. Have the first couple stay in the classroom, toward the front. For the other couple, hand the *male* the "Student B" card and the *female* the "Student A" card for the second role-play, and have them go into the hall and close the door. While they are in the hall, both students should read over their respective cards but should *not* share the information with their partner.
3. For the couple in front of the room, give the *male* the "Student A" card and the *female* the "Student B" card for the first role-play. Instruct both students to read over the information on their card, but not to share the information with their partner.
4. Begin the role-play by having Student A tell Student B how he feels. Student B should then respond according to what is on her card.
5. Instruct the class to observe what occurs during the role-play. After the role-play, ask the audience to write their observations in their notebooks. Notes should include characteristics of unhealthy relationships. They will have a chance to respond to and discuss the role-play later in the lesson.
6. After the first role-play has finished, have the two students in the hallway come in and repeat the process, except this time the female will be Student A and will speak first.
7. Again, ask the audience to write their observations in their notebooks.
8. After both role-plays, allow the class to discuss their observations. Ask processing questions 5 through 12, correcting any misinformation.

9. Conclude the lesson by assigning the homework, in which students must find two available resources for the following:

   a. Assisting teenagers in abusive relationships

   b. Helping teenagers learn how to effectively communicate

   Resources can be from local organizations, the Internet, or both. Students should correctly write each resource's name and where it can be found, as well as a brief paragraph describing the services provided.

Processing

1. Do you think people sometimes feel trapped in a relationship? If so, why do they stay in the relationship?
2. Why is it sometimes difficult to end a relationship?
3. What are some of the signs that a relationship is no longer healthy for both partners?
4. What are some of the characteristics of healthy and unhealthy relationships?
5. What type of relationship was shown in the role-plays? Why? What were some of the signs that they were unhealthy or abusive?
6. How difficult was it for Student B to break up with his or her partner? Why do you think this is?
7. Who was the victim in the relationship?
8. What difference does it make whether the victim was a male or a female? How successful was each in breaking off the relationship? If there were differences, what were they?
9. Would it matter if the relationship were between individuals of the same sex? Explain.
10. How well did Student B communicate his or her thoughts and feelings to his or her partner? What assertiveness techniques were used? What were the tone of voice and body language like?
11. What did Student B do to increase his or her safety during the breakup? What else should he or she have done?
12. If Student A, the person abusing his or her partner, refused to accept the breakup or threatened Student B, what would be the best course of action? What resources are available at home, at school, or in the community to assist someone in an abusive relationship?

Assessment

- Students participate in the string game.
- Students take notes while listening to and observing the role-plays.
- Students participate in the follow-up discussion about characteristics of healthy and unhealthy relationships. Students mention appropriate resources (people or places) to assist someone in an abusive relationship.
- Students complete the homework assignment.

Relationship Role-Plays

Role-Play 1: Student A (Male)

You and **Student B** have been dating for two months. You are both seventeen. You have become closer and feel your relationship is one of the best things in your lives. You love being with your partner and look forward to spending time with her. You enjoy texting and talking on the phone when you are not together. Your relationship has had its ups and downs, but hey . . . that is normal, right?

You have decided you are ready to take your physical relationship to a new level. You feel you really love her and, if you are both responsible about preventing possible STIs and pregnancy, a sexual relationship will only make things better. Up until now, she has resisted, saying she is not ready. But today, you will try to be more "persuasive." You are meeting with her after school at her house. You are planning on explaining how you feel.

When you begin the role-play, you will speak first.

Role-Play 1: Student B (Female)

You and **Student A** have been dating for two months. You are both seventeen. At the beginning you liked this person. Lately, however, you have felt differently. You have begun to feel like you are spending every waking minute with him. He acts jealous and sometimes exhibits aggressive behavior toward you. He also texts you constantly, and if you do not answer immediately, he becomes angry—asking where you are and what you are doing. He is jealous and possessive about the time you spend with your friends and family. When **Student A** gets angry, he calls you names and belittles you.

Yesterday, when you were talking to one of your friends in the hallway, he got angry and pushed you up against the locker. He immediately begged for forgiveness and promised never to do this again. In the past when you have suggested you needed to "take a break" from your partner, he has threatened to hurt himself or others if you break up. Your friends and family have warned you about this person and expressed concern for your safety.

You are meeting with him after school at your house. Your parents know of your plans and will be at home. You are planning on telling your partner how you feel and have decided to break up with him.

When you begin your role-play, **Student A** will speak first.

Role-Play 2: Student A (Female)

You and **Student B** have been dating for two months. You are both seventeen. You have become closer, and feel your relationship is one of the best things in your lives. You love being with your partner and look forward to spending time with him. You enjoy texting and talking on the phone when you are not together. Your relationship has had its ups and downs, but hey . . . that is normal, right?

You have decided you are ready to take your physical relationship to a new level. You feel you really love him and, if you are both responsible about preventing pregnancy, a sexual relationship will only make things better. Up until now, he has resisted, saying he is not ready. But today, you will try to be more "persuasive." You are meeting with him after school at his house. You are planning on explaining how you feel.

When you begin the role-play, you will speak first.

Role-Play 2: Student B (Male)

You and **Student A** have been dating for two months. You are both seventeen. At the beginning you liked this person. Lately, however, you have felt differently. You have begun to feel like you are spending every waking minute with her. She acts jealous and sometimes exhibits aggressive behavior toward you. She also texts you constantly, and if you do not answer immediately, she becomes angry—asking where you are and what you are doing. She is jealous and possessive about the time you spend with your friends and family. When **Student A** gets angry, she calls you names and belittles you.

Yesterday, when you were talking to one of your friends in the hallway, she got angry and pushed you up against the locker. She immediately begged for forgiveness and promised to never do this again. In the past when you have suggested you needed to "take a break" from your partner, she has threatened to hurt herself or others if you break up. Your friends and family have warned you about this person and expressed concern for your safety.

You are meeting with her after school at your house. Your parents know of your plans and will be at home. You are planning on telling your partner how you feel and have decided to break up with her.

When you begin your role-play, **Student A** will speak first.

LESSON 14: UP CLOSE AND PERSONAL

Level: High school

Time: 40 minutes

National Health Education Standards

1. Core Concepts
4. Interpersonal Communication

National Sexuality Education Standards: Performance Indicators

- Describe characteristics of healthy and unhealthy romantic and/or sexual relationships.
- Describe a range of ways to express affection within healthy relationships.
- Demonstrate effective ways to communicate personal boundaries as they relate to intimacy and sexual behavior.
- Demonstrate communication skills that foster healthy relationships.

Rationale

Dating enables people to experience and learn about companionship and intimacy, and to distinguish between healthy and unhealthy relationships. Readiness to date and interest in dating vary among individuals. Gay, lesbian, and bisexual youth, like heterosexual youth, may or may not date. This Up Close and Personal (UCP) activity allows open discussion in a controlled, supportive environment. It also gives students an opportunity to learn more about themselves and students of the opposite sex, and helps them distinguish between healthy and unhealthy relationships.

This Up Close and Personal lesson encourages students to engage in an open, honest discussion by using sentence stems. The objective of this lesson is to integrate the affective (emotional) and cognitive (informational) domains related to the changes at puberty. Students will communicate personal opinions, feelings, and values related to puberty and sexual health. This will occur in an atmosphere of mutual trust and respect for each member of the class.

Note: It is unlikely that you will get through all sentence stems in one class session. You can decide which statements would be most appropriate for your students. Choices may be based on background information discussed in previous lessons, students' developmental level, restrictions you may have concerning what topics *can* and *cannot* be discussed, and your own comfort level in facilitating discussion.

Because UCP lessons deal mainly with the affective or emotional domain, they have a greater potential for personal disclosure on the part of students. You should be aware of and prepared to handle this. Sometimes it simply involves reminding the class that what is said in class stays in class. At other times, it may involve discussing issues with students privately to offer advice, resources, and support.

Materials and Preparation

Small lamp (optional)

Up Close and Personal sheet with several UCP sentence stems. (*Note:* Prior to teaching this activity, you should familiarize yourself with "Facilitating a UCP Session," which can be found at the end of the lesson.)

Procedure*

1. Ask students to form a circle with their chairs. Turning off the overhead lights and using a lamp may make the environment more conducive to an informal discussion.
2. Introduce the activity in the following manner:

   Today we are going to do an activity called Up Close and Personal. It is simple to do, but for it to go smoothly, there are some rules to follow.

   First, understand this is not group therapy. Instead it is an opportunity for you to talk about how you feel about yourself, relationships, likes, dislikes, things that have come up in class, memories, and life in general. Although I will be facilitating the activity, I will also be sitting in the circle and participating along with everyone else.

   The activity is in the following format: I will read an unfinished sentence. Each of you will think about how you would finish this same unfinished sentence. Someone in the circle will then raise his or her hand and state his or her completed sentence. He or she will point to his or her right or left to determine which way around the circle we will proceed.

   When going around the circle, there should be no talking by anyone else. If something is said that you want to respond to or comment on, you must wait until we have gone all the way around the circle. If you cannot think of anything to say, or choose not to respond when it is your turn, you may simply say, "Pass" or "Come back to me." Everyone, including the teacher, is allowed to pass.

   When we have gone around the entire circle, I will ask anyone who passed if he or she would like to respond at this time. I will also ask for any questions or comments about anything that was said when going around the circle. At this point, there can be open discussion.

   Please note that during this activity, no names should be mentioned at any time. Instead, say something like, "I know someone who . . ."

   In addition, as with other lessons, what is said in class stays in class. However, please do not share anything that is too personal, that makes you feel uncomfortable, or that you wish to keep to yourself.

---

*Unfinished sentences have been a useful learning tool for many years. The specific format used in this lesson has been adapted from the book *Up Close and Personal: Effective Learning for Students and Teachers* (Raleigh, NC: Lulu Press, 2007), by teacher, colleague, and friend Robert Winchester. Robert can be contacted at trustinbob@aol.com.

3. Once the rules have been explained and agreed on, read the first sentence stem aloud. After allowing a few moments for reflection, ask a student volunteer to start by stating his completed sentence. That student will then point to his left or right to note in which direction the remaining students will be given a chance to complete the sentence. Students then give their responses until everyone around the circle has spoken or passed.
4. At times, a student may simply not be ready to respond to a particular question. When this happens, remind her to pass, noting that she can answer after everyone else has spoken. It is also not unusual for many students to have the same response to a question or statement. "Repeats" reinforce the important concept that although all people are unique, they often share many of the same thoughts, feelings, and values.
5. After all students have responded, open up the discussion by asking if anyone has any questions or comments about anything that was said. Encourage students to talk in more detail about why they completed the sentence the way they did. Students may also ask others in the circle, including the teacher, to expand on their answer. Students may do so, or they may choose to pass.
6. Continue the circle discussion for as long as it is viable, constantly monitoring and enforcing the rules. When the discussion on a given sentence has run its course, move on to the next unfinished sentence.
7. Share the processing statements.
8. All UCP sessions should end with some brief closure in the form of another unfinished sentence. Examples include the following: "Today I learned . . ." "I learned that I . . ." "Right now I feel . . ." and "Something I want to say to one of my classmates is . . ."
9. Conclude the day's activity by summarizing what occurred in the session, making appropriate connections to the subject matter and curriculum. Then thank the class and say, "This ends our Up Close and Personal class for today."

Processing

1. If anyone has any concerns or questions about what was discussed during our UCP session today, he or she can speak to me privately after class or can bring it up for discussion during our next class session.
2. There are many people, including teachers, coaches, counselors, or school psychologists, who can assist you with any personal issues that you may want to share with them. Keep in mind that these individuals, as mandated reporters, *must* report any verbalization or indication that you may want to hurt yourself or hurt others, or revelations of abuse of any kind, to the appropriate authorities for follow-up and counseling services.

Assessment

- Students actively participate in the UCP activity. Even though some students may decide to pass on one or more questions, as long as they are actively listening and following the ground rules, they are "actively participating."

Facilitating a UCP Session

- Facilitation is a skill that you can improve with practice.
- Silence is not a negative phenomenon. Silence often indicates that higher-level thinking is taking place.
- Going over ground rules at the beginning of each session is a needed and helpful technique to prevent inappropriate behavior.
- Unacceptable behavior should be stopped the moment it is recognized. To do this, pause the activity and point out the offense to the individual. For example, say, "What was just said is a put-down (or personal name), and it is not allowed in the circle discussion. Please do not do it again," or "Please do not talk to your neighbor when you should be listening to the one person who is supposed to be talking."
- If a student persists in breaking the activity's rules, talk to him one-on-one after class. Let the student know that if his behavior continues, he may not be able to participate in the future. This almost always stops the offensive behavior.
- Remind students of the information teachers *must* report if shared:

  1. If they are going to hurt themselves
  2. If they are going to hurt others
  3. If they are being abused

Possible UCP Sentence Stems: Healthy Relationships

1. Today I feel . . .
2. Couples in healthy relationships . . .
3. Chris and Jody are friends who recently started dating. The most important component of their relationship should be . . .
4. Chris and Jody are friends who recently started dating. Chris and Jody are the same sex. The most important component of their relationship should be . . .
5. Chris and Jody are fifty years old. The most important component of their relationship should be . . .
6. As a male or female in a dating relationship, I want . . .
7. One thing I find attractive about a person is . . .
8. One way that males and females can show respect for others is . . .
9. As a man or woman, one thing I've always wanted to ask someone of the opposite sex is . . .
10. An advantage of being a female or male is . . .
11. In the media, heterosexual couples . . .
12. In the media, same-sex couples . . .
13. One way to make school feel safer for gay and lesbian couples would be . . .
14. If a friend confided that his or her boyfriend or girlfriend had hurt him or her, I would . . .
15. If my partner sent me thirty text messages a day, . . .
16. As a male or female, I was surprised about . . .

LESSON 15: HOME-SCHOOL CONNECTION

TALKING ABOUT RELATIONSHIPS

Level: Middle school

Time: Varies

National Health Education Standard

1. Core Concepts

National Sexuality Education Standards: Performance Indicators

- Compare and contrast the characteristics of healthy and unhealthy relationships.
- Describe a range of ways people express affection within various types of relationships.

Rationale

Although the media often portrays unrealistic relationships, young people can develop realistic expectations of romantic relationships by learning about the relationships surrounding them in real life. It is for this reason that this Home-School Connection was created: to give students a chance to receive advice and hear about relationship experiences from trusted adults.

After completing the interview as outlined on the worksheet with the student, parents or guardians are requested to sign the bottom of the page. All responses from teens and parents or guardians on the Home-School Connection activity will be kept confidential. It will not be turned in to the teacher or graded. On the due date, students will be asked to *voluntarily* share any interesting comments or insights they learned or observed by participating in the assignment. Students *and* parents or guardians can choose to pass on any discussion they wish to keep private.

Materials and Preparation

Copies of "Parent or Guardian Interview: Talking about Relationships" worksheet

Procedure

1. Explain to the class they are going to have an assignment to complete with one or more parents or guardians. Distribute the "Parent or Guardian Interview: Talking about Relationships" worksheet.
2. Assign a due date for the assignment.
3. On the day the assignment is due, check if students have completed the assignment by noting if the sheet was signed on the bottom. Do not collect or grade the assignment.
4. Ask for student volunteers to share the results of the discussion they had with the adult or adults they interviewed. Then ask the processing questions.

Processing

1. Were you surprised by any answers from your parents or guardians? Why or why not?
2. Did you learn anything about your parents or guardians that you did not know previously?
3. How do your viewpoints in regard to the questions differ from those of your parents or guardians?
4. In the future, if you became a parent, what advice would you give to your teenager about healthy relationships?

Assessment

- Students complete the assignment, as indicated by at least one adult's signature.
- Students participate in the in-class follow-up discussion.

Parent or Guardian Interview: Talking about Relationships

Directions: Select one or more parents or guardians to interview and ask them to respond to the following questions:

1. What is one of the best relationships you have had in your life, romantic or otherwise? What made it a good relationship?

2. What do you think is the best part of having a close relationship, such as a friendship or a marriage?

3. What traits make a relationship *unhealthy*? Why?

4. What advice would you give to a teenager who likes someone in a romantic way, when the other person "just wants to be friends"?

5. Does *sex* equal *love*? Explain.

6. What advice would you give a teenager about what makes a relationship healthy?

Parent or guardian signature(s): ______________________________

Student signature: ______________________________

Personal Safety

7

This chapter emphasizes the need to create and maintain safe environments for all students. Lessons allow students to discuss various personal safety issues, including the prevention of bullying, sexual harassment, sexual abuse, sexual assault, incest, rape, and dating violence. Although some lessons focus on violence in dating relationships, students should understand that violence in any relationship is inappropriate and there are resources to help people in violent relationships.

Although personal violence is often thought of as incidences that occur face-to-face, cases of teenagers being wrongfully treated through technological sources have been found. Today's teens have become reliant on technology in their everyday lives. This includes the use of cell phones, e-mail, social networking sites, and personal computers. Although there are many benefits to these forms of instant communication, it is not surprising that the use of these technologies increases the chances of cyberbullying, harassment, abuse from dating partners, and contact with online predators.

SPECIAL CONSIDERATIONS FOR TEACHING ABOUT PERSONAL SAFETY

Given the pervasive nature of sexual abuse and various forms of sexual harassment in our society, it is likely that some teens in your class will have been victims of sexual violence. Teachers need to be sensitive to this and to the possibility of disclosure. One of your roles as a health educator is to create an atmosphere of trust in your classroom, and to let it be known that *you* can be one of those caring adults who will listen to students and take the appropriate steps to follow up on any allegations.

You should also be aware of school and community resources that provide intervention and counseling services for these children. There are many trusted adults in the school and community who can assist victims of sexual violence.

Note: Teachers and counselors are *mandated reporters.* If students reveal that they or people they know are being harassed or abused in any way, you are required *by law* to report the situation to your school's administration, the school's counseling department, social services, or law enforcement authorities.

LESSON 1: "STICK 'EM UP" SENTENCE STEMS

Level: Middle school, High school

Time: 35–45 minutes

National Health Education Standards

1. Core Concepts
3. Accessing Information

National Sexuality Education Standards: Performance Indicators

- Describe situations and behaviors that constitute bullying, sexual harassment, sexual abuse, sexual assault, incest, rape and dating violence.
- Identify sources of support such as parents or other trusted adults that they can go to if they are or someone they know is being bullied, harassed, abused or assaulted.

Rationale

Personal safety is a topic students need and want to discuss. You can use this lesson early in a unit to gain insight into students' background knowledge. It also provides students with an opportunity to anonymously refer to situations concerning personal safety: bullying, sexual harassment, sexual abuse, sexual assault, incest, rape, and dating violence.

Materials and Preparation

Four sheets of newsprint and a marker

Masking tape

Front board

Four sticky notes for each student

Box to hold completed sticky notes

Copies of "Personal Safety Definition Sheet" handout

Teacher-constructed quiz developed to assess student knowledge and skills related to personal safety (optional)

Procedure

1. Introduce the topic by informing the class that today's lesson will deal with personal safety.
2. Take the four sheets of newsprint and tape them on a wall in different areas of the room. At the top of each piece of newsprint, write a different sentence stem in large letters with the marker. The sentence stems should be related to the topic of personal safety. Suggested stems include the following:
   a. Something I have heard or a question I have about sexual harassment is . . .
   b. Something I have heard or a question I have about sexual abuse is . . .
   c. Something I have heard or a question I have about bullying is . . .
   d. Something I have heard or a question I have about dating violence or date rape is . . .

3. Hand out four sticky notes to each student.
4. Explain that the displayed sentence stems are open ended so that students can anonymously write responses on their sticky notes. Encourage free thought, allowing students to write whatever they like

   Note: During the course of the activity, students may share personal experiences. Reinforce the rule that personal names cannot be used. Instead, students should write, "I know someone who . . ." or "I heard that someone at another school . . ." Writing statements in this manner is an appropriate way to share personal experiences or stories.
5. Give students a few minutes to write their questions or statements. To maintain anonymity, students should fold their sticky notes in half. You should then walk around the room with a box, into which students should place their completed statements. Once you have collected all of the statements, take them out, open them up, and place the comments or questions on the appropriate sheet of newsprint. For most of the questions or statements it will be obvious on which piece of newsprint to attach the notes. If some are unclear, ask the class on which piece of newsprint they feel the notes should be placed.
6. Discuss the activity by reading (or having a volunteer read) the individual notes on the first piece of newsprint, and asking the processing questions. When all the notes on the first sheet of newsprint have been read and discussed, ask for a second volunteer to read the next set of notes on the second sheet of newsprint. Continue this process with the third and fourth sheets of newsprint. (For the third processing question, formulate a list on the board, with students copying the list down in their notebook.)
7. When all statements and questions have been discussed, distribute the "Personal Safety Definition Sheet" handout. Review the handout, answering any questions students may have.
8. End the lesson with a "class whip," with students stating one "I learned . . ." statement.

Processing

1. From what was read aloud, what information does the class seem to understand about issues related to personal safety?
2. What myths or incorrect information did you hear when the responses were read aloud?
3. In this school, whom can a person talk to if he or she or someone he or she knows is a victim of any of these behaviors? Who is a person from the community he or she may be able to talk with?
4. What can be done by students, teachers, and administrators to prevent or reduce instances of bullying, sexual harassment, sexual abuse, or date rape? Explain.

Assessment

- Students are able to write correct descriptions of specific terms from the "Personal Safety Definition Sheet" handout on a review quiz or test.
- The class generates a list of available resources for those experiencing the discussed situations.
- Students complete a class whip at the close of the session using correct terminology and appropriate statements.

Personal Safety Definition Sheet

Bullying—an act of aggressive behavior intentionally designed to hurt a person physically, mentally, or socially.

Date or acquaintance rape—forced, unwanted sexual intercourse in which the attacker and the victim know each other. Date rape is the most common form of acquaintance rape. In recent years, the use of "date rape" drugs has become more common. These drugs make the victim unconscious or unable to say "no." Two common date rape drugs are Rohypnol, or "roofies," and a drug called GHB. These can be slipped into a drink or food and are tasteless and odorless. You should be cautious of accepting drinks from people, and should never leave a drink unattended at a bar or party. Keeping an eye on your drink is one way of preventing being drugged by a sexual predator and becoming a victim of date or acquaintance rape.

Sexual abuse—the forcing of unwanted sexual activity by one person onto another. *Child sexual abuse* is defined as any contact or interaction between a child and an adult in which the child is used for pleasure or stimulation by the adult. Occasionally, sexual abuse is performed against a minor by an adult whom the child trusts. Because minors cannot legally consent to sexual activity with adults, sexual abuse is a serious crime. A child who has been sexually abused is *never* at fault. Victims of sexual abuse should seek help by reporting the abuse to a trusted adult in school or at home.

Sexual assault—illegal sexual contact that is forced on a person without his or her consent. Sexual assault includes different actions, but usually occurs when someone touches any part of another person's body in a sexual way, even through clothing. Sexual assault can be committed by strangers, acquaintances, friends, dating partners, or family members. Sexual assault is against the law and needs to be reported.

Sexual harassment—unwelcome sexual advances, requests for sexual favors, and other verbal or physical conduct of a sexual nature. Sexual harassment can include sexually suggestive verbal or written comments, slurs, or jokes. It can also include sexually offensive gestures, pictures, cartoons, e-mails, or text messages. Physical forms of sexual harassment may include unwanted touching and blocking movements, whereby someone purposely may try to prevent you from moving or getting away from him or her. Sexual harassment is against school rules and policies as well as against the law. All cases of sexual harassment need to be reported to parents or guardians and school authorities.

Teen dating violence—the control of one teenage partner over the other teenage partner. Teen dating violence includes emotional, verbal, physical, or sexual abuse. Emotional abuse is behavior that harms a person's self-esteem and causes shame. Verbal abuse involves the consistent demeaning of another through put-downs or angry outbursts. Physical abuse is any action causing physical pain or injury. Sexual abuse is any unwanted sexual act or contact.

LESSON 2: FLIRTING OR HURTING? SEXUAL HARASSMENT ROLE-PLAYS

Level: Middle school, High school

Time: 40 minutes

National Health Education Standards

1. Core Concepts
7. Self-Management

National Sexuality Education Standards: Performance Indicators

- Compare and contrast situations and behaviors that may constitute bullying, sexual harassment, sexual abuse, sexual assault, incest, rape and dating violence.
- Describe ways to treat others with dignity and respect.
- Demonstrate ways they can respond when someone is being bullied or harassed.

Rationale

Inappropriate communication is frequently portrayed in the media as "teasing" or flirting. Because of this, students often become confused about the differences between appropriate and inappropriate behaviors. In this activity, students distinguish between flirting and sexual harassment using two different scripted role-plays.

Materials and Preparation

Front board, with the following written down: "In your notebook, please write down ten words, actions, facial expressions, or forms of body language that you think could be interpreted as flirting."

Role-play scripts (included at the end of this lesson): "Tony and Chris Role-Play" (two copies) and "Hector and Anna Role-Play" (two copies)

Copies of "Descriptors of Flirting Versus Sexual Harassment" handout

"In the Eye of the Beholder" chart, displayed in classroom

Copies of "Letter to a Friend" homework

Procedure

1. As students enter the room, ask them to answer in their notebook the question written on the board.
2. While students are answering the question, choose four students (two males and two females) to be actors in two different role-plays. It is advisable to choose volunteers who are comfortable speaking in front of the class. Speak with these students on the side of the room to designate who will play the characters Hector, Anna, Tony, and Chris, and explain their roles. Inform the students that they can change the dialogue so that is sounds more natural, but that they should not change the *intent* of the words. Allow each to read over the script as the rest of the class completes their notebook writing.

3. Have "Tony" and "Chris" come up to the front of the room. Explain to the class that they will be watching a role-play involving communication between two people. Ask students to note anything they see in the role-play using the terms that they wrote in their notebook related to *flirting*.
4. After the role-play, ask the class:
   a. Were these two people flirting?
   b. What specific words or body language gave you the impression that this was or was not flirting?
   c. Did the couple in the role-play demonstrate any of the characteristics of flirting you wrote down? Which ones?
   d. How do you think Tony felt about what went on in the role-play?
   e. How do you think Chris felt about what went on in the role-play?
5. Thank the volunteers and ask them to sit down. Have the next couple, "Hector" and "Anna," come to the front of the room and perform their role-play.
6. After this role-play, ask the same questions as before:
   a. Were these two people flirting?
   b. What specific words or body language gave you the impression that this was or was not flirting?
   c. Did the couple in the role-play demonstrate any of the characteristics of flirting you wrote down? Which ones?
   d. How do you think Hector felt about what went on in the role-play?
   e. How do you think Anna felt about what went on in the role-play?
7. In addition, ask the processing questions.
8. Next distribute the "Descriptors of Flirting Versus Sexual Harassment" handout. Discuss the difference between flirting and sexual harassment. Inquire what the phrase "in the eye of the beholder" means, and what it has to do with sexual harassment. In addition, remind students of the three possible parties who are able to report incidences of sexual harassment: the person doing the harassing, the victim, and any bystanders. Refer to Figure 7.2.1 depicting who can become involved in harassment. Ask students if they have any questions about any of the noted parties.

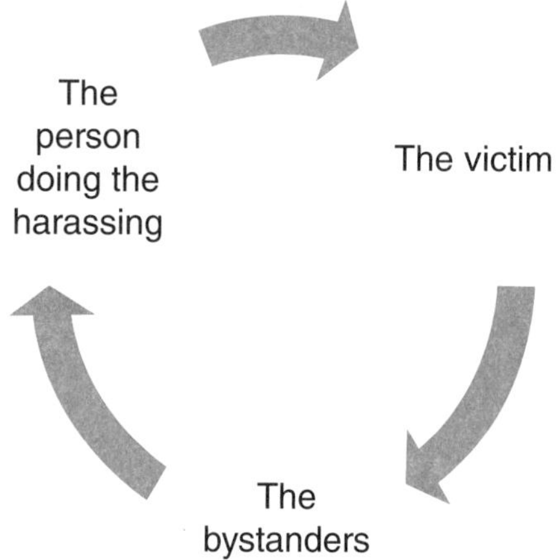

Figure 7.2.1 In the Eye of the Beholder

9. Have students role-play the "Tony and Chris Role-Play" script again, except this time, *both Chris and Tony are guys.* Ask, "Does it change anything? Is it still flirting, or is it now sexual harassment? If a gay person came on to a straight person, would that be considered sexual harassment?"
10. Ask, "What if Chris and 'Toni' were both females? Would that change the situation? How? Would it now be considered sexual harassment?"
11. Have students role-play the "Tony and Chris Role-Play" script again, but this time have a male play Chris and a female play Toni. (*Note:* The only other change to the script beside Toni's name change is that "boyfriend . . . he" should be "girlfriend . . she.") Ask, "How does this change the situation?"
12. To conclude the lesson, assign the "Letter to a Friend" homework.

Processing

1. Hector's comments and actions can be interpreted as *sexual harassment.* Do you think Hector's *intent* was to sexually harass Anna? ("I'm just playin' with you. I try to be nice and you get a real attitude.") If he did not intend to harass her, does this excuse his behavior?
2. What could Hector have done differently to change his harassing behavior to a more acceptable form of flirting?
3. Was there anything more that Anna could have done to prevent being sexually harassed? What should Anna do about this situation? Do you feel that she should report Hector to the principal for sexual harassment? Why or why not?

Assessment

- Students correctly distinguish between "flirting" and "harassing" behaviors.
- Students' role-plays demonstrate assertive behaviors.
- Students participate in a discussion of how the "role reversal" scenarios may have affected their opinions about whether sexual harassment was evident, and give rationales for their responses.
- Students complete the "Letter to a Friend" homework.

Role-Play Student Scripts

Tony and Chris Role-Play

Directions to actors: As you read through your lines, act as though you are glad to see each other and enjoy each other's company.

Setting: The characters are in a high school hallway at dismissal time. Tony, a junior, and Chris, a sophomore, are in the same English class together, but do not really know each other very well.

Tony: Hi, Chris. What's up?

Chris: Hey, Tony. Not much.

Tony: You cut your hair. It looks good.

Chris: Thanks. I got tired of wearing it long so I cut it. Have you started your project for English yet?

Tony: No, that's why I'm staying after. I'm going to the library.

Chris: Oh yeah, me too. Hey, maybe you could help me find some information online. I'm not that great with computers.

Tony: No problem. I'm kind of a computer geek. I'm online all the time.

Chris: I feel like such a dummy around computers. Whenever I try to do something, I always mess up.

Tony: It's not that hard. I'll set you up, no sweat.

Chris: Thanks. I can only stay until 4:00 though. I've got to get the late bus.

Tony: I can give you a ride if you want—as long as your *boyfriend* doesn't mind!

Chris: Oh, I'm not going out with him anymore. We broke up last week.

Tony: (*Smiles*) Oh, really?

Chris: (*Smiles back*) Yeah, really. He was kind of a jerk.

Tony: (*Lightly puts his hand on Chris's shoulder*) You know, not *all* guys are jerks.

Chris: (*Looks at Tony's hand, then looks at Tony's face and smiles*) I know. Hey, are you sure you don't mind taking me home? I'll call my mom and tell her I'll be a little late.

Tony: No, I don't mind at all. Maybe you can return the favor by going out with me this weekend.

Chris: This weekend? (*Smiles*) I'll have to check my "social calendar," but I don't think I've got any plans. I'll give you my cell phone number and we can talk about it later tonight.

Tony: (*Smiles*) Sounds good. (*Both walk off together*)

(*continued*)

Hector and Anna Role-Play

Directions to actors: As you read the role-play, the person who reads Hector's part should act "pushy" and a little annoying. The person who reads Anna's part should be friendly until Hector says, "All the guys in English class like it when you wear those tight sweaters." You should then act annoyed, disgusted, and maybe even a little afraid.

Setting: The characters are in a high school hallway at dismissal time. Hector, a junior, and Anna, a sophomore, are in the same English class, but do not really know each other well.

Hector: Hey, Anna, what's up?

Anna: Hey, Hector. Not much.

Hector: You're looking good today. I really like that sweater.

Anna: Uh, thanks.

Hector: All the guys in English class like it when you wear those tight sweaters, you know what I'm sayin'! (*Smiles at her*)

Anna: (*Gives him a dirty look, but says nothing*)

Hector: Hey, I'm giving you a compliment. You look really good, especially above the waist. (*Smiles again*)

Anna: (*Looks more annoyed, turns, and starts to walk away*)

Hector: Where you goin'? The library? I noticed you go to the library a lot after school.

Anna: (*Doesn't turn around, keeps walking*) No, I'm going home.

Hector: (*Runs after her and tries to put his arm around her shoulder*) You *sure* you're not goin' to the library?

Anna: (*Shoves his arm away, turns to him, and speaks in a loud voice*) Get your arm off me, please.

Hector: Hey, I'm just being friendly. I can be *very* friendly, you know what I'm sayin'. From what I hear, you're friendly with a *lot* of guys! (*Smiles, gives her a "creepy" look, and tries to put his arm around her again*)

Anna: (*Turns around, looks him directly in the eye, and speaks forcefully*) I feel uncomfortable when you talk to me or touch me like you did. I'm not interested in "hookin' up" with you and I want you to please just leave me alone! (*Turns and walks away again*)

Hector: What's your problem? I'm just playin' with you. I try to be nice and you get a real attitude.

Descriptors of Flirting Versus Sexual Harassment

FLIRTING	SEXUAL HARASSMENT
Receivers feel . . .	**Victims feel . . .**
Good	Bad
Happy	Sad, angry, or both
Flattered	Embarrassed
Attractive	Ugly
In control	Helpless
Confident	Powerless
Actions are . . .	**Actions are . . .**
Open	Invading
Mutual	One-sided
Complimentary	Degrading
Desired	Undesired
Motivated by caring	Motivated by power
Empowering	Disempowering
Wanted	Unwanted
Legal	Illegal
Involving positive touch	Involving negative touch
Results in . . .	**Results in . . .**
Higher self-image	Lower self-image

Name: ______________________________

Letter to a Friend

Directions: Imagine you have a friend who has had an experience similar to the one explained in class dealing with harassment.

For the next class, write a letter to this friend, including the following information:

1. The situation your friend is dealing with
2. Your feelings about the harassment
3. What your friend should do about the situation
4. At least three resources your friend can use

The assignment will be graded according to the following rubric:

Letter to a Friend Rubric (8 Points Total)

	2 POINTS	1 POINT	0 POINTS
Description of the situation	The student correctly identified the situation as harassment. A description was provided.	The student correctly identified the situation as harassment, but should have provided more information.	The situation provided was not an example of harassment or any other inappropriate behavior.
Advice	The student provided positive advice about what his or her friend could do regarding the situation.	The student provided some advice for his or her friend, yet information was brief.	Advice was not provided or did not pertain to the situation.
Resources	Three resources were provided; each was an actual resource found within the local area; contact information was also provided.	Fewer than three resources were provided, the contact information was limited, or both.	No resources were provided, or those listed did not pertain to the situation.
Overall	The student wrote the letter in a positive manner. The student included his or her own thoughts and feelings.	The letter was written in a fair manner. More could have been included referring to thoughts and feelings.	The letter was poorly written, and no personal thoughts or feelings were included.

LESSON 3: SEXUAL HARASSMENT? YES, NO, MAYBE SO?

Level: Middle school, High school

Time: 40 minutes

National Health Education Standards

1. Core Concepts
4. Interpersonal Communication
5. Decision-Making

National Sexuality Education Standards: Performance Indicators

- Compare and contrast situations and behaviors that may constitute bullying, sexual harassment, sexual abuse, sexual assault, incest, rape and dating violence.
- Demonstrate effective ways to communicate with trusted adults about bullying, harassment, abuse or assault.
- Apply a decision-making model to various situations relating to sexual health.

Rationale

This lesson is designed as a follow-up to previous discussions about sexual harassment that have included the definition, types, and examples of harassing behaviors.

Materials and Preparation

Five sets of red, green, and yellow cards

Five extra chairs set up in front of the room

Teacher copy of "Scenarios: Sexual Harassment or Not?"

Copies of the school's sexual harassment policy (optional)

Procedure

1. Choose four students (two males, two females) to serve as a "panel of judges." Give each of the four judges a red, green, and yellow card, and ask them to take a chair at the front of the room. Leave the fifth set of cards on the empty chair.
2. Explain that you will be reading scenarios in which people interact with each other in various ways. Based on what they know from earlier discussions and previously given definitions of sexual harassment, individuals on the panel should each hold up either a *red, yellow,* or *green* card to designate what type of behavior the scenario contains.
   - The *red* card indicates that the behavior is clearly an example of sexual harassment.
   - The *yellow* card indicates that the judge is neutral or unsure about what the behavior represents.
   - The *green* card indicates that the behavior is not sexual harassment.

   Explain that any student from the rest of the class who has a strong opinion about a scenario should sit in the empty chair, and hold up the card indicating her opinion. That student can also give an explanation when called on.

Note: An alternative version of this activity involves giving each student in the class a set of red, yellow, and green cards. In this version, students sit in a circle to allow their answers to be seen by all peers.

3. Read the first scenario and allow the panel to indicate their answers. Ask all panel members to voice their opinion. Encourage debate, but stress that all of them should respect the different opinions and values of their peers (no put-downs). When all members of the panel have spoken, if someone sat in the fifth chair, she should return to her seat.
4. Continue with this procedure for each statement. Change the panel after three or four statements.

   Note: Because sexual harassment is not always clearly defined, some of the scenarios can be interpreted differently. The following scenarios, however, are clearly sexual harassment: 1, 3, 4, 6, 9, 10, 11, 13, 14, 16, 17, and 18. Some scenarios (8, 12, and 15) may be considered bullying or harassment, but do not involve sex. Some scenarios, as described, would *not* be considered sexual harassment (2, 5, and 7)—but if the behavior continued and were clearly unwelcome, they then might be considered sexual harassment.
5. Conclude the lesson by asking the processing questions. Remind the class that other people beside the victim are able to report harassment (the harasser, bystanders, and a person the victim confided in).
6. Students can also be assigned one of the following optional homework assignments:
   a. Have students write anonymously about a time when they were the victim of sexual harassment or witnessed sexual harassment in school or online.
   b. Distribute copies of your school's sexual harassment policy to students to read for homework. Students should write a minimum of five "I learned . . ." statements related to any area of the document. Statements should be shared in the next class session.

Processing

1. What indicators tell us that a behavior is sexual harassment? Which tell us that the behavior is harassment overall?
2. Who is the harasser? The victim?
3. What can the victim do?
4. Could anything be done to prevent harassment?
5. If any of these situations happened to you, how do you think you would react?
6. If your mother, sister, or other family member or close friend were being harassed, how would you feel?
7. If you witnessed any of these situations, what would you do?

Assessment

- Students actively participate in the activity and follow-up discussion, giving correct information.
- Students complete the homework assignment (optional).

Scenarios: Sexual Harassment or Not?

1. Matt, a high school junior, has continuously made sexually suggestive comments and gestures to Amanda, a classmate. He often follows her down the hallway at school, telling her off-color jokes. She has asked him repeatedly to stop because his actions are upsetting to her. He responds by saying: "I'm only joking around with you. Can't you take a joke?"

2. Lori, a high school senior, works part-time in a clothing store at the local mall. Her twenty-five-year-old boss, John, asked her out. She refused. He has asked her out on several other occasions over the last month. Lori continuously declined his invitations and explained that he was making her feel uncomfortable. John said he was disappointed but he understood her feelings. He did not ask her out again, and their work relationship continues.

3. Debbie's locker is next to Jack's. He has several centerfold pictures of completely naked women taped to the inside of his locker. Debbie has told him that these pictures are offensive to her and asked him to take them down. Jack told her to mind her own business. He added that she was just jealous because she did not have a body like that.

4. It is the beginning of the school year, and a group of football players are loudly "rating" the freshman girls on a scale of one to ten as they walk by in the hallway.

5. Rebecca's male softball coach gives her a hug after she gets a game-winning hit.

6. Mark repeatedly sends e-mails to Dawn, asking her to send him naked pictures of herself. Dawn has responded several times, informing him that he "creeps her out" and asking him to stop e-mailing her. The next day, Dawn receives another request for a naked picture from Mark.

7. Mr. Peterson, the boys' baseball coach, occasionally slaps his players on the butt on the way back to the dugout after scoring a run. When he does this, he usually says, "Way to go" or "Good hustle."

8. Some of the senior boys in Juan's PE class make fun of him because he is small and not very athletic. He tries to avoid them, but it is difficult to do in the locker room, when the coach is not around. They smack him with their towels and call him "runt" and "wimp."

9. A fifth-grade girl is called "slut," "ho," and other mean words every day by a small group of fifth-grade boys when she gets on the bus. She has told them to stop, but they just laugh at her. When she told the bus driver, he said to just ignore them.

10. A junior high PE teacher became upset with the girls in his coed class because they took a long time to dress for class. Because of this, he told the girls to do jumping jacks in front of the boys. Most of the girls were embarrassed and upset by this.

(continued)

Scenarios: Sexual Harassment or Not? (*continued*)

11. As a senior, Bruce "comes out" and openly admits that he is gay. Rick, a classmate, sends out a text message on his cell phone to over fifty students. The text says, "Bruce Smith is a 'gay faggot' and he better watch his back."
12. Rachel is overweight. Several girls post comments on a social networking site calling her a "fat pig."
13. George and his eighth-grade classmates were happy to go on a special swimming trip sponsored by their school. After swimming for a while, George decided to get out of the water to get a drink at the concession stand. As he walked around the outside of the pool, two of his male friends ran up on either side of him, grabbed the waist of his swim trunks, and pulled them down to his ankles in front of all the other kids.
14. Jason broke up with his girlfriend Diana at the end of the summer. They are both seniors. The first day of school, Diana saw Jason talking to Leigh, a new freshman at the high school. When Diana saw Leigh later that day, she called her a "slut" and blamed her for stealing her boyfriend. Leigh tried to explain that she and Jason were just friends. For the next month, every time Diana saw Leigh, she would loudly call her names and accuse her of performing sexual acts for "all the boys."
15. Abbey has a nose piercing and purple hair, and always wears black army boots. She is constantly teased about how she looks and has gotten nicknamed "the weirdo."
16. Ms. Wilson, the art teacher, sees "Wilson is a gay dyke lesbo" written across the entire chalkboard when she walks into her room.
17. Latisha has just broken up with Nat. The next day, Nat writes the word "slut" on her locker with a Magic Marker.
18. While they are changing in the locker room, Robin uses her cell phone to take a picture of Melissa in her bra and underwear. Melissa was unaware that this picture was taken. Later that day, Robin posts the picture on a social networking site. When Melissa discovers what has happened, she is very upset and embarrassed.

LESSON 4: YOU BE THE JUDGE

Level: Middle school, High school

Time: 45 minutes

National Health Education Standards

1. Core Concepts
8. Advocacy

National Sexuality Education Standards: Performance Indicators

- Describe situations and behaviors that constitute bullying, sexual harassment, sexual abuse, sexual assault, incest, rape and dating violence.
- Compare and contrast situations and behaviors that may constitute bullying, sexual harassment, sexual abuse, sexual assault, incest, rape and dating violence.
- Advocate for safe environments that encourage dignified and respectful treatment of everyone.

Rationale

Thanks to cell phone technology, people are experiencing new challenges having to do with the easy sharing of personal information and pictures. In this lesson, after reading a fictional story involving "sexting," students will evaluate potential legal ramifications of this act. In addition, the emotional, mental, and social consequences of sexting will all also be discussed within small and large groups.

Materials and Preparation

Copies of "You Be the Judge" worksheet

List of applicable laws

Additional paper for the group brainstorm list (one piece per group)

Procedure

1. Begin the lesson by asking students if they can think of any TV shows depicting real personal cases whose outcome is decided by one judge. Most students should be able to refer to one show they have seen, or at least heard of. Explain that for the day's lesson, students will pretend they are judges, similar to judges on TV shows. As a judge, each student will determine who may or may not be charged as guilty in a fictional situation. After first deciding individually, groups of judges will come together to reach an agreement.
2. Distribute copies of the "You Be the Judge" worksheet, one per student. Ask a volunteer to read the story aloud for the class.
3. After the story is read, ask if students need any basic facts clarified.
4. Give students five minutes to answer the questions about the story on their worksheet. Walk around the room to assist them.

5. After all students have completed their worksheet individually, form groups of four or five students, asking groups to arrange themselves away from other groups. Instruct the groups to discuss their answers and attempt to agree on who should receive legal consequences for their actions. Groups should also touch on the emotional, mental, and social consequences involved.
6. After the groups have had ample time to discuss the situation (approximately ten minutes), ask volunteers to share their group's responses. Students should compare and contrast the different viewpoints within the room.

   Note: Although students may not agree on who is at fault, you should be aware of the legal ramifications involved in the story *and* should share the relevant laws. This might mean sharing district rules and state and federal laws. Also, final legal decisions may differ depending on where it occurred, legal counsel, or other factors.
7. To further discussion, ask students the processing questions. Again, you need to ensure that students have the correct information about the relevant laws.
8. To conclude the lesson, explain that because sometimes people do not think about potential negative consequences, like the ones described in the lesson's story, students need to become informed. Allow students to brainstorm on a piece of paper in their small group a list of ways other students can learn about appropriate and inappropriate behaviors in regard to technology use, handing in the completed list as they leave the classroom. Included in their list should be what bystanders can do to stop or prevent inappropriate behaviors.

Processing

1. What legal consequences can result from this situation?
2. Who would be at fault?
3. Without stating names, does anyone know of an actual similar case? What were the consequences?
4. How does "sexting" have an impact on a person's life? Emotionally? Mentally? Socially?
5. People sometimes believe that what they put on their phone and computer is personal, and that no one has the right to know. What is the truth about this?
6. If a picture is placed on a social networking site, who owns it? What can happen with that photo?

Assessment

- Students complete the worksheet individually and then in groups.
- Students discuss legal issues pertaining to social networking sites.
- Groups brainstorm a list of ways students can become informed about appropriate and inappropriate behaviors.

Name: ______________________________

You Be the Judge

Directions: The following story deals with four teenagers. Although the actual story is fictional, aspects of it have occurred in communities throughout the United States. After reading the story, answer the questions on your own. Then, when the teacher asks you to do so, try to agree with the other "judges" in your group about who is at fault.

Bryce and Jessica have been dating for three months. Bryce is a junior, and Jessica is a freshman at the same high school.

One day Bryce asked Jessica to send a "special" picture of her breasts to him for their three-month anniversary. Although she was nervous about sending him a photo like this, she decided it would be a "special" gift for him and sent a photo of herself topless to his cell phone. On receiving it, Bryce showed his best friend, Carlos, who forwarded the photo to his phone without Bryce's knowing.

Later that day Carlos asked his sister, Angela, to hold on to his cell phone during basketball practice. Being a nosy sister, Angela looked through his texts and saw Jessica's photo. Because Angela has never liked Jessica (she has had a crush on Bryce since she was in elementary school), she decided to forward it to her phone and then to her anonymous school blog with Jessica's first and last name next to the photo.

The picture was then discovered by many others, including the local authorities. Someone is now going to be held legally responsible for this "child pornography."

A. Who do you think will be charged with this violation? Explain your answer.

____

____

____

____

B. Rank the four characters in this story (Bryce, Jessica, Carlos, and Angela) from who is most responsible for this violation to who is least responsible:

1. ______________________________ (most responsible for this violation)
2. ______________________________
3. ______________________________
4. ______________________________ (least responsible for this violation)

C. What is the law in our community and state concerning situations like this one?

____

____

____

____

LESSON 5: "A PRETTY GOOD TIME . . ."? A SHORT PLAY ABOUT A FIRST DATE

Level: High school

Time: 45 minutes

National Health Education Standards

1. Core Concepts
3. Accessing Information

National Sexuality Education Standards: Performance Indicators

- Compare and contrast situations and behaviors that may constitute bullying, sexual harassment, sexual abuse, sexual assault, incest, rape and dating violence.
- Explain why a person who has been raped or sexually assaulted is not at fault.
- Demonstrate ways to access accurate information and resources that provide help for survivors of sexual abuse, incest, rape, sexual harassment, sexual assault and dating violence.

Rationale

Dating violence, including sexual assault and date rape, causes emotional, mental, and physical harm for both males and females. In this activity, students will read a play about date or acquaintance rape. Although the characters in the play are describing the same situation from different perspectives, both male and female students should be made aware of what constitutes dating violence and, if it occurs, where a victim or bystander can go for help and support.

Materials and Preparation

Copies of "'A Pretty Good Time . . .'?" handout, one for each of the main characters

Four extra desks, in front of the room on opposite sides

List of available resources (including school personnel)

Procedure

1. Explain to the class that four volunteers (two males and two females) will be acting as the main characters in a short play. These volunteers should be advised to take the script seriously because the lesson focuses on the sensitive topic of date rape. In addition, the volunteers need to read their lines loud enough for the class to hear, and with the appropriate tone and emotion based on what is happening in the play.
2. After choosing the four main characters, give each a copy of the play. Have the boys sit at the two desks on the right side of the room, the two girls at the two desks on left side.
3. Inform the class that they should be absolutely quiet during the reading of the play and observe what is going on. Afterward, they will discuss what they saw.
4. Allow the volunteers to read the script. As this is done, monitor the class, checking for any discomfort from students. (As a skilled educator knows, students who have

experienced dating violence may show certain behaviors and require support and assistance.)

Note: Although the situation focuses on a heterosexual relationship, it applies to other types of relationships also. Be sure to note this to your students.

5. After the script is read, ask the processing questions. Allow for thorough discussion for each. Thank the volunteers, and remind the class that the volunteers were just playing "roles"—their actual attitudes and behaviors are not reflected in the roles they were playing.

   Note: You should leave sufficient time for a full discussion of the written scenario. In addition, a list of resources needs to be available for students.

6. Optional activities for completion after the lesson include students' creating brochures, PSAs, videos, or other products identifying reliable resources for reporting sexual assault or date rape.

Processing

1. Although the names have been changed, this play is based on a true story. What do you think of each of the characters in the play?
2. The definition of date rape is "forced, unwanted sexual intercourse in which the attacker and the victim know each other." Does anyone feel that this was *not* a case of date rape? Explain.
3. Does society play a role in establishing what is the perceived "norm" in regard to dating behaviors or expectations? Do you feel that movies, song lyrics, violent video games, reality shows, and other media sources contribute to dating violence?
4. Mark described Melissa as "wearing a low-cut blouse, short skirt—she was looking pretty hot!" Does this excuse Mark's behavior? Did Melissa make it clear to Mark that she did not want to have sex? What specific actions or words did Melissa employ that should have made Mark stop what he was doing? ("No" means "no.")
5. Do you think that Mark's smoking the marijuana had anything to do with what happened? Why or why not? What role do drugs or alcohol play in date rape?
6. How would you describe the communication between Mark and Melissa?
7. If Melissa decided to pursue legal action against Mark, where could she go for help? What people, places, and other resources are available to assist her? (Parents or guardians, clinics, counselors, and law enforcement officials)
8. Although most sexual violence involves the male as the perpetrator, can a female rape or sexually assault a male? Can a male rape or sexually assault another male? Can a female rape or sexually assault another female?
9. What is something that people of *both* sexes can learn about this play?

Assessment

- Students correctly distinguish between dating violence, date rape, and sexual assault.
- Students complete additional projects (optional).

"A Pretty Good Time . . ."?

A Short Play about a First Date

Directions to actors: You will be playing the role of someone involved in a situation involving date rape. Please take your role seriously, and make every attempt to read your lines with the appropriate tone and volume of your voice. When you are not speaking, you should be quiet and still ("frozen") until it is your turn to speak again.

Characters: Melissa, Jenn, Mark, and Bob

Setting: There are four desks at the front of the room; two on the left side and two on the right. Melissa and Jenn are sitting at the desks on the left, and Mark and Bob are at the desks on the right. The boys "freeze" when the girls talk, and vice versa. The boys are frozen as the girls begin the scene. The remainder of the class should be closely observing what is going on.

Melissa: I can't believe what happened!

Jenn: When?

Melissa: Last night . . .

Jenn: Didn't you go out?

Melissa: Yeah, with Mark . . . he's in our science class.

Jenn: No way . . . he's hot!

Melissa: Well, he got a little overexcited last night.

Jenn: What do you mean?

Melissa: He picked me up around 7:30. We were going to get something to eat and catch a movie. The food wasn't bad, but I felt kinda funny in the restaurant. It was kind of fancy for a first date, and the food was pretty expensive. (***Freeze***)

Bob: (***Unfreezing***) So, who was the lucky girl *last* night?

Mark: Melissa Page.

Bob: Melissa Page? Are you kidding?

Mark: What's wrong with her?

Bob: Nothing! I just didn't think she was your type, if you know what I mean. She seems kinda shy and quiet. Anyway, how was the movie?

Mark: Let's just say we never made it to the movie. (***Freeze***)

Jenn: (***Unfreezing***) What movie did you guys see?

Melissa: Well, we didn't quite make it to the movie.

Jenn: What do you mean you didn't quite make it to the movie? (***Freeze***)

Bob: (***Unfreezing***) So, what happened? Did she ditch you?

Mark: (*Acting cool, smirking*) Not quite!

Bob: You hit it off from the start?

Mark: Don't I always?

Bob: Where did you go if you didn't go to the movie?

"A Pretty Good Time . . ."? (*continued*)

Mark: Well, we started off at this really nice restaurant. I spent a lot of money on her, and she was impressed with the romantic atmosphere.

Bob: So let me guess . . . you "scored" again!

Mark: I can't take all the credit. She was wearing a low-cut blouse, short skirt . . . she was looking pretty hot! (***Freeze***)

Melissa: (***Unfreezing***) When we left the restaurant, the movie he wanted to see had already started. I asked him what he wanted to do, and he suggested taking a walk on the beach. I've gone to the beach on other dates; I didn't think that was a big deal. We hung out for a while and talked . . .

Jenn: Then what happened? (***Freeze***)

Bob: (***Unfreezing***) I don't know, Mark, Melissa seems kind of quiet.

Mark: That's the way they all seem until they get to know me.

Bob: Sounds like she got to know you pretty well last night!

Mark: Yeah, I guess the restaurant put her in a good mood. As a matter of fact, she got pretty friendly after dinner when we drove down to the beach. (***Freeze***)

Melissa: (***Unfreezing***) We went for a walk on the beach and talked. It was a warm night and no one was around. At first it was kinda nice. Then he took out a joint and started smoking. He offered me some, but I told him I don't do pot. He held my hand. He had a blanket. We sat down and watched the waves . . .

Jenn: Well . . . ?

Melissa: He kissed me. I liked him, so I kissed him back. Then he kissed me again. . . Then he started to grab me and undo my top. I tried to push him off, but he was too strong. (*Getting more emotional*) He pulled my skirt up. I kept saying "no" but he wouldn't stop. It was like he was a different person. I kept saying "no," but . . . Jenn, he had sex with me!

Jenn: Oh my God, are you all right? Are you sure you're okay?

Melissa: I don't know—I guess so. But I'm scared. Why did this happen to me? What did I do?

Jenn: You didn't do anything, Melissa! It wasn't your fault! You were raped!!!

Melissa: I don't know. He seemed so nice at the beginning. I was having a pretty good time. But all of a sudden, it's like he changed. When it was over, we got back into his car and he drove me home. Neither of us said anything the whole way. I was kind of in shock . . . and I was afraid of him.

Jenn: What are you going to do about it?

Melissa: Do about it? What *can* I do? I just won't go out with him anymore or any other guy for that matter!

Jenn: You could tell your parents . . . or the police.

Melissa: Oh sure, so everybody will know! Are you crazy? And you better not say anything to anybody, either. Okay? (***Freeze***)

Bob: (***Unfreezing***) So, are you gonna take her out again?

Mark: Yeah, I guess so. I think she had a pretty good time last night.

LESSON 6: PERSONAL SAFETY REVIEW GAME

Level: Middle school, High school

Time: 40 minutes

National Health Education Standards

1. Core Concepts
3. Accessing Information
4. Interpersonal Communication

National Sexuality Education Standards: Performance Indicators

- Compare and contrast situations and behaviors that may constitute bullying, sexual harassment, sexual abuse, sexual assault, incest, rape and dating violence.
- Access valid resources for help if they or someone they know are being bullied or harassed, or have been sexually abused or assaulted.
- Demonstrate effective ways to communicate with trusted adults about bullying, harassment, abuse or assault.

Rationale

Reviewing material in a unit or for an upcoming test in a "game" format can be an effective, fun instructional strategy. To set up this lesson, you can download free templates for PowerPoint presentations online, or, if you do not have the technology, you can draw a grid on the board and simply erase the dollar amounts as the questions are used. The game, by incorporating questions related to the specific topic, can serve as a diagnostic, formative, or summative assessment of student knowledge and skills. Its format is based on that of the popular game show *Jeopardy!,* in which contestants are given an answer and need to come up with the correct question.

Materials and Preparation

PowerPoint game template. You can obtain such a template by typing "educational game templates" in your browser's search box. Several sites allow free downloading for nonprofit educational purposes. One resource is the Parade of Games website (http://facstaff.uww.edu/jonesd/games/), where several different educational games can be accessed. All the games on this site are available free of charge for nonprofit educational purposes. If the technology is not available, you can draw a large grid on the front board (similar to the chart of categories and statements in *Jeopardy!*).

Laptop and LCD projector or Smart Board, if using a PowerPoint template

Front board, for keeping score as the game progresses

Answers and questions dealing with personal safety and sexuality, to be inserted into the PowerPoint game template or grid. (Although you should feel free to modify the questions to meet the developmental needs of your students, sample answers and questions have been provided at the end of this lesson.)

Scrap paper for final question responses (optional)

Procedure

1. Tell students that they will be playing a game similar to the popular TV game show *Jeopardy!* The game is set up as a series of five categories, with five questions in each category, plus a final question. The value of the questions in each category ranges from $100 to $500. The categories and questions will deal with the topic of personal safety and sexuality.
2. Because the clues are actually *answers,* student responses should be in the *form of a question.* For example, the clue might be, "This is repeated aggressive behavior intended to hurt someone, either physically, mentally, or socially," and the correct response would be, "What is bullying?" If you choose to devise your own clues and answers, you should attempt to make the $100 answer easier than the $200 answer, and so on up to $500.
3. Divide the class into Team A and Team B, and seat them on opposite sides of the room. Write "Team A" and "Team B" on the board to keep a running total of how much money each team has won as the game progresses. Teams will earn money for correct answers, and will lose money for incorrect answers.
4. Flip a coin to see which team will go first. Choose a student on that team to pick a category and a dollar amount. If you are using a PowerPoint game template, use the cursor to click on the corresponding square, and a statement will appear. The student will have to come up with the correct *question* to win the money for that square. Only the student who has chosen the box can respond, without any assistance from other team members. The contestant will have thirty seconds to come up with a response.
5. If the contestant responds correctly, her team is awarded the money for that square. If she gets it wrong, that dollar amount will be deducted from her team's total. If an answer is "questionable" or incomplete, you have the final say in determining if it is acceptable.
6. To make the game more equitable, each team will take turns. A student will now be chosen from the other team to be the next contestant. That student will select a category and dollar amount, and the game will progress from there as previously described.
7. Continue playing the game, each time alternating teams, choosing new contestants, and keeping a running total of the money each team has compiled. All team members must have a chance at answering a question before a teammate can go a second time.
8. If using the game template, there is a separate PowerPoint slide for the final question. If not, it can simply be read orally, with one contestant from each team writing the team's response on a piece of scrap paper.

9. The game ends when all the boxes have been used and the final question has been asked. At your discretion, you may choose to offer a few extra credit points on the next quiz or a free pass on a future homework assignment to members of the winning team.
10. To conclude the lesson, ask the processing questions.

    Note: If this game is being used as a diagnostic assessment (to see what students know and do not know *before* a unit), students can be asked what they knew about the topic of personal safety before playing the game. If the game is being used as a formative assessment (a check for understanding *during* the learning process), it can provide you with information needed to adjust teaching and learning based on student feedback and observations from playing the game. It can guide you in making decisions about future instruction.

Processing

1. How much did you know about issues related to personal safety before playing the game? (Diagnostic assessment)
2. What have you learned about personal safety today that you did not know before playing the game? (Formative assessment)

Assessment

- Students actively play and follow the rules of the game.
- Students respond to processing questions related to diagnostic assessment, formative assessment, or both.

Personal Safety and Sexuality: Categories, Clues, and Responses

Category 1: Online Safety

$100—Children or teens should never send anyone a picture of themselves without first checking with these people. (*Response:* Who are parents or guardians?)

$200—When going online, you should never give these to anyone, except maybe your parents or guardians (not even your friends). (*Response:* What are passwords?)

$300—Someone you have been chatting with online wants to meet you. If you choose to do so, you should definitely *not* meet this person here. (*Response:* What is this person's apartment; his or her home; or a private, secluded place?)

$400—These are two things you should never give out to someone you meet online. (*Response:* What is your first and last name, your address, your phone number, a photo of yourself, or the school you attend?)

$500—This type of adult exploits or "preys on" children or teens online, usually for sexual or abusive purposes. (*Response:* What is a predator?)

Category 2: Social Networking

$100—This is the most common risk young people face online. (*Response:* What is peer harassment?)

$200—Thirteen years old is the minimum legal age for someone to join this social networking site. (*Response:* What is Facebook?)

$300—This term is used to describe online bullying. (*Response:* What is "cyberbullying"?)

$400—When it comes to your date of birth, this should not be displayed. (*Response:* What is year of birth?)

$500—This person is the founder of Facebook. (*Response:* Who is Mark Zuckerberg?)

(*continued*)

Personal Safety and Sexuality: Categories, Clues, and Responses (*continued*)

Category 3: Definitions

$100—This refers to any sort of unwanted sexual contact, often over a period of time. (*Response:* What is sexual abuse?)

$200—This type of sexual assault involves forced vaginal, anal, or oral sex. (*Response:* What is rape?)

$300—Unwelcome sexual advances, requests for sexual favors, and other verbal or physical conduct of a sexual nature are all examples of this. (*Response:* What is sexual harassment?)

$400—This is the term used to describe sending or receiving sexually explicit images or messages through a cell phone or other personal mobile device. (*Response:* What is "sexting"?)

$500—Sexual contact between close family members or relatives is referred to as this. (*Response:* What is incest?)

Category 4: Dating Violence

$100—If you are being harassed or abused by a boyfriend or girlfriend, these are the people to whom you should go. (*Response:* Who are parents or guardians, counselors, teachers, administrators, or other adults you trust?)

$200—This form of abuse happens to approximately one out of every five girls. (*Response:* What is being physically or sexually abused by a dating partner?)

$300—This is a street name for Rohypnol, a common "date rape" drug. (*Response:* What are "roofies"?)

$400—Isolating you from friends and family, outbursts of anger, extreme jealousy, controlling behavior, and numerous text messages sent to you throughout the day to "check up" on you are all examples of these. (*Response:* What are signs of an abusive relationship?)

$500—LoveIsRespect.org, BreaktheCycle.org, and ThatsNotCool.com are examples of these. (*Response:* What are websites where teens can get information or help related to dating violence?)

Personal Safety and Sexuality: Categories, Clues, and Responses (*continued*)

Category 5: Life Skills and Sexuality

$100—Stacey has to write a report on date rape, and she wants to access valid information about this issue from the Internet. She knows that the most reliable sites have URLs ending in .gov, .org, or .edu. Yet some people may choose to seek information from sites that end with a different URL and may be biased or trying to sell something. This URL ending indicates a type of site that may not be a reliable source. (*Response:* What is .com?)

$200—Emma is using this interpersonal communication method when she tells Jason, "*I feel* uncomfortable *when you* tell dirty jokes at the cafeteria table *because* I find them disgusting and degrading to women. *I want* you to stop, or I will complain to the principal." (*Response:* What is assertiveness or using "I" messages?)

$300—This is the final step in the decision-making model. (*Response:* What is "Evaluate your decision"?)

$400—In the following interaction, Laura is using this form of interpersonal communication skills*:*

Nick: C'mon baby, you know everybody is doin' it.

Laura: No, they aren't. And I don't care if other people are having sex. My answer is "no."

Nick: But you know I love you.

Laura: The answer is still "no."

Nick: But I'll be careful. I'll even use a condom if you want me to.

Laura: What part of "no" don't you understand? I'm just not ready to have sex, and if you can't respect that, than maybe we should break up.

(*Response:* What are refusal skills, or resistance skills?)

$500—Leon's older brother died from an AIDS-related infection. Leon writes a letter to the school newspaper asking the administration to have an informational AIDS Awareness Day, with guest speakers who are HIV positive. He meets with the administration and convinces them that it is a good idea. His actions are an example of this. (*Response:* What is advocacy?)

Final Question

Most parents or guardians would not be likely to be familiar with the text message abbreviation "LMIRL," which means this. (*Response:* What is "let's meet in real life"?)

LESSON 7: HARASSMENT AND CYBERBULLYING

RANK THE CHARACTERS

Level: High school

Time: 40 minutes

National Health Education Standards

1. Core Concepts
3. Accessing Information
4. Interpersonal Communication

National Sexuality Education Standards: Performance Indicators

- Compare and contrast situations and behaviors that may constitute bullying, sexual harassment, sexual abuse, sexual assault, incest, rape and dating violence.
- Access valid resources for help if they or someone they know are being bullied or harassed, or have been sexually abused or assaulted.
- Demonstrate effective ways to communicate with trusted adults about bullying, harassment, abuse or assault.

Rationale

In this activity, students will read a story about a teen who is being bullied and sexually harassed, both at school and online. The story is fictional, but it is based on a compilation of newspaper articles detailing real-life accounts of students who have been bullied to the point of suicide.

Materials and Preparation

Copies of "Who's Responsible?" worksheet

Five manila folders or large cards. Each folder or card should have the name of one of the characters in the story (Jeanne, Melissa, Seth, Mr. Richards, and Rob) written in large letters.

Procedure

1. Give a copy of the "Who's Responsible?" worksheet to each student. Allow five to seven minutes for students to read the story. When they have finished reading, have them *individually* rank the characters (Jeanne, Melissa, Seth, Mr. Richards, and Rob) from 1 (*most responsible* for what happened) to 5 (*least responsible* for what happened).
2. When they have completed their rankings, hold up the card reading "Melissa." Ask students who ranked this character as most responsible for what happened (number 1) to raise their hand. Have these students form a group in one area of the room. Give one of the group members the "Melissa" folder (or card). This person will be the group spokesperson.

3. Follow the same procedure for the remaining characters. If a character gets no votes, place the folder with the character's name on the front board. It is also possible to have a "group" of one student.
4. After all groups have been formed, tell the groups that they have three minutes to discuss why they felt that person was most responsible for what happened.
5. After the three minutes, have each group spokesperson take a maximum of one minute to justify the group's selection to the class. No other groups or students may respond at this time. When all groups have justified their selection, say: "You have heard why your classmates ranked the characters the way they did. I am now going to allow you to switch groups if you wish." (Students may get up and switch groups at this time.)
6. If any students switched groups, ask them to share why they decided to do so.
7. Tell students that they will now form new groups based on who they felt was least responsible for what happened (number 5). Follow the same procedure as that just given.
8. After all group spokespeople have spoken, ask other students to justify why they rated certain characters high or low on the list in terms of responsibility. Students may disagree, but they should be respectful of each other's values and opinions. Allow about five minutes for this open discussion.
9. Conclude the activity by asking the processing questions.
10. As an optional assignment, students can complete an advocacy project related to bullying, online safety, or other personal safety issues. You may design your own rubric, tailored to the specific requirements you choose to incorporate into the advocacy projects. The following are examples of possible projects:
    a. Design an antibullying poster for the classroom or school hallway.
    b. Create a PowerPoint presentation dealing with online safety and "textual harassment."
    c. Write a letter to your school or local newspaper advocating safe school environments that encourage dignified and respectful treatment of everyone.

Processing

1. Was it easy or hard to rank the characters? Were some characters easier to rank than others?
2. What was realistic or unrealistic about this story? What are the rules in your school or laws in your state about harassment and bullying? Does your school have a written sexual harassment policy? How many of you have seen it? What does it say?
3. Was there any peer pressure in the story? If so, give an example.
4. Do you feel that Mr. Richards might have felt some pressure not to pursue Jeanne's claims with the administration? If so, why?
5. When you were allowed to switch groups, did you feel any peer pressure to stay with the group you started with? Why or why not?

6. Jeanne did not feel comfortable discussing her troubles with her parents. How many of you feel that you could talk to your parents or guardians if you were being bullied or harassed? If Jeanne were your younger sister and she had confided in you about what was going on, what would you have done?
7. Can males be victims of bullying or sexual harassment? Have you ever witnessed boys in your school being bullied or harassed? Without mentioning names, can you briefly describe what you witnessed? If you were a witness to bullying or sexual harassment, what do you think you would do or say?
8. Although Jeanne was the obvious victim in this story, do you feel she could have done more to stop the harassment? Who are some trusted adults in your school you could confide in if you were being bullied, abused, or harassed? How might they help you?

Assessment

- Students complete the "Who's Responsible?" worksheet and participate in the follow-up activity and discussion.
- Students complete an advocacy project (optional).

Name: ______________________________

Who's Responsible?

Directions: The names and details in the following scenario have been changed, but it is based on a compilation of true stories related to cyberbullying and sexual harassment. Read the story quietly to yourself. You will then be asked to rank the characters in the story from who you feel is **most responsible** for what happened (number 1) to who you feel is **least responsible** for what happened (number 5). Do not discuss or share your answers with anyone else. Once you have come up with your list, turn your paper over, and wait for further instructions.

It was a warm spring day when **Jeanne,** a junior at Smalltown West High School, approached **Melissa,** also a junior, and asked if they could talk. Jeanne had just discovered that they had both been dating **Seth,** the captain of the basketball team.

When the handsome basketball star first asked Jeanne out, Seth told her that he and Melissa had broken up, and he was single again. In reality, he and Melissa were broken up for a while, but had recently gotten back together.

Jeanne explained the situation, apologized to Melissa, and said she wanted nothing more to do with the two-timing Seth. Melissa was upset, but said, "I'm glad you told me. I have more respect for you than I do for my so-called 'boyfriend.'" When Melissa got home, she immediately sent a text to Seth, saying, "I just found out you've been cheating on me. It's over!"

When summer vacation came, Melissa discovered that Seth was working as a lifeguard at the neighborhood pool. The first time Melissa went to the pool, Seth came over to her, told her he was sorry about what happened, and said he wanted to see her again. He claimed that Jeanne had known that he and Melissa were still seeing each other but "came on to him" anyway.

Melissa didn't know whom to believe, but was still attracted to Seth. She starting dating Seth again, and thought that maybe he was telling her the truth. Over time, she felt herself becoming more and more angry at and jealous of Jeanne, and decided she wanted revenge.

Melissa started spreading rumors about Jeanne, calling her a "slut" and a "whore." Melissa was one of the "popular" kids, and got a bunch of her friends to send Jeanne threatening and abusive texts and e-mails over the summer. The harassment and bullying got worse once school started in the fall. Seth joined in, getting his friends to harass Jeanne as she walked by in the hallways, in the cafeteria, and just about everywhere she went.

Jeanne became more and more depressed. She was uncomfortable and embarrassed talking to her parents about this, but finally went to see **Mr. Richards,** the school counselor, who was also the assistant basketball coach. He said that he would look into it. He called Seth into his office and

(*continued*)

Name: ______________________________

Who's Responsible? (*continued*)

told him of Jeanne's accusations. Seth denied everything, claiming Jeanne was a "nutcase" and that *she* was "stalking" *him.* Seth immediately sent a text to Melissa, and "coached" her on what to say. When Melissa went to see Mr. Richards, she backed up Seth's story.

Mr. Richards called Jeanne down to his office and said that there was nothing he could do. Because there were no witnesses to the harassment that he knew of, it was her word against Seth's word.

Seth then convinced his best friend **Rob** to post a naked picture of Jeanne on a popular social networking site. Rob was good with computers, and he "photoshopped" Jeanne's yearbook head shot onto a naked body. Jeanne now felt that the whole world was against her. People she didn't even know started posting horrible comments about her. This turned out to be the last straw.

The next day, when Jeanne's mom came home from work, she found her beautiful daughter in her room. Jeanne had committed suicide. She left a brief note, saying simply, "Dear Mom and Dad. I am so sorry, but I just can't take it anymore."

Think about the characters in the story. Rank the characters from 1 (the person you feel is **most responsible** for what happened) to 5 (the person you feel is **least responsible** for what happened). Be prepared to discuss in class why you ranked the characters the way you did.

Most Responsible for What Happened

1. ______________________________
2. ______________________________
3. ______________________________
4. ______________________________
5. ______________________________

Least Responsible for What Happened

LESSON 8: UP CLOSE AND PERSONAL

Level: Middle school, High school

Time: 40 minutes

National Health Education Standards

1. Accessing Information
2. Interpersonal Communication
3. Self-Management

National Sexuality Education Standards: Performance Indicators

- Describe ways to treat others with dignity and respect.
- Identify ways in which they could respond when someone else is being bullied or harassed.
- Identify sources of support such as parents or other trusted adults that they can go to if they are or someone they know is being bullied, harassed, abused or assaulted.

Rationale

When people are being bullied, sexually harassed, or abused, or when they witness these threatening acts, they can have many conflicting emotions. This Up Close and Personal (UCP) activity encourages students to share personal opinions, feelings, and values in a safe, nonthreatening environment. Teens may sometimes be more comfortable discussing issues related to personal safety with peers than they are with their parents or guardians. By communicating their knowledge and attitudes concerning these issues in a supportive environment, teens who experience or witness sexual violence will become empowered to turn to a trusted adult for help. All people have the right to maintain boundaries that will help prevent unwanted behaviors, sexual or otherwise.

Note: Due to the personal nature of this topic, it is best to advise students to reveal only those opinions and experiences that they are comfortable with sharing. Although confidentiality is encouraged, it cannot always be adhered to. As mandated reporters, teachers are required by law to report any suspected cases of abuse, bullying, harassment, dating violence, or other personal safety concerns.

Note: When dealing with issues concerning personal safety, it is extremely important for teachers to be sensitive to the fact that some students in the classroom may have been victims of or witnesses to bullying, sexual harassment, sexual abuse, sexual assault, incest, rape, or dating violence. Remind students of the confidentiality rules in Up Close and Personal sessions, and caution them about revealing issues of a very personal nature that they might later regret sharing. As always, it is incumbent on you to refer students to the proper school or community authorities if revelations about bullying, sexual harassment, sexual abuse, sexual assault, incest, rape, or dating violence come to light during class.

Materials and Preparation

Small lamp (optional)

Up Close and Personal sheet with several UCP sentence stems. (*Note:* Prior to teaching this activity, you should familiarize yourself with "Facilitating a UCP Session," which can be found at the end of the lesson.)

Procedure*

1. Ask students to form a circle with their chairs. Turning off the overhead lights and using a lamp may make the environment more conducive to an informal discussion.
2. Introduce the activity in the following manner:

   Today we are going to do an activity called Up Close and Personal. It is simple to do, but for it to go smoothly, there are some rules to follow.

   First, understand this is not group therapy. Instead it is an opportunity for you to talk about how you feel about yourself, relationships, likes, dislikes, things that have come up in class, memories, and life in general. Although I will be facilitating the activity, I will also be sitting in the circle and participating along with everyone else.

   The activity is in the following format: I will read an unfinished sentence. Each of you will think about how you would finish this same unfinished sentence. Someone in the circle will then raise his or her hand and state his or her completed sentence. He or she will point to his or her right or left to determine which way around the circle we will proceed.

   When going around the circle, there should be no talking by anyone else. If something is said that you want to respond to or comment on, you must wait until we have gone all the way around the circle. If you cannot think of anything to say, or choose not to respond when it is your turn, you may simply say, "Pass" or "Come back to me." Everyone, including the teacher, is allowed to pass.

   When we have gone around the entire circle, I will ask anyone who passed if he or she would like to respond at this time. I will also ask for any questions or comments about anything that was said when going around the circle. At this point, there can be open discussion.

   Please note that during this activity, no names should be mentioned at any time. Instead, say something like, "I know someone who . . ."

   In addition, as with other lessons, what is said in class stays in class. However, please do not share anything that is too personal, that makes you feel uncomfortable, or that you wish to keep to yourself.

---

*Unfinished sentences have been a useful learning tool for many years. The specific format used in this lesson has been adapted from the book *Up Close and Personal: Effective Learning for Students and Teachers* (Raleigh, NC: Lulu Press, 2007), by teacher, colleague, and friend Robert Winchester. Robert can be contacted at trustinbob@aol.com.

3. Once the rules have been explained and agreed on, read the first sentence stem aloud. After allowing a few moments for reflection, ask a student volunteer to start by stating his completed sentence. That student will then point to his left or right to note in which direction the remaining students will be given a chance to complete the sentence. Students then give their responses until everyone around the circle has spoken or passed.
4. At times, a student may simply not be ready to respond to a particular question. When this happens, remind her to pass, noting that she can answer after everyone else has spoken. It is also not unusual for many students to have the same response to a question or statement. "Repeats" reinforce the important concept that although all people are unique, they often share many of the same thoughts, feelings, and values.
5. After all students have responded, open up the discussion by asking if anyone has any questions or comments about anything that was said. Encourage students to talk in more detail about why they completed the sentence the way they did. Students may also ask others in the circle, including the teacher, to expand on their answer. Students may do so, or they may choose to pass.
6. Continue the circle discussion for as long as it is viable, constantly monitoring and enforcing the rules. When the discussion on a given sentence has run its course, move on to the next unfinished sentence.
7. Share the processing statements.
8. All UCP sessions should end with some brief closure in the form of another unfinished sentence. Examples include the following: "Today I learned . . ." "I learned that I . . ." "Right now I feel . . ." and "Something I want to say to one of my classmates is . . ."
9. Conclude the day's activity by summarizing what occurred in the session, making appropriate connections to the subject matter and curriculum. Then thank the class and say, "This ends our Up Close and Personal class for today."

Processing

1. If anyone has any concerns or questions about what was discussed during our UCP session today, he or she can speak to me privately after class or can bring it up for discussion during our next class session.
2. There are many people, including teachers, coaches, counselors, or school psychologists, who can assist you with any personal issues that you may want to share with them. Keep in mind that these individuals, as mandated reporters, *must* report any verbalization or indication that you may want to hurt yourself or hurt others, or revelations of abuse of any kind, to the appropriate authorities for follow-up and counseling services.

Assessment

- Students actively participate in the UCP activity. Even though some students may decide to pass on one or more questions, as long as they are actively listening and following the ground rules, they are "actively participating."

Facilitating a UCP Session

- Facilitation is a skill that you can improve with practice.
- Silence is not a negative phenomenon. Silence often indicates that higher-level thinking is taking place.
- Going over ground rules at the beginning of each session is a needed and helpful technique to prevent inappropriate behavior.
- Unacceptable behavior should be stopped the moment it is recognized. To do this, pause the activity and point out the offense to the individual. For example, say, "What was just said is a put-down (or personal name), and it is not allowed in the circle discussion. Please do not do it again," or "Please do not talk to your neighbor when you should be listening to the one person who is supposed to be talking."
- If a student persists in breaking the activity's rules, talk to him one-on-one after class. Let the student know that if his behavior continues, he may not be able to participate in the future. This almost always stops the offensive behavior.
- Remind students of the information teachers *must* report if shared:

  1. If they are going to hurt themselves
  2. If they are going to hurt others
  3. If they are being abused

Possible UCP Sentence Stems: Personal Safety

1. Right now, I feel . . .
2. In this school, sexual harassment . . .
3. If I knew someone who was sexually assaulted, I would . . .
4. If I received a sexually explicit text or picture, I would . . .
5. To prevent violence from happening, people should . . .
6. One way to make dating safe is to . . .
7. If I were in an abusive relationship, I would probably talk to . . .
8. Something that makes someone a great partner is . . .
9. If a friend confided in me that he or she was sexually abused, I would advise him or her to . . .
10. An adult whom I would feel comfortable talking to about threats to my personal safety would be . . .
11. My opinion of social networking sites is . . .
12. When it comes to sending text messages, I . . .
13. One thing I would never do while online is . . .
14. One thing I learned today is . . .

LESSON 9: HOME-SCHOOL CONNECTION

TALKING ABOUT ONLINE SAFETY—TIPS FOR PARENTS OR GUARDIANS

Level: Middle school

Time: Varies

National Health Education Standard

8. Advocacy

National Sexuality Education Standards: Performance Indicator

- Advocate for safe environments that encourage dignified and respectful treatment of everyone.

Rationale

It is important for parents or guardians to be aware of the latest threats facing children online.

After completing the assignment, parents or guardians are requested to sign on the bottom. All responses from teens and parents or guardians on the Home-School Connection activity will be kept confidential. It will not be turned in to the teacher or graded. On the due date, students will be asked to *voluntarily* share any interesting comments or insights they learned or observed by participating in the assignment. Students *and* parents or guardians can choose to pass on any discussion they wish to keep private.

Materials and Preparation

Copies of "Talking about Online Safety: Tips for Parents or Guardians" worksheet

Procedure

1. Explain to the class that they are going to have an assignment to complete with one or more parents or guardians.
2. Distribute the worksheet and assign a due date.
3. On the day the assignment is due, check if students have completed the assignment by noting whether or not the worksheet has been signed on the bottom. The assignment should not be collected or graded.
4. Ask for student volunteers to share results of the discussion they had with the adult or adults they interviewed. Do so using the processing questions, bearing in mind that all student comments and contributions should be voluntary.

Processing

1. What were the reactions of the parents or guardians who completed this assignment with you? How do you feel about their reactions?
2. What comments were made that you agreed with? That you disagreed with?
3. Were any new rules for Internet or phone use created as a result of completing this assignment? Explain.
4. Why do we have to talk about this assignment's issues?
5. If you were in your parents' or guardians' position, what would you do about this topic?

Assessment

- Students complete the assignment, as indicated by one or more parent or guardian signatures.
- Students participate in the follow-up discussion in class related to Internet safety, bullying, harassment, "sexting," and online predators.

Talking about Online Safety: Tips for Parents or Guardians

Unfortunately, as technology has expanded, so have some of the potential dangers. It is crucial that parents or guardians establish rules and procedures to keep their kids safe online.

Directions: Please read the online safety tips that follow. The objective is to initiate a conversation with your child and establish ground rules for the safe use of his or her computer and personal mobile devices. After you have discussed this information with your teen, please respond to the final question, and sign your name so that your son or daughter can receive credit for this assignment. If you need more room for comments, you may continue on a separate sheet if necessary. Thank you.

Online Safety Tips for Parents or Guardians

1. You should talk to your teen about a "code of conduct" outlining what you expect from him or her when he or she is online or on a cell phone. Parents or guardians have a right and an obligation to check in on their teen's computer and cell phone use. You are not doing this to invade privacy. You are doing it because you care about your teen, his or her safety, and his or her future.
2. Teens should not give out personal information, such as their full name, their home address, their phone number, or where they go to school. They should protect their computer passwords and should not give them out to friends. People on the Internet are not always who they say they are. Online predators may pretend to be someone they are not.
3. Teens should not go into "chat rooms" with people they do not know, they should be wary of anyone who asks them for personal information or pictures, and they should never agree to meet someone in person that they met online without first clearing it with a parent or guardian.
4. Teens should not post anything hurtful online. They should not spread rumors about, make fun of, or harass someone. This is called "cyberbullying." If teens are being bullied or harassed online, they should tell a parent or guardian, a teacher, or another adult they trust.
5. "Sexting" is defined as sending sexually explicit text messages or photographs to someone else electronically, often from one cell phone to another. Sending, saving, or forwarding these photos is illegal in most states under child pornography laws. Once a picture is out in cyberspace, it is there for anyone to see. Sexting has drawn a lot of attention, as well as concern, from parents or guardians, schools, and law enforcement officials.

Parent or Guardian Response

In regard to online safety, I feel that some of the most important issues for my son or daughter to be aware of are . . .

____

____

Parent or guardian signature(s): ______________________________

Student signature: ______________________________

LESSON 10: PERSONAL SAFETY PUBLIC SERVICE ANNOUNCEMENT

Level: High school

Time: Varies

National Health Education Standards

1. Core Concepts
3. Accessing Information
8. Advocacy

National Sexuality Education Standards: Performance Indicators

- Compare and contrast situations and behaviors that may constitute bullying, sexual harassment, sexual abuse, sexual assault, incest, rape and dating violence.
- Access valid resources for help if they or someone they know are being bullied or harassed, or have been sexually abused or assaulted.
- Advocate for safe environments that encourage dignified and respectful treatment of everyone.

Rationale

This project or group performance task can be used to assess students' learning about personal safety. The project can be assigned after you feel sufficient information has been taught from past lessons. Students may be assigned this project in class and complete it during school and after school with their group. The primary objective of this group performance task is to research information related to personal safety issues and create a public service announcement (PSA) that makes others aware of the serious nature of bullying or other forms of harassing behaviors.

Materials and Preparation

Copies of "Advocacy PSA Rubric" handout

Computers with Internet access

Procedure

1. For this project, students will form groups of two or three to write the script for a forty-five- to sixty-second PSA. The topic of the PSA may be
   a. Bullying or cyberbullying
   b. Sexual or "textual" harassment
   c. Dating violence

2. Distribute the "Advocacy PSA Rubric" handout. Groups will be assessed based on the rubric, which should be reviewed with and explained to them:
   - The PSA should clearly take a health-enhancing stance and should advocate for every individual's right not to be bullied, harassed, or abused.
   - Students must research their topic by visiting and referencing one or more credible websites (with a URL ending in .org, .edu, or .gov). A minimum of five accurate facts or statistics must be incorporated into the PSA.
   - The script and message in the PSA should have a clear theme that is appropriate for high school students and that encourages peers to make healthy choices.
   - The message in the PSA should be organized and memorable, and the class presentation should demonstrate conviction.
3. Explain that groups will have one class period to research the topic of their choice in the media center or on multiple classroom computers (if available). The remainder of the project is to be completed outside of class. Students may meet in person after school or communicate via e-mail.
4. Give students approximately one week to research, create, and practice their PSA. Assign student groups a due date on which they will present their PSA to the class.
5. On the due date, have student groups present their respective PSAs to the class. At the conclusion of each presentation, the entire class will participate in a discussion and critique of the PSA, based on the criteria in the rubric.
6. Conclude by asking the processing questions.

Processing

1. Which of the PSAs did you feel was most effective in advocating for the group's personal safety topic? What components made the PSA effective?
2. What suggestions for improvement could you make for some of the presentations?
3. What makes a PSA effective? Can you think of any PSAs that you have heard or seen that were effective in getting their message across?
4. One of the objectives of this assignment was to encourage respectful and dignified treatment for all, regardless of race, religion, ethnicity, or sexual orientation. What are some other ways to create a safer and more respectful school environment?

Assessment

- Student groups use reliable resources in researching their personal safety topic.
- Students participate in a critique and discussion of group presentations, assessing each group based on the rubric provided.
- Students actively participate in a discussion of the processing questions.

Advocacy PSA Rubric (16 Points Total)

	4 POINTS	3 POINTS	2 POINTS	1 POINT
Health-enhancing stance	The PSA took a clear health-enhancing stance. All information presented was accessed from reliable Internet sources.	The PSA's health-enhancing stance was generally clear. Most information was accessed from reliable Internet sources.	The PSA's health-enhancing position was not clear or obvious. Some information was accessed from a reliable source.	There was no evidence of a health-enhancing stance, or the PSA's position was not health enhancing. Information was not accessed from a reliable source, or no relevant information was presented.
Support for the audience	Students were proficient in the skill of advocacy. The PSA thoroughly supported its position with accurate facts from credible sources.	Adequate facts were presented, but the PSA contained some inaccuracies.	There was limited support for the PSA's position. The source or sources of information were questionable.	Support for the PSA's position was weak. Students did not provide any accurate facts from a credible source or sources.
Position awareness	Students demonstrated a strong awareness of the target audience.	Students demonstrated some awareness of the target audience.	Students demonstrated little awareness of the target audience.	Students demonstrated no awareness of the target audience.
Conviction	Students convinced their audience with a relevant and passionate argument that displayed a strong personal interest.	Students convinced their audience with a relevant argument.	Students presented a minimal argument for the position.	Students presented an argument that was weak or confusing. There was no evidence of a personal interest.

ONLINE RESOURCES FOR EDUCATORS, PARENTS OR GUARDIANS, AND TEENS

There are many organizations that provide information and support for educators looking to implement a comprehensive approach to sexuality education. The following list is intended to be a resource for educators, parents or guardians, and teens. Resources are provided for informational purposes only, and do not represent an endorsement of specific organizations or materials. Before assigning a website for students to use when undertaking research or completing projects, teachers should log on to the website to determine whether it is developmentally appropriate for their student population as well as aligned with community standards.

Advocates for Youth

Advocates for Youth is an organization that encourages young people to make responsible decisions about their sexual health. It includes resources for teachers, parents or guardians, and youth activists.

www.advocatesforyouth.org

Alan Guttmacher Institute

The Alan Guttmacher Institute is a nonprofit organization that provides research data and policy analysis on reproductive health issues.

www.guttmacher.org

American Red Cross Association HIV/AIDS Education

The American Red Cross provides information, resources, and services pertaining to HIV/AIDS.

www.redcross.org/services/hss/youth/AIDS.html

Answer

This national organization is dedicated to providing and promoting comprehensive human sexuality education for young people and educators or other adults who teach them. Associated with Rutgers University, Answer also helps to oversee Sex, Etc.

http://answer.rutgers.edu/

BNetSavvy

This online-based program has resources and tools to promote safe and smart Internet behaviors among tweens and teens. The site contains links to lessons plans, resources, and videos.

www.neahin.org/bNetSavvy/

Break the Cycle

Break the Cycle is one of the leading nonprofit agencies addressing teen dating violence.

www.breakthecycle.org

Campaign for Our Children

Campaign for Our Children spearheads education programs designed to address teen pregnancy prevention and encourage responsible decisions among adolescents. The organization's website includes a teen guide, parent resource center, educator resource center, and media campaign toolbox.

www.cfoc.org

Centers for Disease Control and Prevention (CDC), Division of Adolescent and School Health

The mission of the CDC's Division of Adolescent and School Health (DASH) is to prevent HIV, other STIs, and teen pregnancy, and to promote lifelong health among youth. In addition to providing resources for sexual health, the CDC conducts the Youth Risk Behavior Surveillance System (YRBSS) to note six types of health risk behaviors that are associated with leading causes of death and disability for youth. These include sexual behaviors leading to unintended pregnancy and STIs, including HIV infection.

http://www.cdc.gov/HealthyYouth/

ETR Associates

ETR Associates is a nonprofit corporation whose mission is to maximize the physical, mental, emotional, and social health of all individuals, families, and communities. It provides information resources, health education materials, publications, training, and programs.

www.etr.org/recapp

Gay, Lesbian & Straight Education Network (GLSEN)

GLSEN is the leading national education organization focused on ensuring safe schools for all students. GLSEN envisions a world in which every child learns to accept all people, regardless of sexual orientation or gender identity and expression. In addition, the organization hopes to provide support in protecting students from bullying and harassment.

www.glsen.org

Go Ask Alice!

Go Ask Alice! is a health question-and-answer Internet source produced by Alice! Health Promotion at Columbia University—a division of Columbia Health. You can find information using the Go Ask Alice! archives, which house thousands of previously posted questions and answers, along with reader responses. The site also gives you the chance to ask and submit a question to Alice!

www.goaskalice.columbia.edu

Healthy Lifestyle Choices (HLC)

This nonprofit organization advocates for comprehensive health education. Age-appropriate lessons address violence and injury prevention; emotional and mental health; nutrition and physical activity; tobacco, alcohol, and other drugs; family health and sexuality; HIV/AIDS; and personal and consumer health. The HLC website includes information about HLC programming for educators as well as parents or guardians, along with resources for kids.

www.hlconline.org

Kaiser Family Foundation

This independent philanthropic organization focuses on the major health issues facing the nation. Students can take the organization's updated HIV/AIDS quiz to see how much they know about HIV/AIDS, the people it affects, and the efforts to address the epidemic both globally and in the United States.

www.kff.org

Love Is Not Abuse

This website provides information on dating violence, including current research statistics on this topic, lesson plans for educators, support for places of work to provide resources for employees, and apps for iPhones on dating abuse facts.

www.loveisnotabuse.com/

LoveIsRespect.org

Loveisrespect.org is a collaboration of Breaking the Cycle and the National Dating Abuse Hotline to reach as many young people as possible in regard to healthy relationships. This website provides information on dating and relationships, sexting, and warning signs of abuse, as well as support for people in unhealthy relationships.

www.loveisrespect.org

National Campaign to Prevent Teen Pregnancy

The National Campaign to Prevent Teen Pregnancy is a private, nonprofit organization that seeks to improve the lives and future prospects of children and families, and, in particular, to help ensure that children are born into a stable family that is committed to and ready for the demanding task of raising a child. The organization's specific strategy is to prevent teen pregnancy and unplanned pregnancy among single young adults.

www.teenpregnancy.org

National Education Association (NEA) Health Information Network

The mission of the NEA's Health Information Network (HIN) is to improve the health and safety of the school community through the dissemination of information, which empowers school professionals to have a positive impact on the lives of their students.

www.neahin.org

Planned Parenthood Federation of America (PPFA)

PPFA promotes health and well-being, based on each individual's right to make informed, independent decisions about health, sex, and family planning. PPFA provides reliable health care, helping to prevent unplanned pregnancies, reducing the spread of STIs through prevention and treatment, and screening for cervical and other types of cancers. PPFA's website also provides up-to-date information for teens and tools for parents or guardians and educators.

www.plannedparenthood.org

Rape, Abuse and Incest National Network (RAINN)

RAINN is an anti–sexual assault organization working with local rape crisis centers across the United States. This organization provides assistance in the prevention of sexual violence, education on this topic, as well as support for victims.

www.rainn.org

Rubistar

This is a free tool to assist teachers in creating and using rubrics to assess student work.

www.rubistar.forteachers.org

Scenarios USA

Scenarios USA is a nonprofit organization using writing and film to foster youth leadership, self-expression, and advocacy among students across the country. The Scenarios USA REAL DEAL education programs include standards-based curricula and a series of films written by students and produced by professional Hollywood filmmakers that help students in grades six through twelve identify the social norms shaping their individual identity as well as learn about healthy decision making.

www.scenariosusa.org/films/

Sex, Etc.

Sex, Etc. is overseen by Answer and Rutgers University and provides sexuality education for teenagers and young adults. The website allows teens to obtain real, honest sexuality education as well as real-life stories written by teens.

www.sexetc.org

Sexuality Information and Education Council of the United States (SIECUS)

SIECUS provides accurate information, comprehensive education about sexuality, and sexual health services. The SIECUS library (www.sexedlibrary.org) is a resource for educators who teach about sexuality, supplying them with the tools they need to reach young people effectively. The SIECUS library includes lessons, curricula, research, and professional development opportunities.

www.siecus.org

Stop It Now

Stop It Now prevents the abuse of children by encouraging families and communities to take action in protecting children before they are harmed. It provides direct help to individuals with questions or concerns about child sexual abuse. It also provides organizations, communities, and professionals with prevention advocacy and prevention training.

www.stopitnow.org

Teaching Sexual Health Now

This is a resource for sexuality educators that is based out of Alberta, Canada. It provides lesson plans and activities as well as comprehensive resources.

www.teachingsexualhealth.ca

That's Not Cool

This national public education campaign focuses on increasing awareness of teenage dating abuse—specifically behaviors dealing with social media and cell phone use. The website includes digital examples for student and classroom use.

www.thatsnotcool.com